Approach to Hepatocellular Carcinoma (HCC) Management in Low/Middle-Income Countries

Reda Elwakil • Mohamed Kamal Shaker
Ashraf Omar
Editors

Approach to Hepatocellular Carcinoma (HCC) Management in Low/Middle-Income Countries

Springer

Editors
Reda Elwakil
Tropical Medicine Department
Ain Shams University
Cairo, Egypt

Mohamed Kamal Shaker
Tropical Medicine Department
Ain Shams University
Cairo, Egypt

Ashraf Omar
Departments of Hepatology
and Tropical Medicine
Cairo University
Cairo, Egypt

ISBN 978-981-96-3893-2   ISBN 978-981-96-3894-9 (eBook)
https://doi.org/10.1007/978-981-96-3894-9

This Springer imprint is published by the registered company Springer Nature Singapore Pte Ltd.
The registered company address is: 152 Beach Road, #21-01/04 Gateway East, Singapore 189721, Singapore

Preface

This book addresses the management of hepatocellular carcinoma (HCC) in low- and middle-income countries. A predicted 1.3 million people could die from liver cancer in 2040 (56.4% more than in 2020). The number of cases and deaths from liver cancer is predicted to increase by more than 50% over the next 20 years. This book aims to discuss the management of HCC in low- and middle-income countries in the context of limited resources of this category of countries with low health care budgets, which means that algorithms for early diagnosis and prioritization of treatment modalities based on the costs were highly considered in the book chapters.

The three key features of this book are: Highlighting the burden of HCC globally and in low- and middle-income countries besides discussing the disease epidemiology, addressing early detection, diagnosis and stratification methods for HCC cases focusing on low-resource setting and discussing different modalities for the treatment of HCC.

The chapter titled 'Introduction: Global Burden of Hepatocellular Carcinoma (HCC)' discusses the burden of hepatocellular carcinoma from both patients and health care provider's perspective in high-, middle- and low-income countries. The chapter titled 'Hepatocellular Carcinoma Epidemiology' addresses the risk factors and epidemiology in low- and middle-income countries. The chapter titled 'Molecular Basis for Hepatocellular Carcinoma Development in Low-/Middle-Income Countries' discusses the molecular basis of HCC development in low- and middle-income countries. The chapter titled 'Environmental Carcinogens for Development of Hepatocellular Carcinoma' focuses on the carcinogens related to HCC development and the impact of ecological factors in low- and middle-income countries, including climate change. The chapter titled 'Imaging of HCC' details the methods of diagnosis and stratification of HCC cases.

The chapter titled 'Surgical Management of Hepatocellular Carcinoma' presents surgical methods for the treatment of HCC including hepatic resection and liver transplantation with a focus on available options in low-resource setting, while the chapter titled 'Interventional Radiology for HCC management' addresses interventional radiology methods available for HCC management in low- and middle-income countries. Conversely, the chapter titled 'Systemic Therapy for HCC' highlights the available lines of systemic therapy for HCC, focusing on their availability in low- and middle-income countries, prioritization and cost-effectiveness of systemic therapies.

The chapter titled 'Palliative Therapy and Supportive Care for HCC' details the options available for the management of advanced cases of HCC in low-resource setting where curative treatment is not accessible.

The chapter titled 'Prevention of HCC' discusses the available methods for the prevention of HCC, including primary, secondary or tertiary methods in low- and middle-income countries. The last chapter of this book which is titled 'Prospects and Unmet Needs of HCC management'. addresses the future prospects and unmet needs in the management of HCC.

This book is suitable for students, trainees and examinees, as it can be used for both teaching and examination purposes.

Cairo, Egypt Reda Elwakil
Cairo, Egypt Mohamed Kamal Shaker
Cairo, Egypt Ashraf Omar

Acknowledgement To: Patients suffering from HCC, in the hope that progress in early diagnosis and treatment of HCC in the future helps to decrease their suffering.

Contents

1 Introduction: Global Burden of Hepatocellular Carcinoma (HCC)

Ashraf Breedy and Reda Elwakil

Abstract

Hepatocellular carcinoma (HCC) ranks as the fourth leading cause of cancer-related deaths globally. It is the only solid organ malignancy with a rising incidence, typically developing in the setting of chronic liver disease. In addition to its high mortality, patients with HCC often experience substantial challenges that negatively impact their quality of life (QoL). The burden of HCC is greatest in Asian countries, with China reporting the highest incidence rates worldwide. In Africa, HCC is the fourth most common cancer, while in Europe, approximately 47,000 deaths are attributed to HCC each year. In North America, incidence rates are roughly one-third of those observed in East Asia, although a recent increase has been noted in Australia.

The significant global burden of HCC is reflected not only in morbidity and mortality statistics but also in the substantial costs associated with diagnosis and treatment, affecting both individual patients and healthcare systems at large. This chapter aims to explore the worldwide burden of HCC, examining morbidity, mortality, economic impacts, and the broader consequences from the perspectives of patients, healthcare providers, and society. Particular attention will be given to the influence of economic factors on the delivery of treatment, especially within low- and middle-income countries (LMICs).

A. Breedy (✉)
Tropical Medicine Department, Faculty of Medicine, Ain Shams University, Cairo, Egypt

R. Elwakil
Tropical Medicine Department, Ain Shams University, Cairo, Egypt

R. Elwakil et al. (eds.), *Approach to Hepatocellular Carcinoma (HCC) Management in Low/Middle-Income Countries*,
https://doi.org/10.1007/978-981-96-3894-9_1

Keywords
Hepatocellular Carcinoma · HCC · Liver Cancer · HCC Burden · LMICs

Abbreviations

ASDRs	Age-standardized death rates
DALYs	Disability-adjusted life years
DECDG	Development Economics and Data Group
GBD	Global burden of disease
GDP	Gross domestic product
GNI	Gross national income
HBV	Hepatitis B virus
HCC	Hepatocellular carcinoma
HCV	Hepatitis C virus
LMICs	Low- and middle-income countries
IMF	International monetary fund
NAFLD	Nonalcoholic fatty liver disease
NASH	Nonalcoholic steatohepatitis
SEER	Surveillance, epidemiology, and end results
SES	Socioeconomic Status
USA	United States of America
US	Ultrasonography
WHO	World Health Organization

1.1 Introduction

Hepatocellular carcinoma (HCC) ranks as the fourth leading cause of cancer-related deaths globally (El-Serag and Rudolph 2007), accounting for more than 80% of primary liver cancer cases worldwide (Global Burden of Disease Cancer Collaboration 2017). Liver cancer is among the top three causes of cancer mortality in 46 countries and ranks among the top five in 90 countries (Liver Cancer Statistics 2018). Future projections by Rumgay et al. (2022) suggest that both the incidence and mortality of liver cancer will continue to rise by 2040, largely driven by global population growth. Importantly, many primary liver cancers are preventable if targeted prevention strategies are implemented, which could help mitigate the anticipated increase in resource demands associated with liver cancer management.

Hepatitis B virus (HBV) remains the leading cause of HCC in most parts of the world, whereas hepatitis C virus (HCV) has historically been the dominant etiology in the USA. More recently, nonalcoholic fatty liver disease (NAFLD), particularly nonalcoholic steatohepatitis (NASH), has emerged as a significant and rapidly growing contributor to the global HCC burden. Across all regions, HCC stands out for its extremely high fatality rate among cancers (Yang et al. 2019; Kulik and El-Serag 2019) and continues to represent a major cause of cancer-related mortality.

Research into the etiological factors associated with liver cancer—including HBV, HCV, alcohol consumption, NASH, and other causes—reveals notable variations across countries, regions, genders, and age groups (Liu et al. 2022). Despite rising overall incidence rates, the predominant risk factors for liver cancer differ substantially depending on demographic and geographic factors.

Beyond mortality, patients with HCC experience a wide range of symptoms that negatively impact their quality of life (QoL), including pain, fatigue, sleep disturbances, alopecia, and unintended weight loss (Gill et al. 2018). Prognosis, treatment options, and patient experience are closely linked to the extent of liver dysfunction and the stage at diagnosis. In addition to its clinical toll, HCC imposes substantial financial burdens on both patients and healthcare insurers (White et al. 2012; Beste et al. 2015).

Socioeconomic status significantly influences HCC outcomes. Individuals with lower incomes face higher mortality rates compared to their wealthier counterparts. In a cohort of Korean adults newly diagnosed with HCC between 2004 and 2008, low income was associated with markedly poorer 5-year survival rates, with middle-aged men identified as a particularly vulnerable group (Kim et al. 2021). Treatment discontinuation is also common among patients deemed ineligible for curative options such as liver transplantation or surgical resection, largely due to the high cost and limited effectiveness of alternative therapies (Aly et al. 2020).

In the USA, patients living in lower-income areas or those covered by Medicaid—or uninsured—tend to experience worse health outcomes related to HCC (Wang et al. 2018). Economic hardship and restricted healthcare access contribute to shorter survival times and higher disease risk. Moreover, low socioeconomic status increases the likelihood of liver-related mortality among adults with chronic liver disease (Desai et al. 2018). Social disadvantages, including financial instability, housing insecurity, reduced perceived benefits of healthy behaviors, and pessimistic expectations about aging, further exacerbate these health disparities (Petrovic et al. 2018).

This chapter aims to explore the global burden of HCC, encompassing morbidity, mortality, and the economic, social, and healthcare system burdens associated with the disease. Special attention will be given to examining the role of economic factors in influencing treatment access and outcomes, particularly in low- and middle-income countries (LMICs).

1.2 Definition of Low/Middle-Income Countries (LMICs)

For analytical purposes, the World Bank (WB) classifies countries' economies into four income groups: low, lower-middle, upper-middle, and high income. This categorization is based on gross national income (GNI) per capita, calculated in U.S. dollars and converted from local currencies using the World Bank Atlas method (The World Bank Atlas Method—Detailed Methodology 2023).

World Bank demographers estimate national population sizes using various data sources, including the United Nations' biennial World Population Prospects report.

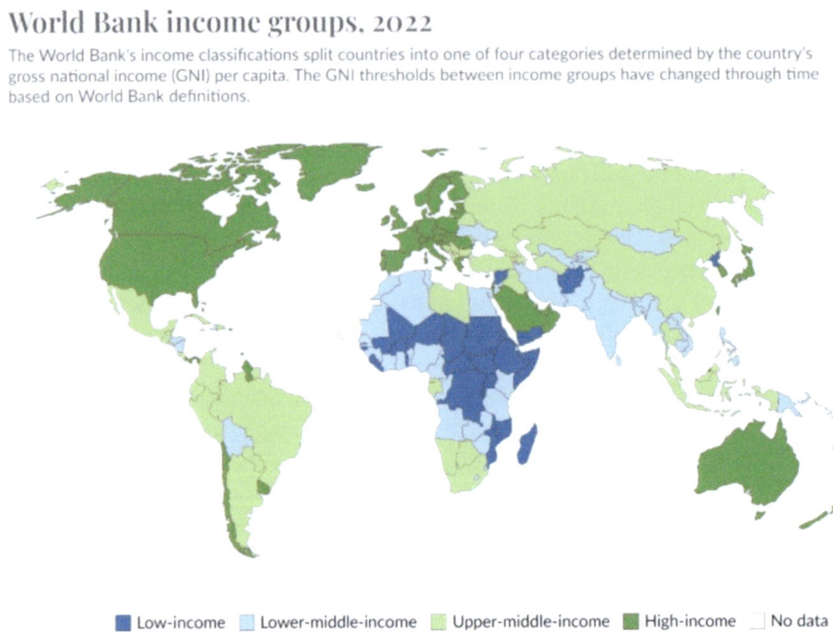

Fig. 1.1 The world map by income 2022. Source: World Bank (2023)—with major processing by Our World in Data. "World Bank income groups" {dataset}. World Bank, "income classifications" {original data}. Retrieved April 11, 2024, from https://ourworldindata.org/grapher/world-banks-income-groups

At the same time, economists in WB country offices primarily derive GNI estimates from official government data. Each year, on July 1st, countries are reclassified based on updated GNI per capita figures from the preceding year. Once determined, these income classifications remain in effect for the entire World Bank fiscal year, ending on July 1st of the following year, even if interim updates to GNI estimates occur.

As of the fiscal year 2024, lower-middle-income economies are defined as those with a GNI per capita between $1136 and $4465. (World Bank Country and Lending Groups 2023) (Fig. 1.1).

1.3 Global Burden of HCC

1.3.1 Global HCC Morbidity and Mortality Burden

According to estimates from the Global Cancer Observatory (Globocan 2020), HCC accounted for approximately 905,677 new cases worldwide in 2020. Asia dominated the global burden, contributing 72.5% of all cases. In terms of mortality, HCC caused around 830,180 deaths globally, with Asia again representing the majority, accounting for 73.3% of all deaths.

1.3.1.1 Burden in Asia

Asia bears the heaviest global burden of HCC, with China reporting particularly high incidence rates (Sayiner et al. 2019). Mongolia registered the world's highest liver cancer incidence in 2020, followed closely by Egypt (World Cancer Research Fund 2020).

The high HCC rates across Asia are primarily linked to widespread chronic hepatitis B (HBV) and hepatitis C (HCV) infections (Sayiner et al. 2019). Additionally, aflatoxin exposure—a toxin produced by mold-contaminated foods—remains a significant risk factor in the region (Wild and Gong 2010). Fan et al. (2013) found that in China in 2005, about 86% of liver cancer cases and deaths were attributed to five preventable risks: HBV, HCV, aflatoxin exposure, alcohol use, and smoking. Their study reported that HBV alone accounted for 65.9% of liver cancer deaths in men and 58.4% in women, while HCV was responsible for 27.3% and 28.6%, respectively. Aflatoxin exposure contributed to 25% of cases in both sexes. Alcohol played a more substantial role among men (23.4% of deaths) than women (2.2%), while smoking was linked to 18.7% of deaths in men and 1% in women. Combined, these factors explained 88% of liver cancer deaths in men and 78% in women.

Beyond infectious causes, lifestyle transitions have begun reshaping HCC epidemiology in Asia. Rising obesity rates and associated metabolic conditions have led to an increasing burden of nonalcoholic fatty liver disease (NAFLD) and nonalcoholic steatohepatitis (NASH). Vongsuvanh et al. (2013) observed that the progression of NASH-related cirrhosis to HCC rivals that of HCV-induced cirrhosis, signaling a major future shift in the region's liver cancer landscape.

1.3.1.2 Burden in Africa

HCC ranks as the fourth most prevalent cancer across Africa, although incidence rates and underlying causes vary between North Africa and Sub-Saharan Africa (SSA) (Parkin et al. 2014). In North Africa, particularly in Egypt, HCC incidence is roughly double that observed in SSA, largely due to Egypt's high prevalence of HCV infection, affecting about 4.6% of men (Bahri et al. 2011).

A study by El-Zayadi et al. (2005) tracking two 5-year periods (1993–1997 and 1998–2002) noted a sharp increase in HCC cases among patients with chronic liver disease. The proportion rose from 4.0% in 1993 to 7.2% in 2002 ($P = 0.000$). The study also recorded a demographic shift toward younger male patients (increase from 82.5% to 87.6% male dominance; $P = 0.009$), particularly in the 40–59 age range. Schistosomiasis, rural living, and a history of blood transfusion were all associated with higher HCC risk. Although the prevalence of hepatitis B surface antigen (HBsAg) positivity decreased significantly, HBV remained a major risk factor for HCC. Elevated α-fetoprotein levels and smaller tumor sizes were increasingly detected during the second period (El-Zayadi et al. 2005).

Outside of Egypt, lower HCC rates are reported in North African countries, including 0.2% in Morocco and Algeria and 0.7% in Libya (Parkin et al. 2014), likely reflecting reduced viral hepatitis prevalence, limited aflatoxin exposure, and lower alcohol use (Bahri et al. 2011).

In SSA, HCC is the second most common cancer among men and third among women (Wiredu and Armah 2006). Key contributing factors include HBV, HCV, chronic aflatoxin exposure, alcohol intake, and iron overload (Tognarelli et al. 2015). Twelve African countries are listed among the top 25 globally for highest liver cancer incidence (Liver Cancer Statistics 2018).

The high disease burden in SSA is exacerbated by weak healthcare systems, with many countries ranking in the lowest third worldwide according to WHO assessments (WHO 2000). HBV and HCV, along with aflatoxins, are the leading causes of HCC, while NAFLD plays a relatively minor role (Liu and Wu 2010; Chimed et al. 2017). Alcohol accounts for approximately 20% of cases, HCV for 23%, and HBV for 47% (Mokdad et al. 2014).

Egypt presents a distinct profile, with HCV contributing to 84% of HCC cases compared to HBV's 55% share elsewhere in Africa (Michael 2013). HCC is now the most prevalent cancer among Egyptian men and a leading cause of cancer deaths (Omar et al. 2023). Access to curative treatments is significantly better in Egypt, with 76% of patients receiving such therapies versus only 3% elsewhere in Africa (Yang et al. 2017).

Despite advances in antiviral treatments and vaccination programs, cost and accessibility continue to limit HCC control in SSA (Spearman and Sonderup 2015). Egypt's national HCV eradication campaigns offer hope for future reductions in HCC incidence (Sayiner et al. 2019).

1.3.1.3 Burden in Europe

Europe records approximately 47,000 deaths due to HCC annually (Ascione et al. 2017). Although HCC incidence is lower than in Asia or Africa, considerable variations exist between European nations. Western Europe ranks third globally for liver cancer incidence and fourth for liver cancer-related mortality (Global Burden of Disease Liver Cancer Collaboration 2017).

Since the 2000s, France, Italy, and Switzerland have had the highest HCC rates in Europe, while Scandinavian countries like Norway and Sweden report the lowest (Bertuccio et al. 2013; Bosetti et al. 2008). Mortality rates have become more homogeneous across the continent, though Western and Southern Europe still have comparatively higher death rates.

Historically, HBV dominated as a risk factor for HCC, but its impact has declined in Europe. In Italy, HCV remained a leading cause until the early 2000s, after which alcohol-related liver disease rose in prominence (Santi et al. 2012). Southern Europe sees more HCV-linked cases, whereas alcohol use, especially spirits, is more common in Northern Europe (Ramstedt 2001).

In contrast to Asia and Africa, Europe's HCC burden is increasingly influenced by alcohol abuse and the rising prevalence of NAFLD (Global Burden of Disease Liver Cancer Collaboration 2017). As a result, NAFLD and alcohol-related liver disease are expected to drive future trends.

1.3.1.4 Burden in North and South America

While East Asia reports the highest number of HCC cases globally, North America also carries a significant burden (Global Burden of Disease Liver Cancer Collaboration 2017). In the USA, HCC incidence has nearly tripled over the last two decades. Golabi et al. (2017a, b) highlighted that HCC is among the few solid tumors with consistently rising incidence in the USA, and mortality from primary liver cancer has been increasing faster than any other malignancy (Espey et al. 2007).

In 2012, 22,252 deaths were attributed to primary liver cancer in the USA, with alcohol-related liver disease responsible for about 37% of cases (Global Burden of Disease Liver Cancer Collaboration 2017). Other leading causes included HCV and HBV infections. Age-adjusted incidence rates have tripled since the early 1980s, and African Americans experience two to three times higher rates compared to Caucasians. Asians, Pacific Islanders, and Native Americans have even higher rates, though proportional increases are most notable among white populations.

Ethnic disparities significantly affect HCC incidence: Asian Americans and African Americans are diagnosed at twice the rate of whites (El-Serag 2012). While NAFLD-associated HCC is growing, HCV and alcohol-related cirrhosis remain the primary drivers (Zhu 2013).

Linkage studies between SEER registry data and Medicare records (2004–2009) identified NAFLD as the third leading cause of HCC and linked it to higher one-year mortality (Younossi et al. 2015).

Demographic shifts, immigration from HBV/HCV-endemic regions, and the aging "baby boomer" cohort with chronic HCV infections have all contributed to rising HCC rates (Mitchell et al. 2011; Kim et al. 2018; Sayiner et al. 2016). Simultaneously, obesity and diabetes have fueled a NAFLD epidemic, further increasing HCC risk (Younossi et al. 2016).

Similarly, Canada mirrors the U.S. trend. In 2012, 1962 HCC-related deaths occurred in Canada, with alcohol, HCV, HBV, and other causes contributing 31%, 34%, 9%, and 27%, respectively (Global Burden of Disease Liver Cancer Collaboration 2017; Kachuri et al. 2013). Migration and growing NAFLD prevalence continue to shape Canada's HCC landscape (Chen et al. 2008; Jiang et al. 2011).

In South America, available data remain sparse. A Peruvian study noted reductions in HCC deaths among women following HBV vaccination, while pediatric rates remained stable (Ramírez-Soto et al. 2017). Regional rates are generally lower than in East Asia (Petrick et al. 2016).

In South Texas, research has shown Hispanics carry the highest HCC burden compared to other ethnic groups (Ha et al. 2017).

1.3.1.5 Burden in Australia and Oceania

Although Australia reports liver cancer incidence rates about one-third lower than the global average, rates have been climbing steadily. A study using South Australian cancer registry data found that incidence and mortality tripled between 1977 and 2007. Men were disproportionately affected, with an incidence three times higher than in women, and risk sharply increased with age (Luke et al. 2010).

The growing HCC burden in Oceania is linked to increased immigration from HBV-endemic Asia-Pacific countries (Zhu et al. 2016). Wallace et al. (2018) documented a 7.5-fold rise in HCC incidence from 1982 to 2014. Waziry et al. (2016) noted that HCV-related HCC cases surged while HBV-related cases stabilized, thanks to improved antiviral therapies.

In New Zealand, though data are limited, census-linked analysis showed relatively high HCC rates compared to Europe, suggesting a substantial burden (Meredith et al. 2012).

1.3.2 Economic Burden of the Disease

Cost-effectiveness analysis (CEA) is widely regarded as the "gold standard" for generating objective evaluations of the value of health interventions to inform decision-making (Siegel et al. 1996). Although there are established guidelines and best practices for conducting CEAs, final estimates can vary significantly depending on researchers' methodological decisions and data sources. Traditionally, CEAs have been encouraged to adopt a "societal perspective," which includes non-healthcare costs such as productivity losses (from absenteeism and presenteeism) and informal caregiving (including caregiver time and travel costs). However, most evaluations focus narrowly on payer perspectives, considering only formal healthcare costs like inpatient, outpatient, pharmacy, and laboratory expenses (Kim et al. 2020).

Researcher-level decisions regarding study population, comparator selection, time horizon, and the choice of health outcome measures can also substantially affect CEA results. Evaluating these methodological factors is crucial for developing appropriate standards tailored specifically to HCC, enabling meaningful comparisons of innovations in prevention, diagnosis, and treatment. Notably, approximately 85% of global HCC cases occur in low- and middle-income countries, particularly in Eastern Asia and sub-Saharan Africa (El-Serag 2012; Tang et al. 2018).

Yuen et al. (2022) conducted a systematic review of economic evaluations for HCC treatments. Analyzing 27 primary studies, they found a median intervention cost of $53,954 and a median incremental cost of $6546. Of the 20 studies utilizing the quality-adjusted life-year (QALY) metric, 11 determined that the interventions were cost-effective using a $100,000/QALY threshold. However, there was significant heterogeneity among study outcomes, and only a minority incorporated indirect costs. The authors concluded that, despite the considerable variability and limited inclusion of indirect costs, the majority of HCC interventions were deemed cost-effective.

In a recent U.S.-based study, Karim et al. (2023) examined healthcare expenditures for Medicare beneficiaries diagnosed with HCC. Using data from the SEER-Medicare database, they identified 4525 adult patients diagnosed between 2011 and 2015 to assess HCC-specific incremental costs beyond those related to cirrhosis. The analysis focused on Medicare payments and patient out-of-pocket liabilities during the first year following diagnosis. Findings indicated that patients with HCC incurred significantly higher Medicare expenditures and patient liabilities compared to cirrhotic patients without HCC, with physician, inpatient, and outpatient services accounting for much of the difference ($P < 0.001$ for all comparisons).

Moreover, patients with early-stage HCC bore lower incremental liabilities than those with advanced disease. Multivariable median regression analysis showed that higher National Cancer Institute comorbidity scores, NAFLD etiology, ascites, and hepatic encephalopathy were independently associated with increased costs. In the year after diagnosis, median Medicare payments and patient liabilities for HCC patients exceeded $65,000 and $10,000, respectively. Even after adjusting for cirrhosis-related costs, the incremental financial burden remained substantial, with median excess Medicare payments surpassing $50,000 and patient liabilities exceeding $7000 (Karim et al. 2023).

1.3.3 Disease Burden: Patient Perspective

1.3.3.1 Gender Burden

Males are more affected by HCC than females. Liver cancer had a standard incidence of 10.1 per 100,000 persons (15.3 in men and 5.3 in women). The nations of East Asia had the highest recorded mortality rates. Liver cancer had a standardized death rate of 9.5 per 100,000 individuals, with a gender difference of 14.3 for males and 5.1 for females (Mohammadian et al. 2018).

Egypt has a significant 45.9% male predominance for HCC compared to 22.7% female. The higher exposure of males to HCV is probably the cause of the male predominance. Some investigators explained this discrepancy by pointing out that males were more susceptible to schistosomiasis. As a result, parenteral anti-schistosomal therapy campaigns primarily targeted men, resulting in iatrogenic infection transmission (Ibrahim and Shash 2022).

Tan et al. (2023) evaluated global sex-based differences in liver cancer incidence across 204 countries and territories between 2010 and 2019. They reported annual figures and age-standardized rates (ASRs) for incidence, mortality, and disability-adjusted life years (DALYs) related to liver cancer. In 2019, men accounted for 376,483 new cases, 333,672 deaths, and 9,048,723 DALYs, while women accounted for 157,881 new cases, 150,904 deaths, and 3,479,699 DALYs. Over the study period, female ASRs for incidence, mortality, and DALYs declined, whereas among males, incidence ASRs increased while mortality and DALYs remained largely unchanged. The Americas was the only region where mortality ASRs increased for both sexes; elsewhere, rates either stabilized or decreased.

Regarding causes, HBV and HCV remained the leading contributors to liver cancer deaths in both sexes in 2019. However, nonalcoholic steatohepatitis (NASH) demonstrated the most rapid increase in death ASRs for both men and women over the decade. In 2019, the lowest female-to-male death ASR ratio was observed for HBV (0.2), while NASH had the highest ratio (0.9). The study highlighted that although the burden of liver cancer remains greater among men, the gap between sexes is narrowing for NASH-associated liver cancer.

Similarly, Zhang et al. (2021) conducted a comprehensive analysis of the burden of liver cancer and cirrhosis attributable to NASH from 1990 to 2017, using data from the Global Burden of Disease (GBD) 2017 study. Socioeconomic status was assessed through the socio-demographic index (SDI). An autoregressive integrated moving average (ARIMA) model projected future trends, while gender disparities were evaluated through the Kruskal-Wallis test and Pearson correlation analysis.

Their results showed that the number of DALYs attributable to NASH-related liver cancer worldwide doubled from 0.71 million in 1990 to 1.46 million in 2017. A negative correlation was identified between SDI and age-standardized DALY rates for NASH-related liver cancer ($r = -0.409$, $p < 0.001$), indicating a higher burden in regions with lower socioeconomic development. Australia and parts of Asia recorded the largest proportional increase in age-standardized DALYs rates, with a 143.54% rise over the study period. The burden peaked for men aged 60–64 and for women aged 65–69. Overall, males experienced a higher burden than females. A positive correlation between SDI and the male-to-female ratio in age-standardized DALYs ($r = 0.303$, $p = 0.011$) was also observed, suggesting wider gender disparities in higher SDI regions. Zhang et al. concluded that the global burden of NASH-associated liver cancer has increased substantially since 1990, with significant disparities by age, sex, and region, emphasizing the need to strengthen public health awareness and prevention strategies targeting NASH-related liver disease.

1.3.3.2 Age Burden

To adjust to the progressive loss of organs and functions, aging entails a progressive reprogramming of the metabolism and physiology. Defense mechanisms against pre-malignant transformations are included in this. Hence, older patients are more liable to develop certain tumors. This pertains to HCC and intrahepatic cholangiocarcinoma (iCCA). Thus, aging-related characteristics like telomere attrition, altered proteostasis, mitochondrial dysfunction, cellular senescence, stem cell niche exhaustion, impaired intracellular communication, and dysregulated nutrient sensing can all have an important role in the appearance of the liver cancer in the elderly. Furthermore, weakened liver tissue dictates a poorer reaction to risk factors. The late diagnosis of HCC and iCCA tumors, which typically affect patients aged 60 and 70 years, respectively, can be attributed to this, besides the challenge of early detection. In addition, there is a great deal of disagreement regarding the best course of action for treating elderly patients with HCC and iCCA. Several studies investigating the safety and feasibility of different therapeutic approaches for liver tumors in older populations suggest that advanced age should not automatically exclude individuals from treatment options. However, the presence of multiple comorbid conditions should be taken into account during treatment planning, as these can influence patient outcomes (Macias et al. 2021).

Liu et al. (2021) aimed to better understand the epidemiological patterns of HCC in China, analyzing the disease's prevalence, incidence, and mortality, while considering the effects of age, period, and birth cohort. Their study utilized data from the

Tianjin Urban Employee Basic Medical Insurance claims database (2003–2017), which includes health information from approximately 5.95 million individuals. The findings revealed that HCC prevalence significantly increased starting at age 25, peaked at age 60, and began to decrease after age 70. The period analysis showed a gradual rise in prevalence between 2008 and 2016, followed by a slight decline in 2017. Furthermore, the prevalence rate dropped in a near-linear fashion across cohorts from the 1925 cohort to the 1990 cohort. The incidence and prevalence trends were closely aligned, while the mortality rate exhibited a slight increase, rising consistently from age 45 to 85. However, mortality declined when comparing earlier cohorts (Liu et al. 2021).

In Sub-Saharan Africa (SSA), HCC ranked as the second leading cause of cancer deaths among men and the fourth among women in 2020. The disease typically affects younger individuals in this region, and the median survival period is short, often ranging from three to 4 months (Mak and Kramvis 2021).

In the USA, an examination of cancer registry data from 1992 to 2015 highlighted a decrease in HCC incidence rates among younger and middle-aged adults, regardless of sex, race, or ethnicity. The study found that from 1992 to 2010, the incidence rate of HCC increased by 4.8% annually (from 4.1 to 9.4 per 100,000). However, from 2010 onward, the incidence rate began to stabilize, with an annual decline of 0.7%. Notably, all racial and ethnic groups saw a rise in HCC incidence in individuals aged 60 and older, except for Asian/Pacific Islanders in the 70–79 age range. Conversely, for those younger than 60, incidence rates began to decline in the mid-2000s. For individuals aged 40–49, rates fell by 6.2% annually, while for those aged 50–59, the decrease was more pronounced at 10.3% annually. Among Black adults, the incidence dropped at a rate of 17.2% per year starting in 2012, whereas declines in other racial/ethnic groups were less significant (Rich et al. 2020).

1.3.4 HCC Burden on Health Care Systems

The growing demand for more sophisticated diagnostic techniques for HCC, combined with the high expenses associated with new treatments such as targeted therapies, has significantly driven up the cost of cancer care. Advances in cancer treatment have also led to an increased number of patients who require ongoing maintenance therapies, often for extended periods, contributing further to the rising costs. Additionally, due to the complex nature of care required, the need for a multidisciplinary approach in managing HCC patients has added to the financial burden (Attia et al. 2022).

In Egypt, the mortality rate due to HCV infection is estimated at 0.6% (Mostafa et al. 2016). The rising rates of HCC in Egypt can largely be attributed to HBV and HCV, both of which are primary risk factors for cirrhosis (Lehman and Wilson 2009).

A study analyzing the cost-effectiveness of sorafenib as a first-line treatment for HCC in military hospitals in Egypt, where healthcare budgets are limited, showed a slight reduction in mortality for the sorafenib group (99.96%) compared to the best supportive care (BSC) group (99.99%). The sorafenib group achieved an additional 3.96 quality-adjusted life years (QALYs), with a total of 46.24 QALYs, compared to 42.27 QALYs for the BSC group. The overall costs for the sorafenib and BSC groups were $4,229,940 and $3,092,886, respectively, with a difference of $1,137,054 in costs (Elsisi et al. 2019).

Furthermore, the proportion of Egyptian HCC patients with chronic liver disease has increased significantly, from 4.0% to 7.2% over the last decade (El-Zayadi et al. 2005). This rise presents critical questions for policymakers: How can healthcare systems afford to treat a growing number of patients? What is the impact of these treatments on the overall disease burden? And how do they affect patients' quality of life? In light of these challenges, healthcare policymakers must develop innovative strategies for treatment reimbursement and prioritize therapies based on comprehensive criteria to mitigate the financial strain of these treatments.

1.3.5 Social Burden of HCC

In a study conducted by Wang et al. (2016), data from the surveillance, epidemiology, and end results (SEER) database were analyzed to examine the changes in relative survival rates (RSRs) among HCC patients in the USA from 1983 to 2012. The study also aimed to determine whether age, sex, race, and socioeconomic status (SES) influenced these survival rates. The data revealed that the incidence rates of HCC in the USA increased over the three decades, from 1.9 per 100,000 in 1983 to 3.1 per 100,000 in 2002, and 4.9 per 100,000 in 2012. A total of 63,640 cases of HCC were examined to evaluate survival trends. The relative six-month survival rates improved steadily, from 31.0% in the early period to 42.9% in the middle, and 57.2% in the most recent decade, with the largest improvements observed in the past two decades. Importantly, the study found that survival rates were lower among Black patients and those in high-poverty groups, highlighting significant disparities based on race and socioeconomic status. This study provides valuable insights into the trends in survival rates and could inform strategies to address disparities in healthcare access and outcomes across different demographic groups.

A separate nationwide study conducted in Korea by Yang et al. (2022) also explored the impact of socioeconomic status (SES) on mortality rates in patients with HCC. The research used data from the National Health Insurance Service-National Sample Cohort, which included 3032 patients diagnosed with HCC between 2003 and 2013. The study revealed that SES was an independent risk factor for mortality, particularly among patients receiving non-curative treatment. The relationship between SES and mortality was found to be non-linear, with a stronger association observed at lower SES levels compared to those in higher SES brackets. Patients from the lowest income group, especially those ineligible for curative treatments, faced a higher mortality risk. This finding underscores the importance of considering SES in healthcare planning and highlights the need for targeted interventions for lower-income patients to reduce health inequities.

1.4 Conclusion

HCC is the only solid organ malignancy with a rising incidence worldwide, most often emerging against a background of chronic liver disease. Across many regions, HBV remains the predominant underlying cause. In addition to facing a high risk of mortality, individuals diagnosed with HCC often endure significant challenges that negatively impact their overall quality of life. Economic disparities play a major role, as lower-income populations are disproportionately affected by higher rates of HCC-related deaths.

Treatment options for HCC can be both limited and financially burdensome. Patients who are not eligible for potentially curative interventions, such as liver transplantation or surgical resection, frequently discontinue therapy due to the high costs and modest clinical benefits associated with alternative treatments. Notably, approximately 85% of global HCC cases occur in low- and middle-income countries (LMICs), where access to care is often constrained. The global surge in cancer care costs poses a serious threat to health systems worldwide, with LMICs being particularly vulnerable. Factors driving these costs include the necessity for advanced diagnostic technologies, the high price of innovative therapies like targeted agents, and the growing number of patients requiring expensive, long-term treatment strategies. Together, these pressures are overwhelming healthcare infrastructures that are already struggling with limited resources.

References

Aly A, Ronnebaum S, Patel D, et al. Epidemiologic, humanistic and economic burden of hepatocellular carcinoma in the USA: a systematic literature review. Hepat. Oncologia. 2020;7(3):HEP27. https://doi.org/10.2217/hep-2020-0024.

Ascione A, Fontanella L, Imparato M, et al. Mortality from cirrhosis and hepatocellular carcinoma in Western Europe over the last 40 years. Liver Int. 2017;37:1193–201. https://doi.org/10.1111/liv.13371.

Attia A, Siala I, Azribi F. General oncology care in Libya. In: Al-Shamsi HO, Abu-Gheida IH, Iqbal F, Al-Awadhi A, editors. Cancer in the Arab world. Singapore: Springer; 2022. https://doi.org/10.1007/978-981-16-7945-2_9.

Bahri O, Ezzikouri S, Alaya-Bouafif NB, et al. First multicenter study for risk factors for hepatocellular carcinoma development in North Africa. World J Hepatol. 2011;3(01):24–30.

Bertuccio P, Bosetti C, Levi F, et al. A comparison of trends in mortality from primary liver cancer and intrahepatic cholangiocarcinoma in Europe. Ann Oncol. 2013;24:1667–74. https://doi.org/10.1093/annonc/mds652.

Beste LA, Leipertz SL, Green PK, et al. Trends in burden of cirrhosis and hepatocellular carcinoma by underlying liver disease in US veterans, 2001–2013. Gastroenterology. 2015;149:1471–1482.e5.

Bosetti C, Levi F, Boffetta P, et al. Trends in mortality from hepatocellular carcinoma in Europe, 1980–2004. Hepatology. 2008;48:137–45. https://doi.org/10.1002/hep.22312.

Chen Y, Yi Q, Mao Y. Cluster of liver cancer and immigration: a geographic analysis of incidence data for Ontario 1998–2002. Int J Health Geogr. 2008;7:28.

Chimed T, Sandagdorj T, Znaor A, et al. Cancer incidence and cancer control in Mongolia: results from the National Cancer Registry 2008–12. Int J Cancer. 2017;140:302–9.
Desai AP, Mohan P, Roubal AM, et al. Geographic variability in liver disease related mortality rates in the United States. Am J Med. 2018;131(7):728–34. https://doi.org/10.1016/j.amjmed.2018.01.047.
El-Serag HB. Epidemiology of viral hepatitis and hepatocellular carcinoma. Gastroenterology. 2012;142:1264–1273.e1. https://doi.org/10.1053/j.gastro.2011.12.061.
El-Serag H, Rudolph KL. Hepatocellular Carcinoma: Epidemiology and Molecular Carcinogenesis. Gastroenterology. 2007;132(7):2557–76. https://doi.org/10.1053/j.gastro.2007.04.061.
Elsisi G, Yousery NY, Rashad N, et al. Cost-effectiveness of sorafenib versus best supportive care in advanced hepatocellular carcinoma in Egypt. J Med Econ. 2019;22(2):163–8. https://doi.org/10.1080/13696998.2018.1552432.
El-Zayadi AR, Badran HM, Barakat EM, Attia MED, Shawky S, Mohamed MK, Selim O, Saeid A. Hepatocellular carcinoma in Egypt: a single center study over a decade. World J Gastroenterol. 2005;11(33):5193–8. https://doi.org/10.3748/wjg.v11.i33.5193.
Espey DK, Wu X-C, Swan J, et al. Annual report to the nation on the status of cancer, 1975–2004, featuring cancer in American Indians and Alaska Natives. Cancer. 2007;110:2119–52. https://doi.org/10.1002/cncr.23044.
Fan JH, Jian-Bing W, Yong J, et al. Attributable Causes of Liver Cancer Mortality and Incidence in China. Asian Pacific J Cancer Prevent Asian Pacific Organ Cancer Prevent. 2013; https://doi.org/10.7314/apjcp.2013.14.12.7251.
Globocan 2020. https://gco.iarc.fr/today/data/factsheets/cancers/11-Liver-fact-sheet.pdf
Golabi P, Jeffers T, Younoszai Z, et al. Independent predictors of mortality and resource utilization in viral hepatitis related hepatocellular carcinoma. Ann Hepatol. 2017a;16:555–64. https://doi.org/10.5604/01.3001.0010.0290.
Golabi P, Fazel S, Otgonsuren M, et al. Mortality assessment of patients with hepatocellular carcinoma according to underlying disease and treatment modalities. Medicine. 2017b;96:e5904.
Ha J, Chaudhri A, Avirineni A, et al. Burden of hepatocellular carcinoma among hispanics in South Texas: a systematic review. Biomark Res. 2017;5:15.
Ibrahim AH, Shash E. General oncology care in Egypt. In: Al-Shamsi HO, Abu-Gheida IH, Iqbal F, Al-Awadhi A, editors. Cancer in the Arab world. Singapore: Springer; 2022. https://doi.org/10.1007/978-981-16-7945-2_4.
Gill J, Baiceanu A, Clark PJ, et al. Insights into the hepatocellular carcinoma patient journey: results of the first global quality of life survey. Future Oncol. 2018;14:1701–10.
Jiang X, Pan SY, de Groh M, et al. Increasing incidence in liver cancer in Canada, 1972–2006: age-period-cohort analysis. J Gastrointest Oncol. 2011;2:223–31.
Kachuri L, De P, Ellison LF, et al. Advisory Committee on Canadian Cancer Statistics. Cancer incidence, mortality and survival trends in Canada, 1970–2007. Chronic Dis Inj Can. 2013;33:69–80.
Karim M, Ramezani M, Leroux T, et al. Healthcare costs for Medicare patients with hepatocellular carcinoma in the United States. Clin Gastroenterol Hepatol. 2023;21(9):2327–2337.e9. https://doi.org/10.1016/j.cgh.2022.11.015.
Kim DJ, Yoo JW, Chang JW, et al. Does low income effects 5-year mortality of hepatocellular carcinoma patients? Int J Equity Health. 2021;20:151. https://doi.org/10.1186/s12939-021-01498-z.
Kim DD, Silver MC, Kunst N, et al. Perspective and costing in cost-effectiveness analysis, 1974–2018. PharmacoEconomics. 2020;38:1135–45.
Kim D, Li AA, Perumpail BJ, et al. Changing trends in etiology- and ethnicity-based annual mortality rates of cirrhosis and hepatocellular carcinoma in the United States. Hepatology. 2018; https://doi.org/10.1002/hep.30161.
Kulik L, El-Serag HB. Epidemiology and management of hepatocellular carcinoma. Gastroenterology. 2019;156:477–491.e1.
Lehman EM, Wilson ML. Epidemic hepatitis C virus infection in Egypt: estimates of past incidence and future morbidity and mortality. J Viral Hepat. 2009;16(9):650–8.
Liu Y, Zheng J, Hao J, et al. Global burden of primary liver cancer by five etiologies and global prediction by 2035 based on global burden of disease study 2019. Cancer Med.

2022;11(5):1310–23. https://doi.org/10.1002/cam4.4551. Epub 2022 Feb 4. PMID: 35118819; PMCID: PMC8894698

Liu C, Wu J, Chang Z. Trends and age-period-cohort effects on the prevalence, incidence and mortality of hepatocellular carcinoma from 2008 to 2017 in Tianjin, China. Int J Environ Res Public Health. 2021;18(11):6034. https://doi.org/10.3390/ijerph18116034.

Liu Y, Wu F. Global burden of aflatoxin-induced hepatocellular carcinoma: a risk assessment. Environ Health Perspect. 2010;118:818–24. https://doi.org/10.1289/ehp.0901388.

Liver Cancer Statistics. World Cancer Research Fund. Published August 22, 2018. Available at: https://www.wcrf.org/dietandcancer/cancer-trends/liver-cancer-statistics. Accessed August 29, 2023.

Luke C, Price T, Roder D. Epidemiology of cancer of the liver and intrahepatic bile ducts in an Australian population. Asian Pac J Cancer Prev. 2010;11(6):1479–85. PMID: 21338184

Macias RI, Monte MJ, Serrano MA, et al. Impact of aging on primary liver cancer: epidemiology, pathogenesis and therapeutics. Aging (Albany NY). 2021;13:23416–34. https://doi.org/10.18632/aging.203620.

Mak D, Kramvis A. Epidemiology and aetiology of hepatocellular carcinoma in Sub-Saharan Africa. Hepatoma Res. 2021;7(39) https://doi.org/10.20517/2394-5079.2021.15.

Meredith I, Sarfati D, Ikeda T, et al. Cancer in Pacific people in New Zealand. Cancer Causes Control. 2012;23:1173–84.

Michael C. Kew, epidemiology of hepatocellular carcinoma in sub-Saharan Africa. Ann Hepatol. 2013;12(2):173–82. https://doi.org/10.1016/S1665-2681(19)31354-7.

Mitchell T, Armstrong GL, Hu DJ, Painter JA. The increasing burden of imported chronic hepatitis B—United States, 1974–2008. PLoS One. 2011;6:e27717.

Mohammadian M, Neda M, et al. Liver cancer in the world: epidemiology, incidence, mortality and riskfactors. WCRJ. 2018;5(2):e1082.

Mokdad AA, Lopez AD, Shahraz S, et al. Liver cirrhosis mortality in 187 countries between 1980 and 2010: a systematic analysis. BMC Med. 2014;12:145. https://doi.org/10.1186/s12916-014-0145-y.

Mostafa A, Shimakawa Y, Medhat A, et al. Excess mortality rate associated with hepatitis C virus infection: a community-based cohort study in rural Egypt. J Hepatol. 2016;64:1240–6.

Omar A, Kaseb A, Elbaz T, et al. Egyptian Society of Liver Cancer Recommendation Guidelines for the Management of Hepatocellular Carcinoma. J Hepatocell Carcinoma. 2023;10:1547–71. https://doi.org/10.2147/JHC.S404424.

Parkin DM, Bray F, Ferlay J, et al. Cancer in Africa 2012. Cancer Epidemiol Biomarkers Prev. 2014;23(6):953–66. https://doi.org/10.1158/1055-9965.EPI-14-0281. Epub 2014 Apr 3. PMID: 24700176

Petrick JL, Braunlin M, Laversanne M, et al. International trends in liver cancer incidence, overall and by histologic subtype, 1978–2007. Int J Cancer. 2016;139:1534–45.

Petrovic D, de Mestral C, Bochud M, et al. The contribution of health behaviors to socioeconomic inequalities in health: a systematic review. Prev Med. 2018;113:15–31. https://doi.org/10.1016/j.ypmed.2018.05.003.

Ramírez-Soto MC, Ortega-Cáceres G, Cabezas C. Trends in mortality burden of hepatocellular carcinoma, cirrhosis, and fulminant hepatitis before and after roll-out of the first pilot vaccination program against hepatitis B in Peru: an analysis of death certificate data. Vaccine. 2017;35:3808–12.

Ramstedt M. Per capita alcohol consumption and liver cirrhosis mortality in 14 European countries. Addiction. 2001;96(Suppl. 1):S19–33. https://doi.org/10.1046/j.1360-0443.96.1s1.2.x.

Rich NE, Yopp AC, Singal AG, et al. Hepatocellular carcinoma incidence is decreasing among younger adults in the United States. Clin Gastroenterol Hepatol. 2020;18(1):242–248.e5. https://doi.org/10.1016/j.cgh.2019.04.043. Epub 2019 Apr 28. PMID: 31042582; PMCID: PMC6817412

Rumgay H, Arnold M, Ferlay J, et al. Global burden of primary liver cancer in 2020 and predictions to 2040. J Hepatol. 2022;77(6):P1598–606. https://doi.org/10.1016/j.jhep.2022.08.021.

Santi V, Buccione D, Di Micoli A, et al. The changing scenario of hepatocellular carcinoma over the last two decades in Italy. J Hepatol. 2012;56:397–405. https://doi.org/10.1016/j.jhep.2011.05.026.
Sayiner M, Golabi P, Younossi ZM. Disease burden of hepatocellular carcinoma: a global perspective. Dig Dis Sci. 2019;64:910–7. https://doi.org/10.1007/s10620-019-05537-2.
Sayiner M, Wymer M, Golabi P, Ford J, Srishord I, Younossi ZM. Presence of hepatitis C (HCV) infection in Baby Boomers with Medicare is independently associated with mortality and resource utilisation. Aliment Pharmacol Ther. 2016;43:1060–8.
Siegel JE, Weinstein MC, Russell LB, et al. Recommendations for reporting cost-effectiveness analyses. JAMA. 1996;276:1339–41.
Spearman CW, Sonderup MW. Health disparities in liver disease in sub-Saharan Africa. Liver Int. 2015;35:2063–71. https://doi.org/10.1111/liv.12884.
Tan DJ, Setiawan VW, Ng C, et al. Global burden of liver cancer in males and females: changing etiological basis and the growing contribution of NASH. Hepatology. 2023;77(4):1150–63. https://doi.org/10.1002/hep.32758. Epub 2022 Sep 12. PMID: 36037274
Tang A, Hallouch O, Chernyak V, et al. Epidemiology of hepatocellular carcinoma: target population for surveillance and diagnosis. Abdom Radiol (NY). 2018;43:13–25.
Tognarelli J, Ladep NG, Crossey MM, et al. Reasons why West Africa continues to be a hotbed for hepatocellular carcinoma. Niger Med J. 2015;56(04):231–5.
Vongsuvanh R, van der Poorten D, Ge orge J. Non-alcoholic fatty liver disease-related hepatocellular carcinoma: a sleeping tiger in the Asia Pacific. Hepatol Int. 2013;7(Suppl 2):823–32. https://doi.org/10.1007/s12072-013-9453-0.
Wallace MC, Preen DB, Short MW, et al. Hepatocellular carcinoma in Australia 1982–2014: increasing incidence and improving survival. Liver Int. 2018; https://doi.org/10.1111/liv.13966.
Wang J, Ha J, Lopez A, et al. Medicaid and uninsured hepatocellular carinoma patients have more advanced tumor stage and are less likely to receive treatment. J Clin Gastroenterol. 2018;52(5):437–43. https://doi.org/10.1097/MCG.0000000000000859.
Wang S, Sun H, Xie Z, et al. Improved survival of patients with hepatocellular carcinoma and disparities by age, race, and socioeconomic status by decade, 1983-2012. Oncotarget. 2016;7(37):59820–33. https://doi.org/10.18632/oncotarget.10930. PMID: 27486977; PMCID: PMC5312351
Waziry R, Grebely J, Amin J, et al. Trends in hepatocellular carcinoma among people with HBV or HCV notification in Australia (2000–2014). J Hepatol. 2016;65:1086–93.
White LA, Menzin J, Korn JR, et al. Medical care costs and survival associated with hepatocellular carcinoma among the elderly. Clin Gastroenterol Hepatol. 2012;10:547–54.
Wild C, Gong Y. Mycotoxins and human disease: a largely ignored global health issue. Carcinogenesis. 2010;31(1):71–82. https://doi.org/10.1093/carcin/bgp264.
Wiredu EK, Armah HB. Cancer mortality patterns in Ghana: a 10- year review of autopsies and hospital mortality. BMC Public Health. 2006;6:159.
WHO. The World Health Organization Report 2000. Health Systems: Improving Performance. Available at: https://www.who.int/whr/2000/media_centre/press_release/en/. Accessed December 12, 2023.
World Bank Country and Lending Groups. https://datahelpdesk.worldbank.org/knowledgebase/articles/906519-world-bank-country-and-lending-groups accessed 20 December 2023.
World Bank Atlas method - Detailed Methodology. https://datahelpdesk.worldbank.org/knowledgebase/articles/378832-what-is-the-world-bank-atlas-method. Last accessed 15 December 2023.
Yang WJ, Kang D, Song MG, et al. The impact of socioeconomic status on mortality in patients with hepatocellular carcinoma: a Korean National Cohort Study. Gut Liver. 2022;16(6):976–84. https://doi.org/10.5009/gnl210567. Epub 2022 Apr 22. PMID: 35466091; PMCID: PMC9668501
Yang JD, Hainaut P, Gores GJ, et al. A global view of hepatocellular carcinoma: trends, risk, prevention and management. Nat Rev Gastroenterol Hepatol. 2019;16:589–604.
Yang JD, Mohamed EA, Aziz AOA, et al. Characteristics, management, and outcomes of patients with hepatocellular carcinoma in Africa: a multicountry observational study from the

Africa Liver Cancer Consortium. Lancet Gastroenterol Hepatol. 2017;2:103–11. https://doi.org/10.1016/S2468-1253(16)30161-3.

Younossi ZM, Koenig AB, Abdelatif D, et al. Global epidemiology of nonalcoholic fatty liver disease-meta-analytic assessment of prevalence, incidence, and outcomes. Hepatology. 2016;64:73–84.

Younossi ZM, Otgonsuren M, Henry L, et al. Association of nonalcoholic fatty liver disease (NAFLD) with hepatocellular carcinoma (HCC) in the United States from 2004 to 2009. Hepatology. 2015;62:1723–30.

Yuen SC, Amaefule AQ, Kim HH, et al. A systematic review of cost-effectiveness analyses for hepatocellular carcinoma treatment. Pharm Econ Open. 2022;6:9–19. https://doi.org/10.1007/s41669-021-00298-z.

Zhang T, Xu J, Ye L, et al. Age, gender and geographic differences in global health burden of cirrhosis and liver cancer due to nonalcoholic steatohepatitis. J Cancer. 2021;12(10):2855–65. https://doi.org/10.7150/jca.52282. https://www.jcancer.org/v12p2855.htm

Zhu RX, Seto W-K, Lai C-L, et al. Epidemiology of hepatocellular carcinoma in the Asia-Pacific region. Gut Liver. 2016;10:332–9.

Zhu AX. Current status of hepatocellular carcinoma in the United States. Chin Clin Oncol. 2013;2:45.

Hepatocellular Carcinoma Epidemiology 2

Mohamed Kamal Shaker and Heba Mohamed Abdella

Abstract

Hepatocellular carcinoma (HCC) stands as the most prevalent type of primary liver cancer, with projections indicating over one million new cases by 2025. It ranks as the sixth most frequently diagnosed cancer worldwide and is the fourth leading cause of cancer-related mortality on a global scale. The underlying causes of HCC vary by region and are usually linked to chronic liver disease, with fewer instances arising in healthy liver tissue. Hepatitis B and C infections remain the predominant contributors to HCC onset. However, in Western countries, non-alcoholic steatohepatitis—often associated with metabolic syndrome or type 2 diabetes—is becoming increasingly significant. The burden of HCC, in terms of both incidence and death rates, is heaviest in East Asia and Sub-Saharan Africa. This chapter focuses on the epidemiology of HCC, particularly in low- and middle-income regions.

Keywords

Hepatocellular carcinoma · Primary liver cancer · HCC burden · Risk factors · Low- and middle-income countries · Sub-Saharan Africa · MENA region

Abbreviations

ART	Antiretroviral Therapy
ASR	Age-Standardized Rate
HBV	Hepatitis B Virus

M. K. Shaker · H. M. Abdella (✉)
Tropical Medicine Department, Ain Shams University, Cairo, Egypt

R. Elwakil et al. (eds.), *Approach to Hepatocellular Carcinoma (HCC) Management in Low/Middle-Income Countries*,
https://doi.org/10.1007/978-981-96-3894-9_2

HIV	Human Immunodeficiency Virus
HCV	Hepatitis C Virus
DRC	Democratic Republic of the Congo
DAAs	Direct-Acting Antiviral Drugs
GCO	Global Cancer Observatory
GLOBOCAN	Global Cancer Statistics Database
HCC	Hepatocellular Carcinoma
HH	Hereditary Hemochromatosis
IDU	Injection Drug Use
IQR	Interquartile Range
IARC	International Agency for Research on Cancer
LMICs	Low- and Middle-Income Countries
MENA	Middle East and North Africa
MOH	Ministry of Health
NAFLD	Non-Alcoholic Fatty Liver Disease
NASH	Non-Alcoholic Steatohepatitis
PLC	Primary Liver Cancer
PLWH	People Living with HIV
SSA	Sub-Saharan Africa
WHO	World Health Organization

2.1 Overview

Hepatocellular carcinoma (HCC) ranks as the fifth most common cancer among men and the ninth among women. According to the World Health Organization (WHO), approximately 900,000 new cases of HCC are diagnosed each year, with 69.8% occurring in males. This results in a male-to-female ratio of 2.66 (Table 2.1) (Wong et al. 2015).

2.1.1 Prevalence of HCC

Globally, around 995,000 individuals are living with a diagnosis of HCC, corresponding to approximately 12.8 cases per 100,000 people. The majority of these cases are observed in males (69.8%) and originate from Asia (73.6%) (Table 2.1). Cure rates for HCC remain low, with only 5% of men and 7% of women achieving a cure (Kristensen et al. 2014).

2.1.2 Incidence of HCC

The incidence of HCC varies significantly depending on geographic location (Fig. 2.1).

Table 2.1 Incidence, mortality, and prevalence of hepatocellular carcinoma in 2020 (Ettorree 2023)

	Incidence rate[a]	New cases (rank[b])	Mortality rate[a]	Deaths (rank[b])	Prevalence (proportion[c])
Asia	11.6	656,992(5)	10.7	608,898(2)	732,048(15.8)
Africa	8.8	70,542(4)	8.5	66,944(3)	83,201(6.2)
Oceania	7.2	4419(12)	5.5	3539(6)	4845(11.4)
Latin America and Caribbean	4.8	39,495(9)	4.6	37,566(6)	39,580(6.1)
Northern America	6.8	46,599(13)	4.7	34,818(6)	49,746(13.5)
Europe	5.2	87,630(13)	4.4	78,415(7)	85,119(11.4)
Worldwide	9.5	905,677(6)	8.7	830,180(3)	994,539(12.8)
Males	14.1	632,320(5)	12.9	577,522(2)	693,917(17.7)
Females	4.2	237,357(9)	4.8	252,658(6)	300,622(7.8)

Source: International Agency for Research on Cancer (International Agency for Research on Cancer/World Health Organization 2021)

[a]Rates of incidence or mortality per 100,000 individuals per year are standardized according to the age distribution of the global population. [b]Ranking position based on incidence or mortality rates among all types of cancer. [c]Percentage of individuals diagnosed with hepatocellular carcinoma who are still living within 5 years post-diagnosis, measured per 100,000 individuals

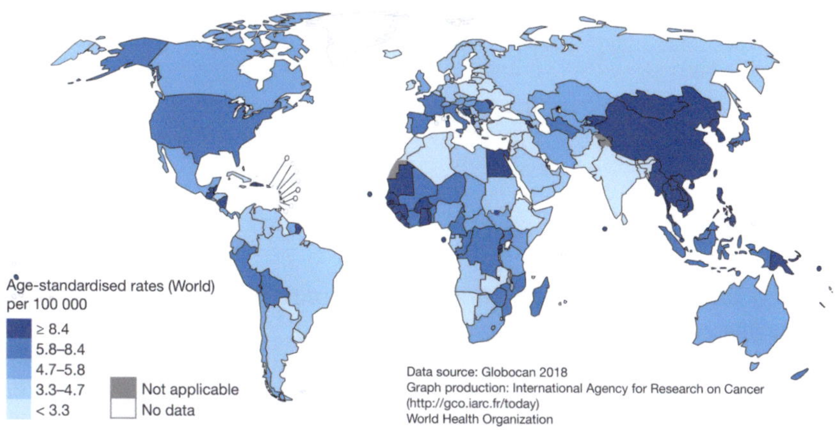

Fig. 2.1 Global estimates of hepatocellular carcinoma. Age-standardized incidence rates for liver cancer in both males and females, based on 2018 data (Rawla et al. 2018)

Asia accounts for about 72.5% of newly diagnosed HCC cases, showing an age-standardized incidence rate of 11.6 cases per 100,000 individuals per year. In Africa, HCC stands as the fourth most prevalent cancer, with an annual standardized incidence of 8.8 cases per 100,000 people, according to the Global Cancer Observatory (GCO) under the International Agency for Research on Cancer (IARC) (Table 2.1).

In contrast, Oceania, Northern America, and Europe report much lower incidence rates, with Europe having the lowest at 5.2 new cases per 100,000 individuals annually.

2.1.3 Mortality of HCC

On a global scale, HCC ranks as the third leading cause of cancer-related deaths, resulting in over 830,000 fatalities each year. Among males, HCC is the second most frequent cause of oncological death, while among females, it ranks sixth (Table 2.1).

Mortality rates are highest in males (69.6%), with 12.9 deaths per 100,000 individuals annually. Regionally, HCC represents the second leading cause of cancer death in Asia, third in Africa, and falls to the seventeenth position in Oceania, Northern America, and Europe (Table 2.1).

2.2 Risk Factors for Hepatocellular Carcinoma

Chronic liver disease underlies more than 90% of HCC cases (EASL 2018; Marrero et al. 2018).

The principal risk factors include chronic alcohol use, non-alcoholic steatohepatitis (NASH) related to diabetes or obesity, and infections with hepatitis B virus (HBV) or hepatitis C virus (HCV).

Additional, less common risk factors are cirrhosis secondary to primary biliary cholangitis, hereditary haemochromatosis, and α1-antitrypsin deficiency (Fracanzani 2001).

Among these, cirrhosis from any cause is the strongest predictor for HCC, with an annual incidence ranging from 1% to 6% (Trinchet et al. 2015).

2.2.1 Hepatitis B Virus (HBV) Infection

Infection with HBV is responsible for about 60% of HCC cases in Asia and Africa and roughly 20% of cases in Western countries.

HBV is a DNA virus capable of integrating into the host genome, causing insertional mutagenesis and activation of oncogenes, thereby promoting HCC development, sometimes even without the presence of cirrhosis (Wang et al. 1990). Nonetheless, the majority of HBV-associated HCC patients present with cirrhosis.

In East Asia, the high endemicity of HBV results in a sufficiently elevated HCC risk that warrants surveillance programs starting at 40 years of age for men and 50 years for women (Kew 2003).

Notably, HBV vaccination campaigns have contributed to a reduction in HCC incidence in several Asian regions (Chang et al. 2016).

Hepatitis C Virus (HCV) Infection

The risk of HCV-associated HCC is mainly confined to patients who develop cirrhosis as a result of chronic HCV infection, since HCV is an RNA virus that does not integrate into the host's genome. In North America, Europe, and Japan, chronic

HCV infection is the leading cause of liver disease among HCC patients (Akinyemiju et al. 2017).

Among individuals who achieve a sustained virologic response (SVR) through interferon-based therapies, the risk of HCC drops from 6.2% to 1.5% (Eyraud et al. 2002).

The advent of direct-acting antivirals (DAAs) has further lowered HCC risk by 50–80% in patients attaining SVR (Kanwal et al. 2017). Despite these advances, many individuals remain undiagnosed and unaware of their HCV status (Jain et al. 2019).

Importantly, even after SVR, patients with cirrhosis continue to face a significant HCC risk (>2% annually) and should therefore remain under regular surveillance (Ioannou et al. 2019; Llovet and Villanueva 2016).

2.2.2 Alcohol Consumption

Cirrhosis linked to alcohol use stands as the second leading cause of HCC in Europe and North America.

Annual incidence rates for HCC among those with alcohol-related cirrhosis range from 1% to 3% (Jepsen et al. 2012).

The likelihood of developing HCC rises with both the quantity and duration of alcohol intake, beginning even at low levels (<10 g/day).

According to the World Cancer Research Fund, each additional 10 g/day of alcohol consumed is associated with a 4% increase in HCC risk (Li et al. 2014).

Moreover, alcohol's contribution to HCC development is amplified when combined with other factors like HBV or HCV infection, older age, and obesity (Jones et al. 1998).

2.2.3 Hepatitis D Virus (HDV) Infection

HDV is an RNA virus that requires HBV surface antigens to replicate and cause infection. Globally, it is estimated that between 20 and 40 million individuals are infected with HDV.

Compared to HBV infection alone, HDV leads to a more aggressive progression of liver disease, including greater risks of fibrosis, cirrhosis, and HCC (Puigvehí et al. 2019).

2.2.4 Non-Alcoholic Steatohepatitis (NASH)

Since 2010, the share of HCC cases attributable to NASH has risen rapidly, now accounting for 15–20% of cases in Western countries (Estes et al. 2018a, b).

Although the annual incidence of HCC among patients with NASH-related cirrhosis is lower (1–2%) compared to viral-related cirrhosis (3–5%), the risk remains significant (>1.1 per 100 person-years), supporting the cost-effectiveness of routine surveillance (Kanwal et al. 2018).

Conversely, for individuals with non-cirrhotic NASH, the annual HCC incidence remains below thresholds that would justify surveillance (Kanwal et al. 2018; Mittal et al. 2016).

2.2.5 Age, Sex, and Additional Risk Factors

Advancing age is a strong risk factor for HCC, with incidence rates peaking in individuals over 70 years old (Rich et al. 2020).

The male-to-female ratio for HCC is approximately 2–3:1, attributed both to a higher prevalence of risk factors among men and possible hormonal differences (Bray et al. 2018).

Among ethnic groups, Hispanics show a higher incidence of HCC compared to white populations, largely linked to NASH-associated liver cancer (GLOBOCAN 2018; Rich et al. 2019).

Epidemiological studies have also demonstrated that smoking increases HCC risk (Lee et al. 2009).

Although some evidence suggests that coffee and aspirin consumption may have a protective effect, the role of diet in HCC prevention remains uncertain (Bravi et al. 2013).

2.3 Hepatocellular Carcinoma in Africa

Africa accounts for about 12% of the global population, with 83.6% (approximately 1.1 billion people) residing in sub-Saharan Africa (SSA), where most inhabitants are of Black African descent.

In contrast, populations in North Africa are more Mediterranean in racial, cultural, and traditional characteristics (Kew 2013).

According to the most recent Global Cancer Statistics, liver cancer accounts for 7.8% of all cancers in Africa, with an equivalent 7.8% mortality rate (Sung et al. 2021).

Figure 2.2 illustrates the incidence and mortality of liver cancer across various African regions for both sexes.

In 2020, SSA recorded the fourth-highest number of primary liver cancer (PLC) cases globally—following South-Eastern Asia, South-Central Asia, and North America—with more than 38,000 newly diagnosed PLC cases, 77% of which were HCC (Mak and Kramvis 2021).

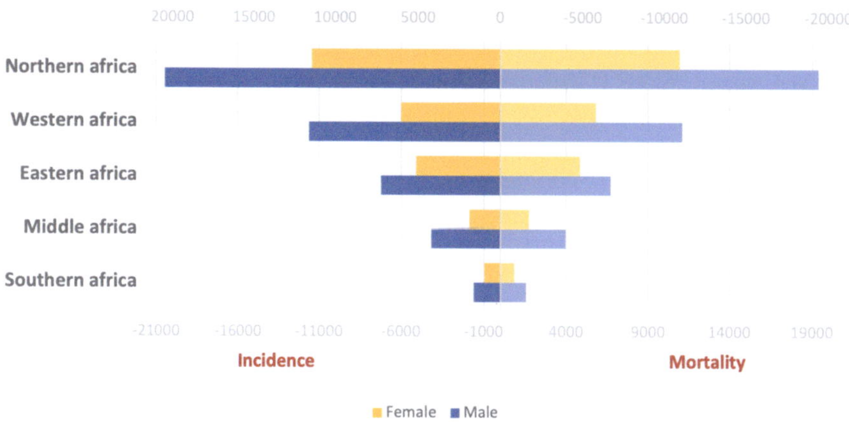

Fig. 2.2 Liver cancer incidence and mortality rates across various African regions (El-Kassas and Elbadry 2022)

2.4 Hepatocellular Carcinoma (HCC) in Sub-Saharan Africa (SSA)

2.4.1 Incidence and Survival Rate of HCC in SSA

HCC incidence in SSA is approximately 46,000 cases per year. It predominantly affects rural and, to a lesser extent, young urban Black Africans, often presenting with a poor prognosis. Men are more frequently affected than women. Around 60% of patients have coexisting cirrhosis (Moonsamy et al. 2022). Published incidences of primary liver cancer (PLC) in SSA are likely underestimated due to underdiagnosis or lack of cancer registry data (Kew 2013).

Survival rates are generally poor compared to East Asia and even worse compared to developed countries (Xu et al. 2016; Allemani et al. 2015; Sankaranarayanan 2011). For example, in North Africa, median survival is 10.9 months in Egypt, compared to just 2.5 months in SSA countries (Yang et al. 2017). In South Africa, rural Black patients survive on average only 6 weeks after diagnosis and 11.2 weeks after symptom onset (Kew 1981).

In SSA, HCC tends to occur at a much younger age, with a median diagnosis age of 45 years, 3 years younger in men than women. Similarly, African-Americans are diagnosed at a younger age compared to Caucasians in the USA (McGlynn et al. 2006).

2.4.2 Etiology and Risk Factors of HCC in SSA

Key risk factors for HCC include chronic HBV or HCV infection, aflatoxin exposure, heavy alcohol use, obesity, type 2 diabetes, and smoking (London et al. 2018). In SSA, about 50% of liver cancers are linked to HBV, 17% to HCV, and approximately 3% of patients are co-infected with both viruses (Parkin et al. 2020; Yang et al. 2017).

2.4.2.1 Hepatitis B Virus (HBV)

Over 50–60% of HCC cases in SSA are HBsAg-positive (Jemal et al. 2012; Yang et al. 2015a, b), with many others having past chronic or occult HBV infections (Kew et al. 2008). HBV prevalence is lower in East and South Africa (6–8%) (Schweitzer et al. 2015). Before the introduction of HBV vaccination, HBsAg prevalence in infants exceeded 10% in countries like Nigeria (Musa et al. 2015), Senegal (Coursaget et al. 1993), and South Africa (Mdlalose et al. 2016; Vardas et al. 1999). Less than 10% of acute HBV infections resolve spontaneously; the rest progress to chronic liver disease or HCC (Elgouhari et al. 2008).

2.4.2.2 Hepatitis D Virus (HDV)

Genotypes 1 and 5–8 predominate in SSA. Genotype 5 is prevalent in West Africa, while Genotypes 6–8 are common in Central Africa (Rizzetto and Hepatitis 2015).

2.4.2.3 Hepatitis C Virus (HCV)

As of 2018, Africa had approximately 18 million chronic HCV carriers (Kamali et al. 2022), with HCV prevalence estimated at 2.1–3.3% in SSA (Nordien et al. 2020). HCV is the primary cause of HCC in Central Africa, such as Cameroon (Andoulo et al. 2014).

2.4.2.4 Aflatoxin B1 (AFB1)

AFB1 is a potent hepatocarcinogen produced by *Aspergillus* species, contaminating foods like peanuts, grains, and corn under unsanitary, humid conditions common in SSA (Mazumder and Sasmal 2001). AFB1 exposure can be detected in urine and serum (Qian et al. 1994; Tang et al. 2009).

2.4.2.5 Iron Overload

Iron overload, linked to the consumption of traditionally brewed beer stored in iron containers, is a known risk factor (Kew and Asare 2007). Although plastic containers have replaced iron drums, recent studies on this change are lacking.

2.4.2.6 Alcohol and Smoking

Alcohol consumption has been increasing in SSA (WHO 2019a, b). In South Africa, heavy drinking is a major HCC risk factor, particularly among older white and urban Black men (Kew et al. 1984; Mohamed et al. 1992).

2.4.2.7 Non-Alcoholic Fatty Liver Disease (NAFLD)/Non-Alcoholic Steatohepatitis (NASH)

Changing lifestyles, including increased obesity and diabetes (possibly linked to antiretroviral therapy use for HIV), have contributed to NAFLD/NASH prevalence (~13.5% in Africa) (Mak et al. 2018; Paruk et al. 2019).

2.4.2.8 Hormonal Contraception

High-estrogen oral contraceptives (>50-μg estrogen) have been associated with increased HCC risk in high-risk Asian and African women. Risk appears to decrease after cessation of use (Brandt et al. 2004; Lindberg 1992; Hannaford et al. 1997; Fiel et al. 1996).

2.5 Hepatocellular Carcinoma in the Middle East and North Africa (MENA Region)

2.5.1 Epidemiology

The MENA region includes diverse countries (Egypt, Libya, Algeria, Saudi Arabia, Iran, etc.) and ethnicities (Arabs, Persians, Kurds, etc.). The total population was 456,707,404 in 2019–2020, about 7% of the global population (PTCMENA 2020). Economic disparities exist, with oil-rich countries (e.g., UAE, Saudi Arabia) having advanced healthcare systems, while war-torn countries (e.g., Yemen, Syria) face devastated infrastructures.

2.5.2 Incidence

HCC incidence has varied over time within the MENA region based on environmental exposures, healthcare practices, and risk factor management (Kaito et al. 1994; Smith et al. 2014). In 2018, there were 37,184 new cases (25,699 males, 11,485 females), with a cumulative risk of 2.18%. Mortality was similarly high with 36,601 deaths (25,267 males, 11,334 females) (Kaito et al. 1994; Smith et al. 2014).

Three patterns of incidence trends exist:

- **Increasing trends**: Egypt, Iran, Libya, UAE, Algeria.
- **Stable incidence**: Saudi Arabia, Kuwait, Bahrain, Oman, Tunisia.
- **Decreasing trends**: Turkey (HCC incidence dropped from 4.2 to 3.5/100,000 between 1990 and 2018) (El-Serag 2012).

Egypt continues to have exceptionally high incidence and mortality rates (Pearson 2008; Thompson et al. 2010; Poynard et al. 2000).

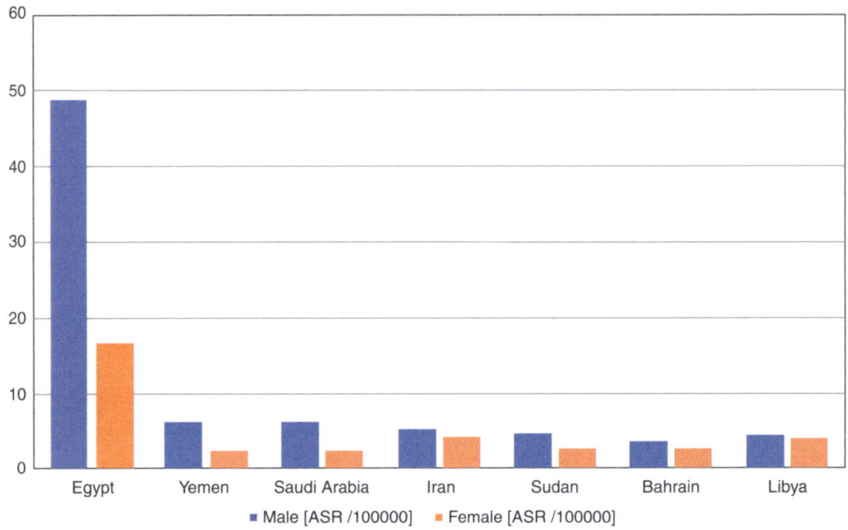

Fig. 2.3 Incidence of Hepatocellular Carcinoma (HCC) in Males and Females in Some MENA Countries (2018). (Adapted from Car 2021; p. 301)

2.5.3 Mortality

HCC-related mortality in the MENA region is rising. The age-standardized mortality rate (ASMR) per 100,000 increased from 5.31 in 1990 to 5.94 in 2018 (Kaito et al. 1994; Smith et al. 2014; Rauch et al. 2010; Thomas et al. 2009) (Fig. 2.3 and Table 2.2).

2.5.4 Risk Factors of Hepatocellular Carcinoma in the MENA Region

Several factors contribute to the development of HCC in the MENA region. These include cirrhosis resulting from chronic infections with hepatitis viruses, alcohol intake, and non-alcoholic fatty liver disease (NAFLD). Other contributors are male sex, consumption of aflatoxin-contaminated foods, exposure to inorganic arsenic and certain chemicals, as well as metabolic conditions such as iron overload and obesity. Additionally, hormonal influences—whether from external sources like oral contraceptives or from endogenous hormone production—have also been implicated (Ringelhan et al. 2017).

2.5.4.1 Hepatitis B Infections in MENA Countries

The MENA region shows a prevalence of chronic HBV infection ranging from low-intermediate levels (2–4%) across most countries, to high-intermediate rates (5–7%) observed in Sudan (Llovet et al. 2003). Chronic HBV infection stands as a key risk

Table 2.2 Hepatocellular Carcinoma (HCC) — New Cases, Mortality, and 5-Year Prevalent Cases in MENA Countries (2018)

		Number of new HCC cases				Deaths mortality rank				Number of prevalent cases (5-years)
Country	Total population	Number	Cum. risk	Rank[a]	(%)[b]	Number	Cum. Risk	Rank	(%)[c]	
Egypt	102,334,403	25,399	3.8	1	19.7	25.084	3.77	1	29.4	19.361
Saudi Arabia	33,554,333	905	0.55	9	3.7	852	0.52	4	8.1	701
Iran	82,011,737	3492	0.48	11	3.0.2	3439	0.48	7	6.2	2671
Sudan	41,511,523	942	0.43	7	3.4	906	0.43	5	5.3	830
Turkey	81,916,866	4362	0.52	15	2.1	4307	0.52	9	3.7	3127
Qatar	2,694,843	42	0.45	11	3.0.3	40	0.44	6	6	32
UAE	9,541,612	97	0.47	15	2.1	96	0.45	8	4.6	82
Yemen	28,915,286	620	0.51	7	4.7	595	0.51	5	6.5	535
Bahrain	1,566,994	30	0.37	12	2.9	22	0.29	12	3.6	108
Syria	18,284,423	380	0.34	18	1.6	380	0.29	18	1.4	514
Lebanon	6,093,510	227	0.38	18	1.3	216	0.37	11	2.4	163
Jordan	9,903,798	188	0.31	16	1.7	178	0.30	10	3.1	142
Iraq	39,339,754	539	0.32	12	2.1	538	0.32	7	3.7	443
Kuwait	4,197,129	121	0.6	8	3.4	114	0.6	4	6.9	90
Oman	4,829,946	117	0.51	10	3.5	111	0.5	5	6.6	98
Libya	6,470,857	191	0.54	12	3.0	147	0.44	7	4.4	148
Tunisia	11,659,175	355	0.29	12	2.2	356	0.30	11	3.5	317
Algeria	42,008,056	563	0.17	21	1.1	544	0.16	17	1.8	486
Morocco	36,191,813	428	0.14	24	0.81	411	0.13	18	1.2	524
Israel	8,452,843	336	0.28	14	1.3	397	0.35	11	3.2	253

Adapted from Car (2021; p. 301)

[a]Rank with respect to other cancers, [b]Percentage from all cancers, [c]Percentage from all cancer deaths

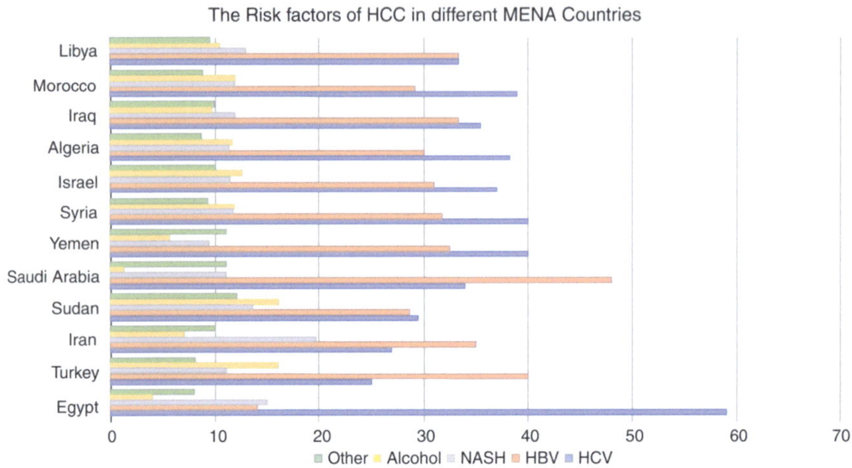

Fig. 2.4 Major Risk Factors for Hepatocellular Carcinoma (HCC) in MENA Countries (2018) (Adapted from Car 2021)

factor for HCC development in nations such as Iran, Saudi Arabia, Lebanon, the UAE, Oman, Qatar, Turkey, and Israel (Kaito et al. 1994; Chuang et al. 2009; Llovet et al. 2003; Koppes 1976; GLMM-Gulf 2020) (Fig. 2.4).

Patients infected with HBV genotype D — the predominant strain in Turkey, Iran, Saudi Arabia, the UAE, and Bahrain — are at a greater risk of developing HCC compared to those with genotype A (Petrick and McGlynn 2019; SPCHBME 2012; Ozdemir et al. 2005; Janahi et al. 2019).

Most countries in the region have introduced mandatory nationwide HBV vaccination programs (WHO 2017; Akyıldız et al. 2019). Although these campaigns have significantly reduced new infections, conflict and political instability in Yemen, Syria, Libya, and Sudan have hampered consistent HBV immunization efforts.

2.5.4.2 Hepatitis C Infections in MENA Countries

Although highly effective direct-acting antiviral (DAA) treatments are available for HCV infection, complete elimination of HCV across MENA countries remains challenging, primarily due to inadequate testing, diagnosis, and treatment coverage (Blach and Sanai 2020; WHO 2016).

Cirrhosis linked to chronic HCV infection is a major risk factor for HCC in Egypt, Sudan, Libya, Syria, Iraq, Yemen, Algeria, Bahrain, Jordan, Kuwait, Morocco, and Tunisia (National Cancer Institute 2015; IARC 2020; Lehman and Wilson 2009; Talaat et al. 2019) (Fig. 2.4).

In an important public health effort, Egypt's Ministry of Health initiated a mass national screening campaign aiming to cover the entire population (Esmat et al. 2018). Individuals diagnosed with HCV were enrolled in a fully government-funded DAA therapy program, which rapidly led to improvements in the nation's HCC statistics (El Kassas et al. 2019).

2.5.4.3 Non-alcoholic Fatty Liver Disease (NAFLD) in the MENA Region

In Kuwait, Saudi Arabia, southern Iran, and northern Iran, the reported prevalence of NAFLD stands at 33.3%, 16.6%, 21.5%, and 43.8%, respectively (Ramezani-Binabaj et al. 2014; Sohrabpour et al. 2010).

In Egypt, the NAFLD prevalence ranges from 16% among children to as high as 50% among adults (Ahmed et al. 2011; El-Koofy et al. 2011; El-Karaksy et al. 2011).

Turkey's NAFLD prevalence falls between 48.3% and 60.1% (Yılmaz et al. 2019) (Fig. 2.5).

The surge in NAFLD rates across the MENA region closely correlates with rising obesity and type 2 diabetes rates, largely driven by sedentary lifestyles, poor dietary habits, and population aging (Boutayeb et al. 2012; Beyhan et al. 2013).

2.5.4.4 Alcohol Consumption

Despite the religious prohibition of alcohol in Islamic-majority MENA countries, alcohol consumption still contributes to HCC risk, given the presence of diverse ethnic and religious populations (Figs. 2.4 and 2.6).

Overall, heavy alcohol use and alcohol-related liver disease are less common causes of HCC in the MENA region compared to other parts of the world.

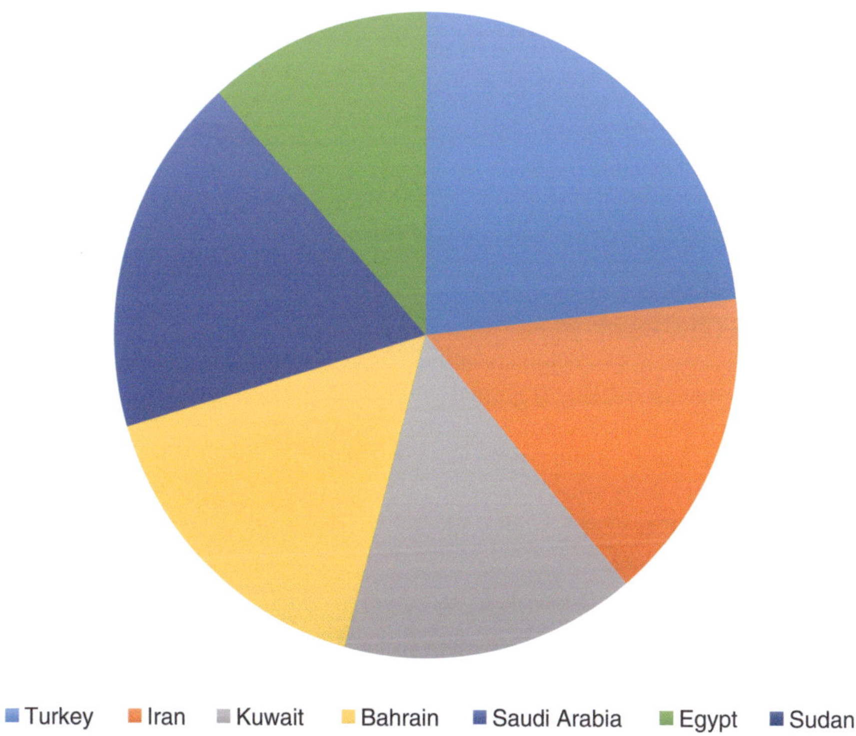

Fig. 2.5 Prevalence of NAFLD in some MENA countries (Car 2021; p. 301)

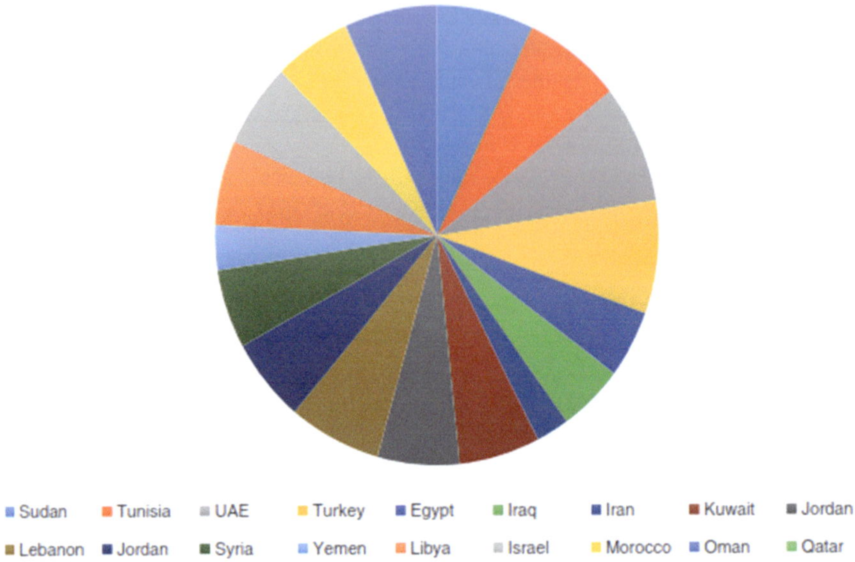

Fig. 2.6 The role of alcohol as a contributing risk factor for HCC in selected MENA countries (Car 2021; p. 301)

2.5.4.5 Aflatoxins in the MENA Region

Research examining the role of aflatoxin exposure in HCC development in MENA countries is limited.

In Egypt, dietary exposure to aflatoxins ranges between 7 and 57 ng/kg body weight per day, indicating relatively high levels (Liu et al. 2012).

Several epidemiological studies have highlighted the co-existence of aflatoxin exposure and HCV infection within the Egyptian population (Abdel-Wahab et al. 2008; Soliman et al. 2010).

2.5.4.6 Iron Overload

In the MENA region, hemoglobinopathies—especially thalassemia—are prevalent and are often managed through repeated blood transfusions, leading to iron overload.

The burden of β-thalassemia is notably significant in countries such as Iran, Lebanon, Syria, Egypt, Saudi Arabia, the UAE, and across North Africa.

Studies, particularly those conducted in Italy and Greece, have documented an elevated incidence of HCC among patients with thalassemias (Kourakli et al. 2018).

2.6 Hepatocellular Carcinoma in Latin America

Latin America comprises 20 nations, collectively housing over 639 million people (Baten 2016).

Substantial disparities exist between urban centers and rural areas across Latin America, with some remote regions (e.g., Haiti, Honduras, Nicaragua, Bolivia) lacking even basic healthcare services (World Bank).

2.6.1 Incidence and Mortality of HCC in Latin America

The male-to-female incidence rates of HCC are reported at 6.7/6.0 per 100,000 in Central America; 5.8/3.5 per 100,000 in South America; and 10.1/3.4 per 100,000 in North America (Mexico).

In 2018, HCC-related deaths across Latin America totaled approximately 840,000, accounting for 4.6% of deaths worldwide.

Mortality rates varied by country, ranging from less than 2.8 to greater than 6.3 per 100,000 individuals (Fig. 2.7).

The incidence-to-mortality ratio being close to 1 emphasizes the high fatality associated with HCC in the region (Table 2.3) (Bray et al. 2018).

Available data on survival outcomes and long-term monitoring is limited. However, reports suggest that around 50% of patients are symptomatic at diagnosis, and 20–41% present with advanced-stage disease. Patients identified through screening programs tend to have better survival rates if treated appropriately (Kikuchi et al. 2017; Piñero et al. 2018; Debes et al. 2018).

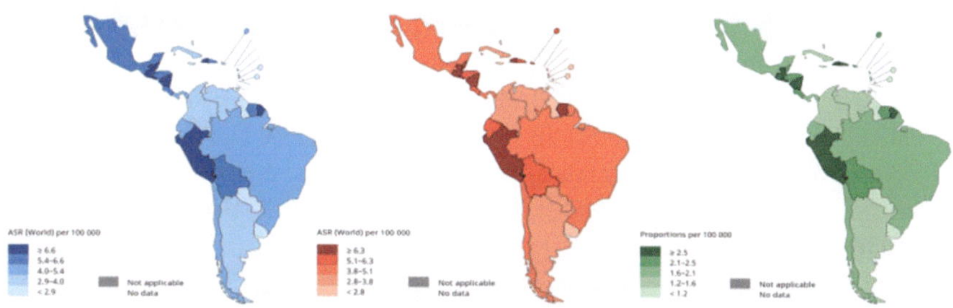

Fig. 2.7 Liver Cancer Epidemiology in Latin America. Data sourced from the International Agency for Research on Cancer (IARC, accessed August 15, 2019). (**a**) Projected age-standardized incidence rates for 2018; (**b**) Projected age-standardized mortality rates for 2018; (**c**) Projected one-year prevalence rates for 2018 (ASR: age-standardized rate per 100,000 individuals)

Table 2.3 Projected New Cases and Deaths from Liver Cancer in 2018 (Both sexes, all ages)

Regions	New cases	ASR (world)	Deaths	ASR (world)
Latin America and the Caribbean	38,400	5.0	36,436	4.7
Asia	609,596	11.4	566,269	10.5
Europe	82,466	5.1	77,375	4.4
Africa	69,779	8.4	63,562	8.3
North America	41,851	6.6	34,339	4.8
Oceania	3988	6.9	3650	5.8

Bray et al. (2018)

2.6.2 Risk Factors for HCC in Latin America

Between 2005 and 2015, a large multinational study was conducted across 14 medical institutions spanning six South American countries. Males accounted for 68% of participants, with a median age of 64 years.

Among the study population, chronic HCV infection emerged as the most common risk factor for HCC, responsible for 48% of the cases. Alcohol-related cirrhosis followed as the second most prevalent cause, accounting for 22% of cases. HBV infection was identified in 14% of patients, NAFLD contributed to 9%, while the remaining 8% were associated with other etiologies including cryptogenic cirrhosis, hemochromatosis, autoimmune hepatitis, HBV/HCV co-infection, schistosomiasis, and primary biliary cholangitis (Debes et al. 2018).

HBV genotype F has been linked to the early onset of HCC among Alaska Native populations (Devesa and Pujol 2007). In Latin America, patients with HBV-associated HCC were diagnosed at a median age of 58 years, whereas HCV-associated cases had a median age of 63 years at diagnosis. Those with NAFLD-related HCC had a median diagnosis age of 67 years, while patients with alcohol-related cirrhosis presented at a median age of 68 years (Debes et al. 2018).

The introduction of direct-acting antivirals (DAAs) across Latin America is anticipated to substantially lower the rates of HCV-associated HCC (Pawlotsky et al. 2018).

Currently, approximately 57% of adults in Latin America are categorized as overweight, with 19% classified as obese. The prevalence of NAFLD in South America has reached an estimated 31% (Younossi et al. 2016).

A 2016 study investigating 110 Brazilian HCC patients with underlying NASH revealed that 73.6% had diabetes, 52.7% were obese, 41.0% had dyslipidemia, and 57.2% exhibited features of metabolic syndrome. Of these patients, 52 (47.2%) had a confirmed histological diagnosis of HCC. Among these, 61.5% had NASH accompanied by cirrhosis, 27% had NASH with fibrosis stages 1 to 3, and 3.8% had NASH without fibrosis (Cotrim et al. 2016).

Molecular studies among 74 Brazilian patients undergoing liver resection or transplantation for HCC identified the aflatoxin-specific TP53 249Ser mutation. This mutation correlated with more aggressive tumor characteristics, including larger tumor size and poorer differentiation (Nogueira et al. 2009).

2.7 Hepatocellular Carcinoma in Asia

In 2020, Asia accounted for approximately 609,596 new liver cancer cases, which represents 72.5% of the global incidence. The Age-Standardized Rate (ASR) was reported at 11.6 per 100,000. During the same period, liver cancer caused 566,269 deaths in Asia, corresponding to 72.4% of worldwide liver cancer deaths, with an ASR of 10.7 (WHO 2020).

2.7.1 Incidence and Mortality of HCC in Asia

Among Asian men, liver cancer ranks fourth in incidence and second in cancer-related deaths. In Asian women, liver cancer ranks as the seventh most common cancer and the sixth leading cause of cancer mortality.

2.7.2 Risk Factors for HCC in Asia

The predominant causes of HCC in Asia are shifting from viral to non-viral origins. Changes in lifestyle and dietary habits have contributed to a rise in NAFLD cases in China (Fan 2013). NAFLD and related conditions now account for roughly 10.5% of liver cancer deaths in China (WHO 2016).

Hepatitis B virus (HBV) infection remains common across the Asia-Pacific region, where approximately 75% of HBV-positive individuals reside (Liaw 2009). However, widespread neonatal HBV vaccination campaigns between 1990 and 2005 have significantly reduced chronic HBV infections (Liang et al. 2009).

The prevalence of HCV varies across the region, being approximately 1% in India, 1.3% in China, 2.7% in Thailand, 6.7% in Pakistan, and as high as 10% in Mongolia (Gower et al. 2014). In 2012, HCV overtook HBV as the leading cause of HCC in Pakistan, accounting for 58% of HCC cases (Butt et al. 2012).

It is projected that implementing widespread HCV screening, treating around 510,000 patients annually, raising public awareness, and improving sterilization practices could dramatically reduce the HCV burden and prevent about 116,000 new liver cancer cases over the next 15 years in Pakistan (Bosan et al. 2010).

There remains a lack of comprehensive data regarding the impact of autoimmune hepatitis, primary biliary cholangitis, primary sclerosing cholangitis, and IgG4-related liver disease on HCC incidence in the Asia-Pacific region.

Several large cohort studies from Taiwan have shown that metabolic syndrome significantly elevates the risk of HCC in individuals infected with HBV or HCV (Yu et al. 2008).

Moreover, diabetes mellitus has been identified as a predictive factor for HCC development. In HCV-infected patients, diabetes worsens HCC progression risk and is associated with higher all-cause mortality rates, both in patients with and without HCC (Chen et al. 2008; Huang et al. 2017).

Chronic low-level exposure to aflatoxins remains a significant environmental risk factor for liver cancer in Asia (McGlynn et al. 2015). Mycotoxins, particularly in foodstuffs such as corn, peanuts, and soybeans, have been implicated in causing liver damage (Magnussen and Parsi 2013).

One major factor contributing to the reduction in liver cancer incidence has been aflatoxin mitigation programs (Sun et al. 2013).

While studies on alcoholic liver disease trends in Asia are limited, available evidence suggests that the incidence is rising among hospitalized patients. Nevertheless, alcohol consumption appears to have a lesser role in HCC development in Asia compared to Europe and North America (Estes et al. 2018a, b; Poustchi et al. 2010).

2.8 Conclusion

HCC remains a significant health burden, particularly in low- and middle-income nations. Comprehensive epidemiological data are crucial for prioritizing liver cancer prevention strategies.

Although viral hepatitis remains the principal risk factor, its impact is expected to decline with the growing influence of metabolic-related liver diseases, due to the widespread use of DAAs and rising rates of obesity and metabolic syndrome.

Expanding HBV vaccination coverage in endemic regions is poised to be transformative. In Western countries, reducing alcohol intake remains an essential component of HCC prevention efforts.

Ongoing work is critical to enhance HCC screening, early diagnosis, and effective management strategies.

References

Abdel-Wahab M, Mostafa M, Sabry M, et al. Afatoxins as a risk factor for hepatocellular carcinoma in Egypt, mansoura gastroenterology center study. Hepato-Gastroenterology. 2008;55:1754–9.

Ahmed AM, Hassan MS, Abd-Elsayed A, et al. Insulin resistance, steatosis, and Fbrosis in Egyptian patients with chronic hepatitis C virus infection. Saudi J Gastroenterol. 2011;17(4):245–51.

Akinyemiju T, Abera S, Ahmed M, et al. The burden of primary liver cancer and underlying etiologies from 1990 to 2015 at the global, regional, and national level. JAMA Oncol. 2017;3:1683–91. https://doi.org/10.1001/jamaoncol.2017.3055.

Akyıldız M, Ahiskli E, Zeybel M, Yurdadin C. Regional epidemiology, burden, and management of hepatitis B virus in the Middle East. Clin Liver Dis. 2019;14(6):212–4.

Allemani C, Weir HK, Carreira H, et al. Global surveillance of cancer survival 1995-2009: analysis of individual data for 25 676 887 patients from 279 population-based registries in 67 countries (CONCORD-2). Lancet. 2015;385:977–1010.

Andoulo FA, Noah DN, Djapa R, et al. Epidemiology of hepatitis C: related hepatocellular carcinoma in Cameroon. Pan Afr Med J. 2014;19:4143. https://doi.org/10.11604/pamj.2014.19.379.4143.

Baten J. International Economic History Association. A history of the global economy: from 1500 to the present. Cambridge University Press; 2016.

Beyhan S, Yildiz O, Kalaca T, et al. Twelve-year trends in the prevalence and risk factors of diabetes and prediabetes in Turkish adults. Eur J Epidemiol. 2013;28(2):169–80.

Blach S, Sanai FM. HCV burden and barriers to elimination in the Middle East. Clin Liver Dis (Hoboken). 2020;14(6):224–7.

Bosan A, Qureshi H, Bile KM, et al. A review of hepatitis viral infections in Pakistan. J Pak Med Assoc. 2010;60:1045–58.

Boutayeb A, Lamlili ENM, Boutayeb W, et al. The rise of diabetes prevalence in the Arab region. Open J Epidemiol. 2012;2:55–60.

Brandt S, Heller H, Schuster KD, Grote J. Tamoxifen induces suppression of cell viability and apoptosis in the human hepatoblastoma cell line HepG2 via down-regulation of telomerase activity. Liver Int. 2004;24:46–54.

Bravi F, Bosetti C, Tavani A, et al. Coffee reduces risk for hepatocellular carcinoma: an updated meta-analysis. Clin Gastroenterol Hepatol. 2013;11:1413–1421.e1.

Bray F, Ferlay J, Soerjomataram I, et al. Global cancer statistics 2018: GLOBOCAN estimates of incidence and mortality worldwide for 36 cancers in 185 countries. CA Cancer J Clin. 2018;68:394–424.

Butt AS, Abbas Z, Jafri W. Hepatocellular carcinoma in Pakistan: where do we stand? Hepat Mon. 2012;12:e6023.

Car BI. Liver cancer in the Middle East: hepatocellular carcinoma in the Middle East: an overview. Springer Nature Switzerland AG; 2021. p. 301.

Chang MH, et al. Long- term effects of hepatitis B immunization of infants in preventing liver cancer. Gastroenterology. 2016;151:472–480.e1.

Chen CL, Yang HI, Yang WS, et al. Metabolic factors and risk of hepatocellular carcinoma by chronic hepatitis B/C infection: a follow-up study in Taiwan. Gastroenterology. 2008;135:111–21.

Chuang SC, La Vecchia C, Boffetta P. Liver cancer: descriptive epidemiology and risk factors other than HBV and HCV infection. Cancer Lett (Internet). 2009;286(1):9–14. https://doi.org/10.1016/j.canlet.2008.10.040.

Cotrim HP, Oliveira CP, Coelho HSM, et al. Nonalcoholic steatohepatitis and hepatocellular carcinoma: Brazilian survey. Clinics (São Paulo). 2016;71(05):281–4.

Coursaget P, Leboulleux D, Yvonnet B, et al. Hepatitis B virus infection and hepatocellular carcinoma in Senegal: prevalence and prevention. J Gastroenterol Hepatol. 1993;8(S1):S128–33.

Debes JD, Chan AJ, Balderramo D, et al. Hepatocellular carcinoma in South America: evaluation of risk factors, demographics and therapy. Liver Int. 2018;38(01):136–43.

Devesa M, Pujol FH. Hepatitis B virus genetic diversity in Latin America. Virus Res. 2007;127(02):177–84.

El Kassas M, Elbaz T, Salaheldin M, et al. Impact of treating chronic hepatitis C infection with direct-acting antivirals on the risk of hepatocellular carcinoma: the debate continues—a mini-review. J Adv Res. 2019;17:43–8. https://doi.org/10.1016/j.jare.2019.03.001.

Elgouhari HM, Abu-Rajab TI, Carey WD. Hepatitis B virus infection: understanding its epidemiology, course, and diagnosis. Cleve Clin J Med. 2008;75:881–9.

El-Karaksy HM, El-Koofy NM, Anwar GM, et al. Predictors of nonalcoholic fatty liver disease in obese and overweight Egyptian children: single center study. Saudi J Gastroenterol. 2011;17(1):40–6.

El-Kassas M, Elbadry M. Hepatocellular Carcinoma in Africa: challenges and opportunities. Front Med. 2022;9:1–4.

El-Koofy NM, El-Karaksy HM, Mandour IM, et al. Genetic polymorphisms in non-alcoholic fatty liver disease in obese Egyptian children. Saudi J Gastroenterol. 2011;17(4):265–70.

El-Serag HB. Epidemiology of viral hepatitis and hepatocellular carcinoma. Gastroenterology (Internet). 2012;142(6):1264–1273.e1. https://doi.org/10.1053/j.gastro.2011.12.061.

Esmat G, El-Sayed MH, Hassany M, et al. One step closer to elimination of hepatitis C in Egypt. Lancet Gastroenterol Hepatol. 2018;3:665. https://doi.org/10.1016/S2468-1253(18)30268-1.

Estes C, Anstee QM, Arias-Loste MT, et al. Modeling NAFLD disease burden in China, France, Germany, Italy, Japan, Spain, United Kingdom, and United States for the period 2016–2030. J Hepatol. 2018a;69:896–904.

Estes C, Razavi H, Loomba R, et al. Modeling the epidemic of nonalcoholic fatty liver disease demonstrates an exponential increase in burden of disease. Hepatology. 2018b;67:123–33.

Ettorree GM. Hepatocellular Carcinoma. Updat Surg. 2023; https://doi.org/10.1007/978-3-031-09371-5_1.

European Association for the Study of the Liver. EASL clinical practice guidelines: management of hepatocellular carcinoma. J Hepatol. 2018;69:182–236.

Eyraud D, Richard O, Borie DC, et al. Hemodynamic and hormonal responses to the sudden interruption of caval low: insights from a prospective study of hepatic vascular exclusion during major liver resections. Anesth Analg. 2002;95(5):1173–8.

Fan JG. Epidemiology of alcoholic and nonalcoholic fatty liver disease in China. J Gastroenterol Hepatol. 2013;28(Suppl. 1):11–7.

Fiel MI, Min A, Gerber MA, et al. Hepatocellular carcinoma in long-term oral contraceptive use. Liver. 1996;16:372–6.

Fracanzani A. Increased cancer risk in a cohort of 230 patients with hereditary hemochromatosis in comparison to matched control patients with non–iron- related chronic liver disease. Hepatology. 2001;33:647–51.

GLMM-Gulf Labour Markets and Migration (Internet). (cited 2020 Oct 30). Available from: https://gulfmigration.org/
Gower E, Estes C, Blach S, et al. Global epidemiology and genotype distribution of the hepatitis C virus infection. J Hepatol. 2014;61(Suppl. 1):S45–57.
Hannaford PC, Kay CR, Vessey MP, et al. Combined oral contraceptives and liver disease. Contraception. 1997;55:145–51.
Huang TS, Lin CL, Lu MJ, et al. Diabetes, hepatocellular carcinoma, and mortality in hepatitis C-infected patients: A population-based cohort study. J Gastroenterol Hepatol. 2017;32:1355–62.
International Agency for Research on Cancer. GLOBOCAN 2018. IARC https://gco.iarc.fr/today/online-analysis-map?
International Agency for Research on Cancer/World Health Organization. Global Cancer Observatory. Cancer Today: Data visualization tools for exploring the global cancer burden in 2020. http://gco.iarc.fr/today Accessed 16 Dec 2021.
Ioannou GN, et al. Increased risk for hepatocellular carcinoma persists up to 10 years after HCV eradication in patients with baseline cirrhosis or high FIB-4 scores. Gastroenterology. 2019;157:1264–1278.e4.
Jain MK, et al. Evaluation of a multifaceted intervention to reduce health disparities in hepatitis C screening: a pre- post analysis. Hepatology. 2019;70:40–50.
Janahi EM, Ilyas Z, Al-Othman S, et al. Hepatitis B virus genotypes in the Kingdom of Bahrain: prevalence, gender distribution and impact on hepatic biomarkers. Medicina (Kaunas). 2019;55(10):622.
Jemal A, Bray F, Forman D, et al. Cancer burden in Africa and opportunities for prevention. Cancer. 2012;118:4372–84. https://doi.org/10.1002/cncr.27410.
Jepsen P, Ott P, Andersen PK, et al. Risk for hepatocellular carcinoma in patients with alcoholic cirrhosis. Ann Intern Med. 2012;156:841.
Jones RM, Moulton CE, Hardy KJ. Central venous pressure and its effect on blood loss during liver resection. Br J Surg. 1998;85(8):1058–60.
Kaito M, Watanabe S, Tsukiyama-Kohara K, et al. Hepatitis C virus particle detected by immunoelectron microscopic study. J Gen Virol (Internet). 1994;75(7):1755–60. https://doi.org/10.1099/0022-1317-75-7-1755.
Kamali I, Shumbusho F, Barnhart DA, et al. Time to complete hepatitis C cascade of care among patients identified during mass screening campaigns in rural Rwanda: a retrospective cohort study. BMC Infectious Dis. 2022;22:1–10. https://doi.org/10.1186/s12879-022-07271-z.
Kanwal F, et al. Risk of hepatocellular cancer in HCV patients treated with direct- acting antiviral agents. Gastroenterology. 2017;153:996–1005.e1.
Kanwal F, Kramer JR, Mapakshi S, et al. Risk of hepatocellular cancer in patients with non-alcoholic fatty liver disease. Gastroenterology. 2018;155:1828–1837.e2.
Kew MC. Clinical, pathologic, and etiologic heterogeneity in hepatocellular carcinoma: evidence from southern Africa. Hepatology. 1981;1:366–9.
Kew MC, Asare GA. Dietary iron overload in the African and hepatocellular carcinoma. Liver Int. 2007;27:735–41.
Kew MC, Song E, Dusheiko GM. Hepatocellular carcinoma in white South Africans-aetiological considerations. S Afr Med J. 1984;66:835–7.
Kew MC. Synergistic interaction between aflatoxin B1 and hepatitis B virus in hepatocarcinogenesis. Liver Int. 2003;23:405–9.
Kew MC. Epidemiology of hepatocellular carcinoma in sub-Saharan Africa. Ann Hepatol 2013;12:173–82.
Kew MC, Welschinger R, Viana R. Occult hepatitis B virus infection in Southern African blacks with hepatocellular carcinoma. J Gastroenterol Hepatol. 2008;23:1426–30.
Kikuchi L, Chagas AL, Alencar RSSM, et al. Adherence to BCLC recommendations for the treatment of hepatocellular carcinoma: impact on survival according to stage. Clinics (São Paulo). 2017;72(08):454–60.

Koppes CR. Captain Mahan, General Gordon, and the origins of the term 'Middle East'. Middle East Stud (Internet). 1976;12(1):95–8. https://doi.org/10.1080/00263207608700307.

Kourakli A, Diamantidis MD, Skafdas ME, et al. Hepatitis C virus infection, but not hepatic iron overload is the dominant risk factor for the manifestation of hepatocellular carcinoma among Greek thalassemic patients. Blood. 2018;132:2347.

Kristensen SD, Knuuti J, Saraste A, et al. 2014 ESC/ESA Guidelines non-cardiac surgery: cardiovascular assessment and management. Eur Heart J. 2014;35(35):2383–431.

Lee YCA, et al. Meta-analysis of epidemiologic studies on cigarette smoking and liver cancer. Int J Epidemiol. 2009;38:1497–511.

Lehman EM, Wilson ML. Epidemiology of hepatitis viruses among hepatocellular carcinoma cases and healthy people in Egypt: a systematic review and meta-analysis. Int J Cancer. 2009;124(3):690–7.

Li Z, Sun YM, Wu FX, et al. Controlled low central venous pressure reduces blood loss transfusion requirements in hepatectomy. World J Gastroenterol. 2014;20(1):303–9.

Liang X, Bi S, Yang W, et al. Epidemiological serosurvey of hepatitis B in China–declining HBV prevalence due to hepatitis B vaccination. Vaccine. 2009;27:6550–7.

Liaw YF. Antiviral therapy of chronic hepatitis B: opportunities and challenges in Asia. J Hepatol. 2009;51:403–10.

Lindberg MC. Hepatobiliary complications of oral contraceptives. J Gen Intern Med. 1992;7:199–209.

Liu Y, Chang CH, Marsh GM, Wu F. Population attributable risk of afatoxin-related liver cancer: systematic review and meta-analysis. Eur J Cancer. 2012;48:2125–36.

Llovet JM, Burroughs A, Bruix J. Hepatocellular carcinoma. Lancet (Internet). 2003;362(9399):1907–17. https://doi.org/10.1016/s0140-6736(03)14964-1.

Llovet JM, Villanueva A. Effect of HCV clearance with direct-acting antiviral agents on HCC. Nat Rev Gastroenterol Hepatol. 2016;13:561–2.

London WT, Petrick JL, McGlynn KA. Liver cancer. In: Thun MJ, Linet MS, Cerhan JR, Haiman CA, Schottenfeld DE, editors. Cancer epidemiology and prevention. New York: Oxford University Press; 2018. p. 635–60.

Magnussen A, Parsi MA. Aflatoxins, hepatocellular carcinoma and public health. World J Gastroenterol. 2013;19:1508–12.

Mak D, Babb de Villiers C, Chasela C, et al. Analysis of risk factors associated with hepatocellular carcinoma in black South Africans: 2000–2012. PLoS One. 2018;13:e0196057.

Mak D, Kramvis A. Epidemiology and aetiology of hepatocellular carcinoma in Sub-Saharan Africa. Hepatoma Res. 2021;7:39. Available online at: https://hrjournal.net/article/view/4046

Marrero JA, et al. Diagnosis, staging, and management of hepatocellular carcinoma: 2018 practice guidance by the American Association for the Study of Liver Diseases. Hepatology. 2018;68:723–50.

Mazumder PM, Sasmal D. Mycotoxins - limits and regulations. Anc Sci Life. 2001;20:1–19.

McGlynn KA, Tarone RE, El-Serag HB. A comparison of trends in the incidence of hepatocellular carcinoma and intrahepatic cholangiocarcinoma in the United States. Cancer Epidemiol Biomarkers Prev. 2006;15:1198–203.

McGlynn KA, Petrick JL, London WT, et al. Global epidemiology of hepatocellular carcinoma: An emphasis on demographic and regional variability. Clin Liver Dis. 2015;19:223–38.

Mdlalose N, Parboosing R, Moodley P. The prevalence of hepatitis B virus infection in HIV-positive and HIV-negative infants: KwaZulu-Natal, South Africa. Afr J Lab Med. 2016;5:283.

Mittal S, et al. Hepatocellular carcinoma in the absence of cirrhosis in United States veterans is associated with nonalcoholic fatty liver disease. Clin Gastroenterol Hepatol. 2016;14:124–131.e1.

Mohamed AE, Kew MC, Groeneveld HT. Alcohol consumption as a risk factor for hepatocellular carcinoma in urban southern African blacks. Int J Cancer. 1992;51:537–41.

Moonsamy S, Suchard M, Pillay P, Prabdial-Sing N. Prevalence incidence rates of laboratory-confirmed hepatitis B infection in South Africa, 2015 to 2019. BMC Publ. Heal. 2022;22:1–13. https://doi.org/10.1186/s12889-021-12391-3.

Musa BM, Bussell S, Borodo MM, et al. Prevalence of hepatitis B virus infection in Nigeria, 2000–2013: a systematic review and meta-analysis. Niger J Clin Pract. 2015;18:163–72.

Nogueira JA, Ono-Nita SK, Nita ME, et al. 249 TP53 mutation has high prevalence and is correlated with larger and poorly differentiated HCC in Brazilian patients. BMC Cancer. 2009;9(01):204.

National Cancer Institute; Surveillance, Epidemiology and End Results Program (SEER) Liver and Intrahepatic Bile Duct Cancer, CSR 1975–2015: (Internet) available at https://seer.cancer.gov/archive/csr/1975_2015/results_merged/sect_14_liver_bile.pdf. Accessed 1 Oct 2020.

Nordien R, Sonderup M, Spearman C. A decade of hepatitis C at the University of Cape Town/Groote Schuur hospital liver clinic, South Africa, in the pre-direct-acting antivirals era. S Afr Med J. 2020;110:106–11. https://doi.org/10.7196/SAMJ.2020.v110i2.14208.

Ozdemir FT, Duman D, Ertem D, et al. Determination of hepatitis B genotypes in patients with chronic hepatitis B virus infection in Turkey. Turk J Gastroenterol. 2005;16(4):183–7.

Parkin DM, Hämmerl L, Ferlay J, Kantelhardt EJ. Cancer in Africa 2018: The role of infections. Int J Cancer. 2020;146:2089–103.

Paruk IM, Pirie FJ, Motala AA. Non-alcoholic fatty liver disease in Africa: a hidden danger. Glob Health Epidemiol Genom. 2019;4:e3. https://doi.org/10.1017/gheg.2019.2.

Pawlotsky J-M, Negro F, Aghemo A, et al. EASL recommendations on treatment of hepatitis C 2018. J Hepatol. 2018;69(02):461–511.

Pearson TA. How to interpret a genome-wide association study. JAMA (Internet). 2008;299(11):1335. https://doi.org/10.1001/jama.299.11.1335.

Petrick JL, McGlynn KA. The changing epidemiology of primary liver cancer. Curr Epidemiol Rep. 2019;6:104–11.

Piñero F, Marciano S, Fernández N, et al. Argentinean Association for the Study of Liver Diseases (A.A.E.E.H). Adherence to Barcelona Clinic Liver Cancer therapeutic algorithm for hepatocellular carcinoma in the daily practice: a multicenter cohort study from Argentina. Eur J Gastroenterol Hepatol. 2018;30(04):376–83.

Population trends and challenges in the Middle East and North Africa (PTCMENA): (Internet) available at https://www.prb.org/resources/population-trends-and-challenges-in-the-middle-east-and-north-africa/. Accessed 4 Oct 2020.

Poustchi H, Sepanlou S, et al. Hepatocellular carcinoma in the world and the middle East. Middle East J Dig Dis. 2010;2:31–41.

Poynard T, Ratziu V, Benmanov Y, et al. Fibrosis in patients with chronic hepatitis C: detection and signifcance. Semin Liver Dis (Internet). 2000;20(01):47–56. https://doi.org/10.1055/s-2000-9258.

Puigvehí M, Moctezuma-Velázquez C, Villanueva A, Llovet JM. The oncogenic role of hepatitis delta virus in hepatocellular carcinoma. JHEP Rep. 2019;1:120–30.

Qian GS, Ross RK, Yu MC, et al. A follow-up study of urinary markers of aflatoxin exposure and liver cancer risk in Shanghai, People's Republic of China. Cancer Epidemiol Biomarkers Prev. 1994;3:3–10.

Ramezani-Binabaj M, Motalebi M, Karimi-Sari H, et al. Are women with polycystic ovarian syndrome at a high risk of nonalcoholic Fatty liver disease; a meta-analysis. Hepat Mon. 2014;14(11):e23235. https://doi.org/10.5812/hepatmon.23235.

Rauch A, Kutalik Z, Descombes P, et al. Genetic variation in IL28B is associated with chronic hepatitis C and treatment failure: a genome-wide association study. Gastroenterology (Internet). 2010;138(4):1338–1345.e7. https://doi.org/10.1053/j.gastro.2009.12.056.

Rawla P, Sunkara T, Muralidharan P, et al. Update in global trends and aetiology of hepatocellular carcinoma. Contemp Oncol (Pozn). 2018;22(3):141–50. https://doi.org/10.5114/wo.2018.78941.

Rich NE, et al. Racial and ethnic differences in presentation and outcomes of hepatocellular carcinoma. Clin Gastroenterol Hepatol. 2019;17:551–559.e1.

Rich NE, Yopp AC, Singal AG, Murphy CC. Hepatocellular carcinoma incidence is decreasing among younger adults in the United States. Clin Gastroenterol Hepatol. 2020;18:242–248.e5.

Ringelhan M, McKeating JA, Protzer U. Viral hepatitis and liver cancer. Philos Trans R Soc Lond Ser B Biol Sci (Internet). 2017;372(1732):20160274. Available from: https://pubmed.ncbi.nlm.nih.gov/28893941

Rizzetto M, Hepatitis D. Virus: Introduction and Epidemiology. Cold Spring Harb Perspect Med. 2015;5:a021576.

Sankaranarayanan R. Cancer survival in Africa, Asia, the Caribbean and Central America. Introduction. IARC Sci Publ. 2011;162:15.

Schweitzer A, Horn J, Mikolajczyk RT, et al. Estimations of worldwide prevalence of chronic hepatitis B virus infection: a systematic review of data published between 1965 and 2013. Lancet. 2015;386:1546–55. https://doi.org/10.1016/S0140-6736(15)61412-X.

Smith DB, Bukh J, Kuiken C, et al. Expanded classifcation of hepatitis C virus into 7 genotypes and 67 subtypes: updated criteria and genotype assignment web resource. Hepatology (Internet). 2014;59(1):318–27. Available from: https://pubmed.ncbi.nlm.nih.gov/24115039

Sohrabpour A, Rezvan H, Amini-Kafabad S, et al. Prevalence of nonalcoholic steatohepatitis in Iran: a population based study. Middle East J Dig Dis. 2010;2(1):14–9.

Soliman AS, Hung CW, Tsodikov A, et al. Epidemiologic risk factors of hepatocellular carcinoma in a rural region of Egypt. Hepatol Int. 2010;4:681–90.

Specialist Panel on Chronic Hepatitis B in the Middle East (SPCHBME). A review of chronic hepatitis B epidemiology and management issues in selected countries in the Middle East. Viral Hepatol. 2012;19(1):9–22.

Sun Z, Chen T, Thorgeirsson SS, et al. Dramatic reduction of liver cancer incidence in young adults: 28-year follow-up of etiological interventions in an endemic area of China. Carcinogenesis. 2013;34:1800–5.

Sung H, Ferlay J, Siegel RL, et al. Global Cancer Statistics 2020: GLOBOCAN Estimates of Incidence and Mortality Worldwide for 36 Cancers in 185 Countries. CA Cancer J Clin. 2021;71(3):209–49. https://pubmed.ncbi.nlm.nih.gov/33538338/

Talaat M, Aff S, Reaves EJ, et al. Evidence of sustained reductions in the relative risk of acute hepatitis B and C virus infections, and the increasing burden of hepatitis a virus infection in Egypt: comparison of sentinel acute viral hepatitis surveillance results, 2001–17. BMC Infect Dis. 2019;19(1):159.

Tang L, Xu L, Afriyie-Gyawu E, et al. Aflatoxin-albumin adducts and correlation with decreased serum levels of vitamins A and E in an adult Ghanaian population. Food Addit Contam Part A Chem Anal Control Expo Risk Assess. 2009;26:108–18.

Thomas DL, Thio CL, Martin MP, et al. Genetic variation in IL28B and spontaneous clearance of hepatitis C virus. Nature (Internet). 2009;461(7265):798–801.

Thompson AJ, Muir AJ, Sulkowski MS, et al. Interleukin-28B polymorphism improves viral kinetics and is the strongest pretreatment predictor of sustained virologic… (Internet). SciVee, Inc; 2010. https://doi.org/10.4016/19518.01.

Trinchet JC, et al. Complications and competing risks of death in compensated viral cirrhosis (ANRS CO12 CirVir prospective cohort). Hepatology. 2015;62:737–50.

Vardas E, Mathai M, Blaauw D, et al. Preimmunization epidemiology of hepatitis B virus infection in South African children. J Med Virol. 1999;58:111–5.

Wang J, Chenivesse X, Henglein B, Bréchot C. Hepatitis B virus integration in a cyclin A gene in a hepatocellular carcinoma. Nature. 1990;343:555–7.

WHO. Data Visualization Tools for Exploring the Global Cancer Burden in 2020. 2020. Available online: https://gco.iarc.fr/today/

Wong RJ, Aguilar M, Cheung R, et al. Nonalcoholic steatohepatitis is the second leading etiology of liver disease among adults awaiting liver transplantation in the United States. Gastroenterology. 2015;148(3):547–55.

World Health Organization (WHO). Global Status Report on Alcohol and Health 2018. Geneva: World Health Organization; 2019a. Available online at: https://www.who.int/publications/i/item/9789241565639

World Health Organization (WHO). Global health sector strategy on viral hepatitis, 2016–2021 towards ending viral hepatitis. Geneva: WHO; 2016.

World Health Organization (WHO): Hepatitis B Fact Sheet, 2017. Available from https://www.who.int/news-room/factsheets/detail/hepatitis-b (Last accessed on 7 May 2021).

World Health Organization (WHO): HIV/AIDS 2019b. Available from https://www.who.int/news-room/fact-sheets/detail/hiv-aids# (Last accessed on 7 May 2021).

World Health Organization (WHO): Regional action plan for the implementation of the global health sector strategy on viral hepatitis 2017–2021; 2017. Available from: http://apps.who.int/iris/handle/10665/258729. Accessed: 12 Oct 2020.

Xu L, Kim Y, Spolverato G, et al. Racial disparities in treatment and survival of patients with hepatocellular carcinoma in the United States. Hepatobiliary Surg Nutr. 2016;5:43–52.

Yang JD, Gyedu A, Afihene MY, et al. Hepatocellular carcinoma occurs at an earlier age in africans, particularly in association with chronic hepatitis B. Am J Gastroenterol. 2015a;110:1629–31. https://doi.org/10.1038/ajg.2015.289.

Yang JD, Gyedu A, Afihene MY, et al. Africa Network for Gastrointestinal and Liver Diseases. Hepatocellular Carcinoma Occurs at an Earlier Age in Africans, Particularly in Association With Chronic Hepatitis B. Am J Gastroenterol. 2015b;110:1629–31.

Yang JD, Mohamed EA, Aziz AOA, et al. Characteristics, management, and outcomes of patients with hepatocellular carcinoma in Africa: a multicountry observational study from the Africa Liver Cancer Consortium. Lancet Gastroenterol Hepatol. 2017;2:103–11.

Yılmaz Y, Kanı HT, Demirtaş CÖ, et al. Growing burden of nonalcoholic fatty liver disease in Turkey: a single-center experience. Turk J Gastroenterol. 2019;30(10):892–8.

Younossi ZM, Koenig AB, Abdelatif D, et al. Global epidemiology of nonalcoholic fatty liver disease-Metaanalytic assessment of prevalence, incidence, and outcomes. Hepatology. 2016;64(01):73–84.

Yu MW, Shih WL, Lin CL, et al. Body-mass index and progression of hepatitis B: a population-based cohort study in men. J Clin Oncol. 2008;26(5576):5582.

Molecular Basis for Hepatocellular Carcinoma Development in Low/Middle-Income Countries

3

Ashraf A. Tabll, Eman A. El-Maadawy, and Roba M. Talaat

Abstract

This chapter aims to analyze in depth the molecular pathways driving the development of hepatocellular carcinoma (HCC) in low- and middle-income countries (LMICs). HCC is a liver cancer that commonly originates from the liver itself. It has a significant global health burden, especially in resource-constrained settings. So, understanding the complicated molecular processes that cause HCC to grow in these situations is very important for making progress in effective ways to prevent it, find it early, and tailor treatment plans. This paper also looks at some important changes that happen at the molecular level during the development of hepatocarcinogenesis. These include alterations in genes and epigenetics, malfunctioning signaling pathways or networks, and risk factors unique to LMICs. It further provides insights into the candidate biomarker identification process and potential therapy targets specific to these sites only. In summary, this article will give readers, whether they are researchers, healthcare providers, or policymakers, an understanding of the different steps involved in the pathogenesis of liver cancer within poor nations, thus enabling them to take care more effectively of patients under their management while at the same time improving outcomes generally in such environments.

A. A. Tabll
Immunology Department, Egypt Center for Research and Regenerative Medicine (ECRRM), Cairo, Egypt

Microbial Biotechnology Department, Biotechnology Research Institute, National Research Center, Giza, Egypt
e-mail: aa.tabll@nrc.sci.eg

E. A. El-Maadawy · R. M. Talaat (✉)
Molecular Biology Department, Genetic Engineering and Biotechnology Research Institute (GEBRI), University of Sadat City, Sadat City, Egypt
e-mail: Eman.anwr@gebri.usc.edu.eg; roba.talaat@gebri.usc.edu.eg

R. Elwakil et al. (eds.), *Approach to Hepatocellular Carcinoma (HCC) Management in Low/Middle-Income Countries*,
https://doi.org/10.1007/978-981-96-3894-9_3

Keywords

Hepatocellular carcinoma · Low/Middle-Income Countries · Signaling pathways · Molecular indicators · Therapeutic targets

Abbreviations

HCC	Hepatocellular carcinoma
LMICs	Low and middle-income countries
NAFLD	Non-alcoholic fatty liver disease
NASH	Non-alcoholic steatohepatitis
HBV	Hepatitis B virus (or HCV—the hepatitis C virus)
CT	Computed tomography
AFP	Alpha-fetoprotein
RB	Retinoblastoma protein
CDKs	Cyclin-dependent kinases
GS	Glutamine synthetase
APC	Adenomatous polyposis coli
TCF	T cell factor
LEF	Lymphoid enhancer-binding protein family
CCA	Cholangiocarcinoma
EMT	Epithelial-mesenchymal transition
CCNY	Cyclin Y
VEGF	Vascular endothelial growth factor
EGFR	Epidermal growth factor receptor
FGFR	Fibroblast growth factor receptor
HGF	Hepatocyte growth factor
PARP	Poly (ADP-ribose) polymerase
TCGA	Cancer Genome Atlas
β-TRCP	β-transducin repeat-containing protein

3.1 Overview of Hepatocellular Carcinoma as a Global Health Burden

HCC is a form of liver cancer that originates from hepatocytes, which are the most common cell types in the liver (Chidambaranathan-Reghupaty et al. 2021). It is the most common type of liver cancer and represents a significant global health problem. Globally, it ranks as the sixth most frequently diagnosed cancer and the fourth leading cause of cancer-related death (Okeke et al. 2020; Rich 2024). HCC has high mortality rates worldwide, with increasing incidences in developing and developed countries. The places where HCC is most common are also places where chronic hepatitis B virus (HBV) and chronic hepatitis C virus (HCV) are most common. These are mostly in sub-Saharan Africa, Southeast Asia, and some parts of Eastern Europe (Kedar Mukthinuthalapati et al. 2021; Cargill et al. 2021; Dakurah et al.

2021; Abdelhamed and El-Kassas 2023). However, industrialized nations, including the USA and Western European countries, have also begun to experience this trend. Increased cases of non-alcoholic fatty liver disease (NAFLD) and non-alcoholic steatohepatitis (NASH), both associated with obesity and metabolic syndrome, are the main cause of this (Rich 2024; Motta et al. 2023).

The main causes of HCC are chronic viral hepatitis, cirrhosis, NAFLD/NASH, alcohol abuse, and aflatoxin exposure. The hepatitis B or C virus causes chronic viral hepatitis, a long-term infection. This kind of infection is the main cause of HCC across the globe (Shadi et al. 2024). Any form of liver cirrhosis, irrespective of its origin, contributes significantly to developing HCC (Attallah et al. 1999; El-Sayed et al. 2004; Elderkin et al. 2023). Non-alcoholic fatty liver disease (NAFLD) and non-alcoholic steatohepatitis (NASH) are becoming more common because of obesity and metabolic syndrome. Both of these conditions can get worse and lead to cirrhosis and then cancer (Rich 2024; Michelotti et al. 2021). HCC risk increases substantially with heavy drinking over time (Singal et al. 2023). Ingesting food contaminated with aflatoxins, especially in low-income regions, raises the chances of getting HCC (Romualdo et al. 2023).

It is important to recognize HCC early on, take preventive measures, and use efficient treatments to reduce its worldwide burden. During its initial stages, HCC often does not show any clear symptoms, which leads to late discovery and a bad prognosis. Common indications are abdominal pain, weight loss, jaundice, and signs of liver malfunction (Piñero et al. 2023). Various imaging techniques, such as ultrasound scans, computed tomography (CT), or magnetic resonance imaging (MRI), can be used for diagnosis alongside blood tests that measure tumor markers like alpha-fetoprotein (AFP) (Omar et al. 2023). However, histological examination of a liver biopsy sample remains the most frequently employed method for diagnosing HCC (Di Tommaso et al. 2019).

Different therapeutic methods for HCC are available depending on the stage of the disease and the general condition of the patient's health (Bruix et al. 2016). Some treatments attempt to cure it; these may involve cutting out part or all of the liver, replacing a diseased liver with a healthy one, or destroying abnormal cells by heat or coldness (Petrowsky et al. 2020). People who have locally advanced or metastatic HCC can get drugs that only work where they're needed. For example, tyrosine kinase inhibitors stop growth signals, and immune checkpoint inhibitors make the immune system attack cancer cells (Raj et al. 2023; Xue et al. 2021). Prevention mainly involves reducing exposure to known risk factors such as hepatitis B vaccination, screening and treating chronic HBV and HCV infections, and promoting healthier lifestyle choices like quitting smoking, and many more (Yang et al. 2019). Early detection through surveillance programs targeted at high-risk groups can lead to earlier treatment before symptoms appear as well as improved overall outcomes (Ezzat et al. 2021). Successful management strategies also include public awareness campaigns about prevention methods alongside education programs plus easy access as well as affordability of healthcare services among others—not forgetting Momin SA's point on cost-effective delivery systems being put into place for better results within limited budgets!

3.2 Significance of Studying the Molecular Basis of HCC in Low/Middle-Income Countries

It is important to investigate the molecular underpinnings of HCC in LMICs. We should conduct this investigation because HCC is a common cause of cancer-related deaths worldwide, with particularly high prevalence rates in low- and middle-income countries. Understanding these mechanisms is critical to tailoring prevention strategies to specific at-risk populations and developing treatment options within resource-constrained settings. Also, looking into the molecular pathways involved in hepatocarcinogenesis might help solve the problem of not having enough money for research on new drugs to fight this malignant tumor, and it might also help make international efforts to get rid of liver cancer fairer (Llovet et al. 2018; Maloberti et al. 2022). There are often different risk factors between LLMICs and high-income countries, such as chronic viral infections like HBV or HCV, non-alcoholic fatty liver disease, metabolic disorders, and aflatoxin exposure, among others. Therefore, we can look into the relationship between these two things to understand how they change at the molecular level as severity sets in during the progression of diseases like hepatocellular carcinoma from an earlier stage to more advanced ones.

Resource limitations often result in a lack of healthcare facilities, diagnostics, and treatment options in low- and middle-income countries (LMICs). Analyzing the molecular basis of HCC in such contexts may lead to the discovery of inexpensive ways to diagnose, predict, and treat the disease (Rashed et al. 2020). This can enable the development of affordable diagnostic tools, accurate drugs, and individualized treatment strategies that are compatible with LMICs' health systems (Horton et al. 2020). Knowledge of the genetic underpinnings of HCC in LMICs could enhance translational research by combining basic science knowledge with practical medical applications (Dhanasekaran et al. 2016; Zucman-Rossi et al. 2015; Wogan et al. 2012). Furthermore, the analysis of HCC's molecular foundation in low- and middle-income countries is consistent with the goal of global health fairness. It deepens our understanding of the ailment, which means that investigations along with medical care solutions should be extensive enough to meet different population needs (Guy and Yee Jr. 2009; Wu et al. 2021). This should reduce worldwide health disparities as well as maximize gains for all patients, regardless of where they are located on earth or their social status, by giving priority to those nations where the HCC burden is high but research facilities are limited (Jensen et al. 2022).

3.3 Basics of Carcinogenesis

Preneoplastic states are the first step in the multi-step process that turns healthy cells into invasive cancer cells. Uncontrolled cell proliferation, longevity, genetic instability, and the ability to affect nearby and distant tissues (metastasis) are among the fundamental characteristics of cancer cells (Rosenberg and Rosenberg 2012).

Somatic mutations, which are caused by a variety of endogenous and environmental variables, including exposure to mutagens, viral infection, and nutrition, are the primary cause of most malignancies (Cha and DeMatteo 2005). The accumulation of DNA mutations, which can occur spontaneously in somatic cells or through germline mutation, leads to genomic instability in cancer cells.

According to Uma Devi (1989), the process of carcinogenesis comprises three key phases: initiation, promotion, and progression. Early mutations cause the start of a tumor, and a variety of other alterations are what cause the tumor to develop (Cha and DeMatteo 2005). Two major gene categories that are frequently changed in cancer are proto-oncogenes and tumor suppressor genes. A disruption in the balance between the activation and deactivation of these two categories of genes is thought to be a significant contributor to the formation of cancer (Chen and Wang 2015).

3.4 HCC and Cirrhosis

Like other neoplasia, HCC develops through a convoluted, multi-step process that is caused by a confluence of environmental and genetic variables. Regardless of the cause, most patients have cirrhosis before HCC. The regenerative nodules formed during cirrhosis provide a favorable environment for the transformation of normal hepatocytes into dysplastic hepatocytes and eventually neoplastic lesions, leading to the development of hepatocellular carcinoma (HCC). This transformation is facilitated by the accumulation of genetic and epigenetic alterations over time (Thorgeirsson and Grisham; 2002; Ramakrishna et al. 2013). When compared to other cancer forms, the neoplastic development of HCC is less clear. Hyperplastic nodules of regenerated hepatocytes may be an early sign of HCC and exhibit normal cytological characteristics. These lesions have the potential to develop into premalignant dysplastic nodules, which are linked to aberrant liver architecture and exhibit aberrant cytological characteristics such as nuclear crowding and clear cell alterations. These dysplastic nodules have the potential to develop into frank HCC, which can occasionally spread metastatically and infect the surrounding fibrous stroma and arteries (Farazi and DePinho 2006).

3.5 Genetic Modifications in HCC

Genetic and epigenetic changes that lead to the dysregulation of important oncogenes and tumor suppressor genes have been revealed by the molecular investigation of human HCC. Changes in the genes and epigenetics that stimulate HCC, are resistant to apoptotic signals, are not affected by growth-inhibitory signals, and are capable of angiogenesis (Aravalli et al. 2008). During the initiation, promotion, and progression phases of HCC development, several genetic and epigenetic alterations accumulate (Liu et al. 2014). New theories of carcinogenesis are put out and the molecular mechanisms of cancer unraveled more swiftly with the advent of modern molecular biology tools. This could ultimately result in improved treatment choices. The molecular pathophysiology of HCC remains unclear despite these developments.

Several risk variables interact to control a complex, long-term process that leads to HCC (Fig. 3.1). Accordingly, HCC represents the net outcome of somatic genetic and epigenomic changes that have accumulated in the original cells. On average, coding areas contain 40–60 somatic mutations, primarily in "passenger" genes but also a small number in "driver" genes for cancer that are involved in triggering important signaling pathways for the development of hepatocarcinogenesis (Llovet et al. 2015, 2016). HCC progression is driven by the aberrant activation of many molecules in several signaling pathways that impact the cell cycle, proliferation, differentiation, cell survival, and apoptosis., according to growing research on tumor signal transduction pathways (Chen and Wang 2015). In the following sections, we tried to shed some light on the most important pathways, focusing on the documented genetic dysregulation associated with hepatocarcinogenesis.

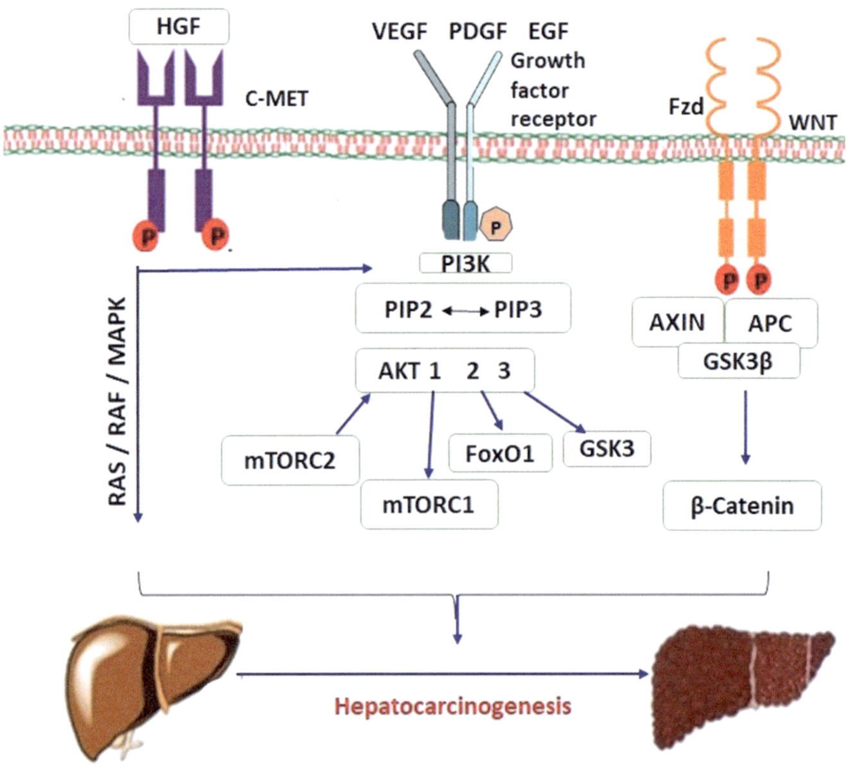

Fig. 3.1 Multiple risk factors work together to regulate the development of liver carcinogenesis

3.5.1 Dysregulated Oncogenic Signaling Pathways in HCC

3.5.1.1 Wnt/β-Catenin Signaling Pathway

One highly conserved and strictly regulated molecular mechanism that controls cellular proliferation, differentiation, and embryonic development is the Wnt/β-catenin signaling system. It is part of the main signaling routes controlling cancer, regeneration, and liver homeostasis. This pathway consists of frizzled receptor, ligand Wnt protein, and regulator proteins such β-catenin and GSK-3 (He et al. 2022).

CTNNB1 encodes β-catenin, which is essential for the development of tumors. It functions as an intracellular signal transducer and is an essential downstream part of the Wnt signaling pathway (Monga 2015; Perugorria et al. 2019). In a healthy liver, β-catenin is found on the cell membrane of hepatocytes. The Wnt/β-catenin pathway is activated specifically in pericentral hepatocytes, as evidenced by the presence of β-catenin-dependent glutamine synthetase (GS) staining (Benhamouche et al. 2006; Monga 2015).

Most of the cellular β-catenin is trapped in the adherents' junctions at the plasma membrane when Wnt ligands are absent. N-terminal phosphorylation of β-catenin is mediated by a complex formed by cytosolic β-catenin, adenomatous polyposis coli (APC), and AXIN1 proteins. As a result, β-catenin is ubiquitinated by the E3 ubiquitin ligase β-transducin repeat-containing protein (β-TRCP), and subsequent proteasomal degradation. Dvl/Dsh is phosphorylated when Wnt ligands attach to the Frizzled receptors. This prevents the formation of the degradation complex by recruiting AXIN1 and GSK3β next to the plasma membrane. Thus, unphosphorylated β-catenin moves into the nucleus and attaches to the transcription factors TCF and lymphoid enhancer-binding protein family (LEF) after eluding detection by β-TRCP. Genes that control cell proliferation and survival are transcribed by the active β-catenin/TCF/LEF complex. Numerous target genes, including MYC, cyclin D1, COX_2, and matrix metalloproteinase 7 (MMP7), are transactivated by this transcription factor complex and control processes important to cancer (He et al. 1998; Shtutman et al. 1999; Angers and Moon 2009; Pate et al. 2014).

Notably, accumulating evidence indicates that abnormal Wnt/β-catenin signaling contributes to the development and/or advancement of liver cancer, including cholangiocarcinoma (CCA) and HCC, the two most common primary liver tumors in adults (He et al. 2022). Research has demonstrated that abnormal Wnt/β-catenin activation in human HCCs is associated with unique clinical, pathological, and molecular characteristics. Genes that encode essential elements of the Wnt/β-catenin signaling pathway are mutated in most liver tumors. Furthermore, multiple additional signaling pathways can interact with β-catenin. Multiple studies have shown that the occurrence of overexpression and β-catenin mutations is more prevalent in HCCs associated to HCV compared to those connected to HBV.

These mutations are also frequently seen in HCC with non-cirrhotic liver when usual HCC risk factors are absent (Audard et al. 2007; Cieply et al. 2009). Some years earlier, Peng et al. (2004) stated that the Wnt/β-catenin cascade is associated with both tumor progression and early-stage HCC.

Between 20% and 40% of HCC cases have mutations in this pathway. According to Waly Raphael et al. (2012), mutations in the N-terminal of β-catenin frequently result in constitutive transcriptional activation of β-catenin/TCF complexes. In HCC, there is also a dephosphorylation of β-catenin and an overexpression of the frizzled-7 gene (Aravalli et al. 2008). Exposure to AFB1 and HCV infection are associated with activation of the Wnt/β-catenin pathway. HBV-related HCC had a decreased frequency of β-catenin mutations. Furthermore, Axin-1 and Axin-2 mutations were found in HCC; these proteins adversely control the Wnt/β-catenin pathway (Aravalli et al. 2008; Waly Raphael et al. 2012; Mao et al. 2016). Thus, all these data point to the Wnt/β-catenin signaling pathway's crucial role in the development of HCC.

Two different Wnt signaling pathways have been identified, non-canonical and canonical pathways, where the former is β-catenin dependent, while the latter is β-catenin independent.

The canonical pathway is initiated by the binding of Wnt ligands to cell surface receptors of the Frizzled family, which then triggers a cascade of events. This process liberates β-catenin from its degradation complex consisting of AXIN, APC, and GSK3, leading to its subsequent movement from the cell membrane to the nucleus. Alterations in several molecules, such as CTNNB1 and AXIN1, enable β-catenin to evade degradation and go into the nucleus, promoting the continuous activation of its target genes (Sia and Villanueva 2011). The canonical Wnt/FZD signaling is a critical contributor to HCC pathogenesis (Peng et al. 2016; Song et al. 2018) as β-catenin activation can be observed in 20–35% of HCC cases (Russell and Monga 2018). It is noteworthy that CTNNB1 has been recognized as one of the most frequently mutated genes in primary HCC (Lu et al. 2014). CTNNB1 mutations impact the serine/threonine site or exon 3 of neighboring amino acids. This hinders the phosphorylation and subsequent breakdown of β-catenin, resulting in its stability and movement into the nucleus (Monga 2015).

On the other hand, the ***non-canonical pathways*** of Wnt signal play a vital role in HCC development. Wnt ligand (Wnt5a) can hinder TCF activation mediated by activated CTNNB1 in HCC cells, which illustrates that canonical Wnt signaling can be antagonized by non-canonical Wnt5a in HCC (Yuzugullu et al. 2009). Wnt11 has the potential to function as an antagonist of canonical Wnt signaling by phosphorylating CTNNB1 and decreasing TCF-mediated transcriptional activity. This effect is triggered by activated PKC (Toyama et al. 2010; Chang et al. 2017). Moreover, non-canonical Wnt5-Frizzled2 could activate STAT3 phosphorylation (Chang et al. 2017). This process regulates epithelial-mesenchymal transition (EMT), and promotes metastasis in HCC (Gujral et al. 2014). Of note, like canonical Wnt signal, non-canonical pathway can also be regulated by upstream molecules such as, PFTK1, a Cdc2-related protein kinase which can interact with cyclin Y(CCNY) to activate non-canonical Wnt signaling in HCC (He and Tang 2020).

β-Catenin

In human HCC, β-catenin mutations and elevated nuclear expression have been found (Edamoto et al. 2003). According to certain publications, β-catenin mutations and overexpression have been linked to HCC progression in the early (Peng et al. 2004) and in late stages (An et al. 2001). Hsu et al. (2000) found that HCV-related HCCs are more likely than HBV-related HCCs to exhibit mutations and overexpression of β-catenin. Furthermore, it has been proposed that HCCs without genomic instability typically have β-catenin mutations. Very few β-catenin mutations are found in human HCCs with high rates of genomic instability (Gross-Goupil et al. 2003). Murin research has shown that considerable genomic instability or significant frequencies of β-catenin mutations are found in HCCs. These results suggest that a different mechanism to hepatocarcinogenesis may include disrupting the Wnt signaling system (Calvisi et al. 2004).

Mutations that activate CTNNB1 are present in 11–41% of liver cancer patients (Takai et al. 2014; Ahn et al. 2014). CTNNB is an essential component of the Wnt canonical signaling pathway. The encoded protein product serves as an anchor for the actin cytoskeleton after the completion of the epithelial sheet. It is likely responsible for transmitting the signal of contact inhibition, which halts cell division (Belinky et al. 2015). In hepatic carcinogenesis mouse model, Delgado et al. (2015) showed a full response following β-catenin inhibition.

Most of missense mutations in CTNNB1 are located at the serine/threonine sites of exon 3 or in nearby amino acids. These mutations prevent the β-catenin protein from being phosphorylated and degraded, which results in its stabilization and unchecked transcriptional activity. Human HCCs frequently have mutations in the β-catenin protein's armadillo repeat domains 5 and 6 (Monga 2015). Research indicates that these changes in amino acids have reduced their binding to APC, which has resulted in increased Wnt/β-catenin signaling (Liu et al. 2020a, b, c).

Additionally, mutations in APC and AXIN1, which encode essential elements of the β-catenin degradation complex, have been detected. In 3–8% of HCC, respectively, mutations in APC and AXIN1 are discovered. Most missense, deletion, and/or truncated mutations affecting APC and AXIN1 result in loss of protein expression and function, which is a hallmark of tumor suppressors. Crucially, it is rare for mutations of APC, AXIN1, or CTNNB1 to co-occur in the same HCC, indicating that these mutations result in shared downstream effectors. Surprisingly, canonical Wnt target genes, such as GLUL, TBX3, AXIN2, LGR5, SP5, and OAT, are significantly upregulated in HCC patients with GOF CTNNB1 mutations (Bugter et al. 2021).

AXIN1

AXINI is a negative regulator of Wnt/β-catenin signaling by regulating the amount of β-catenin. AXIN1 mutations are seen in 5–19% of liver cancer specimens (Takai et al. 2014; Ahn et al. 2014). AXIN1 is a therapeutic target in HCC, as evidenced by the suppression of HCC cell line proliferation and accelerated apoptosis caused by overexpressing wild-type AXIN1, but not mutant AXIN1 (Li et al. 2013). The idea is reinforced by the finding that in HCC cells with increased β-catenin due to APC, AXIN1, or CTNNB1 gene mutations, expression of the wild-type AXIN1 gene induced apoptosis (Satoh et al. 2000). One unique strategy to target the Wnt pathway is to decrease the poly-ADP-ribosylating enzymes tankyrase 1 and 2, which stabilizes AXIN (Huang et al. 2009).

Autophagy and Wnt/β-Catenin Signaling in HCC

Autophagy is a cellular process that degrades and recycles damaged organelles and proteins, helping to maintain cellular homeostasis. It is a closely regulated process in which autophagosomes develop and absorb cytoplasmic components before fusing with lysosomes to degrade them. It has intricated and context-dependent roles in various illnesses, including cancer (Franco-Juárez et al. 2024; Li et al. 2021).

According to studies, autophagy is believed to be crucial to the origin and growth of HCC. Abnormalities in autophagy can either suppress or promote tumors depending on the stage of disease and cellular milieu (Pourbagheri-Sigaroodi et al. 2024; Franco-Juárez et al. 2024). In its early stages, autophagy is believed to restrain neoplastic progression. It helps maintain cellular homeostasis by removing dysfunctional mitochondria and other intracellular materials, limiting toxic substance accumulation, and preventing genetic instability. In addition, it might help cells defend themselves by getting rid of intracellular pathogens and damaged proteins more quickly. This lowers inflammation and increases cell survival (Barbosa et al. 2019; Liu et al. 2017). Nevertheless, with the advancement of HCC, autophagy's role becomes more multifaceted. Sometimes cancer cells may utilize autophagy for their survival advantage. Autophagy at later stages of HCC can supply cancer cells with nutrients and energy under deprived conditions such as low oxygen or nutrient availability. Adaptation to hostile environments allows for metabolic persistence as well as proliferation in cancer, thereby driving tumorigenesis and resistance to therapy (Poillet-Perez et al. 2021; Poillet-Perez and White 2019).

Therefore, autophagy plays a double duty in HCC. In the beginning, it functions as an anti-cancer agent, but at later stages, this can be exploited by cancer cells to foster their survival against therapy (Huang et al. 2018). Recently conducted research reveals that autophagy blocks HepG2 cell growth by restraining Wnt/β-catenin signaling. Furthermore, by activating Wnt/β-catenin signaling, this process causes the expression of monocarboxylate transporter 1 (MCT1), which involves lactic acid transport and clearance of H+ in cancer cells, thus promoting metastasis as well as glycolysis, among other effects on different parts of the body, like the liver, where there are many cases of such diseases, including hepatocellular carcinoma (Fan et al. 2018). A different study showed that HCC is caused by bad control of the v-ATPase proton pump through Wnt/beta-catenin signaling. However, drugs that target v-ATPase/autophagy stop these cells from multiplying (He and Tang 2020).

3.5.1.2 PI3K/AKT/mTOR Pathway

Insulin and other growth hormones trigger the intracellular signaling system known as the PI3K/AKT/mTOR pathway. The transcription of p70 or 4EBP1 is impacted by PI3K activation, which also phosphorylates and activates AKT. In turn, AKT promotes mTOR. Fatty acid synthesis, glycogen synthesis, cell survival, proliferation, autophagy, glycolysis, and protein synthesis are all caused by the signal pathway being activated (Fan et al. 2018).

The liver is an organ that is heavily involved in lipid metabolism under physiological settings. Insulin and enzymes work together to control the PI3K/AKT/

mTOR pathway, which converts glucose into fatty acids in the liver. Crucial normal cellular activities and most cancer hallmarks, such as cell cycle, survival, motility, metabolism, and angiogenesis, are regulated by the PI3K/AKT/mTOR signaling pathway. Phospholipase 3-kinase (PI3K) dysregulation is one of the most common processes in the development of tumors (Fruman and Rommel 2014; Fruman et al. 2017).

PI3K

The human genome has three distinct classes of PI3K: class I, class II, and class III (Fruman et al. 2017). The primary function of Class I PI3K is known to be driving carcinogenesis; when Class I PI3K is activated, it phosphorylates PIP2 to PIP3 (phosphatidylinositol 3,4,5-triphosphate). Three highly similar class IA catalytic isoforms, p110α, p110β, and p110δ, are encoded by the four catalytic units of the Class I PI3Ks, PIK3CA, PIK3CB, PIK3CG, and PIK3CD (Vanhaesebroeck et al. 2010). While the other catalytic isoforms are rarely altered but can be overexpressed in cancer, PI3K catalytic isoform p110α mutations are often the most common in human cancers (Thorpe et al. 2015). The three Class II PI3K isoforms, namely PI3K-C2α, PI3K-C2β, and PI3K-C2γ, have distinct functions. PI3K-C2α is heavily involved in endocytosis, vesicular trafficking, and mitosis. PI3K-C2β is associated with cell migration and the suppression of mTOR signaling. PI3K-C2 controls the activation of AKT2 and the storage of glycogen.

Cellular functions depend on Class III PI3K (PIK3C3) (Ronan et al. 2014). The activation of AMP-activated kinase (AMPK) and SGK3, the promoter of cancer stem cells (CSCs), is blocked by inhibition of PIK3C3, which suppresses the formation of HCC CSCs in mice (Liu et al. 2020a, b, c). There are three isoforms of the serine and threonine kinase AKT family: AKT1, AKT2, and AKT3. AKT dysregulation is the cause of several disorders, including cancer (Vasudevan et al. 2009).

mTOR

The user's text is a single letter "T". The mammalian target of rapamycin (mTOR) kinase is a potent controller of protein synthesis that connects the detection of food to cell growth and is frequently observed in cancer (Hsieh et al. 2012). Two complexes, known as mTOR complex 1 (mTORC1) and mTOR complex 2 (mTORC2), are formed when several proteins attach to mTOR and activate its action (Hara et al. 2002). The process of adding a phosphate group to ribosomal protein S6 kinase 1 (S6K1) and eukaryotic translation initiation factor 4E-binding protein-1 (4E-BP1) results from PI3K and AKT activation, which also activates mTORC1. AKT is phosphorylated by the mTORC2 complex, which also contains Richard, the rapamycin-insensitive mTOR companion, increasing AKT kinase activity (Dancey 2010).

AKT

It has been observed that hepatocytes express AKT1 and AKT2, but not AKT3 (Wang et al. 2016). Research has shown that phosphorylated AKT1 expression and c-MYC activation are closely associated and that patients with HCC who express

AKT1 comparatively more than AKT2 do not fare well (Xu et al. 2019). However according to earlier studies, AKT2 affects HCC patients' prognosis and may encourage cell invasion and proliferation (Xu et al. 2004). In addition, Galicia et al. documented that the activation of PI3K/AKT signaling occurs as a result of the inactivation of the tumor suppressor phosphatase and tensin homolog (PTEN). AKT2's first function in tumor transformation is not to promote the survival or proliferation of tumor cells. Instead, it plays a critical role in regulating metabolism in the HCC model of mice (Galicia et al. 2010).

PI3K/AKT/mTOR in HCC

PI3K is significantly overexpressed in HCC tumor tissue, and the increased expression of PIK3CA is linked to HCC cell growth and is inversely connected to cell death. Furthermore, a strong correlation was observed between elevated PIK3CA expression and a negative prognosis in patients with hepatocellular carcinoma (HCC) (Liu et al. 2022). PI3KC2α downregulation results in impaired vascular endothelial growth factor A (VEGFA)-mediated signaling and reduction in human hepatocellular carcinoma (HCC) cells (Chai et al. 2013). PI3K-C2α is essential for the spread of hepatitis C virus (HCV) in cells of human liver cancer (Maehama et al. 2013).

An increase in the mTOR pathway has been observed in 50% of cases of hepatocellular carcinoma (HCC), highlighting the potential of mTORC1 as a target for therapy (Bhat et al. 2013). Nevertheless, the prolonged use of mTORC1 inhibitors leads to an elevation in the production of interleukin-6 (IL-6), triggers the activation of signal transducer and activator of transcription 3 (STAT3), and promotes the development of hepatocellular carcinoma (HCC) in a mouse model of obesity-related liver disease (Umemura et al. 2014). Hepatic mTORC2 has been identified as a contributor to hepatosteatosis and cancer by promoting the production of new fatty acids and lipids in hepatocellular carcinoma (HCC) (Guri et al. 2017). Both mTOR complexes play a role in the disruption of PI3K/AKT/mTOR signaling in HCC. mTORC1 regulates protein synthesis, autophagy, glucose, and lipid metabolism, whereas mTORC2 contributes to the development of liver cancer. Approximately 40–50% of patients with HCC were found to have increased levels of both mTOR complexes (Sahin et al. 2004).

A persistent HBV or HCV infection is one of the risk factors for HCC. It is common for viruses that translate the host's proteins themselves; they do this by using a variety of methods, such as PI3K/AKT/mTOR. This signal route relates to cap-dependent translation, where the regulation of the eIF4F complex's formation requires 4E-BP. Phosphorylation and viruses both can positively and negatively influence the interaction between eIF4E and 4E-BP. Viral stimulation of this pathway prevents apoptosis and increases the ability of infected cells to survive and proliferate further (Cooray 2004; Roberts et al. 2009).

HCV enters a cell by means of the PI3K/AKT signaling pathway which is activated when the HCV NS5A protein binds to PI3K, according to research (Street et al. 2005). Despite being beneficial to the viruses, the use of PI3K/AKT/mTOR simultaneously inhibits HBV reproduction. This is because reduced RNA transcription and reduced HBV X (HBx) protein play a crucial role in pathogenesis by promoting cell cycle progression, deactivating growth factors, and influencing tumor suppressive genes (Neuveut et al. 2010). According to Wang et al. (2013), the PI3K/AKT/mTOR signal pathway is activated with HBx-transfection, increasing autophagy. When HCV and HBV coexist, HBV replication is inhibited (Guo et al. 2007).

3.5.2 Dysregulated Tumor Suppressor Signaling Pathways in HCC

3.5.2.1 The p53 and Retinoblastoma (RB) Pathways

The p53 transcription factor acts as a key mediator that converts different signals into a range of cellular responses, including DNA repair, cell cycle arrest, or cell death (Levine and Oren 2009). P53 activation can effectively regulate various cellular responses by transactivating certain target genes that play a crucial role in these processes. The primary consequences of p53 activation include the arrest of cell cycle progression, induction of cellular senescence, initiation of DNA repair mechanisms, and promotion of apoptosis. In addition, p53 has the ability to control other cellular processes, including the promotion of autophagy, cellular differentiation, and ferroptosis, as well as the inhibition of invasion and metastasis, metabolic reprogramming, and stem cell self-renewal. TP53 functions as a tumor suppressor by promoting either growth arrest or apoptosis, depending on the specific physiological conditions and cell type (Belinkyet al., 215). One of the most frequent abnormalities in several types of cancers is the genomic aberrations in the p53 pathway which usually correlate with high-grade histology (Ahn et al. 2014).

Ribonucleotide reductase (RB) suppresses the proliferation of cancer cells. When the retinoblastoma protein (RB) is inactivated, the cell cycle progresses without any control, resulting in uncontrolled cell growth. In addition, pRb has exerted regulatory control on numerous cyclin-dependent kinases (CDKs) that play a role in the G1/S cell cycle transition. Approximately 90% of hepatocellular carcinoma (HCC) cases exhibit modified levels of CDK inhibitors, such as p16INK4A, p21WAF1/C1P1, and p27Kip1 (either individually or in combination). p16INK4A is inactive in the early and late phases of hepatocarcinogenesis. Numerous investigations revealed significant pRb pathway disruption in HCC, including either altered pRb expression or total disappearance (Aravalli et al. 2008).

p53 and RB Pathway in HCC

The p53 and RB pathways are essential in inducing senescence arrest, which is a significant indicator of the cirrhosis stage in chronic liver disorders. HCC is infrequently observed in liver tissues without the presence of chronic liver disease. The majority of these malignancies, over 80%, are found in patients with cirrhosis. Given that the emergence of rapidly growing cancerous cells during the senescence stage necessitates the evasion of senescence, the condition of both the p53 and RB pathways in HCC holds significant significance in terms of the molecular elements of hepatocellular carcinogenesis. Although it is widely accepted that p53 deficiency participates in the development of HCC. The p53 gene is encoded by the TP53 gene. Approximately, 13–48% of liver cancers harbor TP53 mutations (Guichard et al. 2012; Takai et al. 14; Ahn et al. 2014). TP53 is subject to mutation or inactivation in many forms of human malignancies, with a mutation frequency exceeding 50%. This occurs regardless of the tissue origin or cause of the malignancy. The DNA-binding domain of the p53 protein is frequently impacted by mutations at five specific amino acid residues: 175, 248, 249, 273, and 282. These residues are considered hotspots (Soussi 2007). Only bigger HCCs exhibited mutations in the p53 gene, indicating that complete genetic inactivation of p53 is linked to the advancement of late-stage illness. Studies on HCCs connected to HBV and HCV have revealed a higher occurrence of p53 mutations in advanced cancer cases (43%) compared to regenerating nodules (about 7%). (Minouchi et al. 2002).

According to Takai et al. (2014), patients with HCC in Western nations who have TP53 mutations are likewise associated with a worse prognosis and clinical stage. VEGF-A expression is one of the many biological processes that the TP53 gene controls (Schwaederlé et al. 2015). Crucially, in patients whose tumors included TP53 mutations, anti-angiogenic drugs like bevacizumab were linked to better progression-free survival (PFS) (Wheler et al. 2016). Furthermore, it has been suggested that tumors harboring TP53 mutations could be susceptible to Wee1 inhibitors, which are currently undergoing clinical trials (Janku et al. 2014). According to Janku et al. (2014), there is a suggestion that cancers with TP53 mutations may be vulnerable to Wee1 inhibitors, which are now being tested in clinical studies. Shi et al. (2000) showed that the p21 gene, which acts as a link between the p53 and RB pathways, was shown to be downregulated in 73% of HCCs. Similarly, Wiemann et al. (2002) observed a reduction in the expression of p21 in HCC lesions compared to cirrhotic hepatocytes.

The two primary participants in the retinoblastoma (RB) pathway that are responsible for halting senescence are pRb and p16. HCC seldom exhibits mutations in these genes. RB has been found to experience loss of heterozygosity; however, there is no evidence to demonstrate its mutational inactivation in HCC. Conversely, ankyrin, a protein that enhances the breakdown of pRb protein through proteosomal degradation, was discovered to be excessively produced in HCC (Higashitsuji et al. 2000). The sole recurring mutation that impacts the RB pathway in HCC is the complete deletion of the INK4a/ARF gene, but this happens at a rate lower than 10% (Liew et al. 1999). A study conducted by Tannapfel et al. (2001) found that mutations in the retinoblastoma pathway genes (p16, p15INK4b, or RB1) were present in 83% of HCCs, while modifications in the p53 pathway genes (p53 or p14ARF) were only observed in 31% of these tumors. 30% of HCCs exhibited modifications in both the RB and p53 pathways. Therefore, it seems that the RB and/or p53 pathway is disrupted in most cases of HCC, and both pathways are impacted in at least 33% of these tumors.

3.5.2.2 Erythroblastic Leukemia Viral Oncogene Homologue (ERBB)

The four members of the ERBB family of receptor tyrosine kinases (ERBB1–ERBB4) share a structural ancestry with the epidermal growth factor receptor, which has been linked to the emergence of several human cancer types. Analyzing these receptor tyrosine kinases has revealed that 68% of HCC cases overexpress ERBB1 (also called epidermal growth factor receptor, or EGFR), 84% overexpress ERBB3, 21% overexpress ERBB2 (also called HER2), and 61% overexpress ERBB4 (although at a reduced level). A more aggressive appearance, including a high proliferation index, intrahepatic metastasis, dedifferentiation, and tumor size, was associated with ERBB1 and ERBB3 expression (Ito et al. 2001). The epidermal growth factor receptor, which has been connected to the genesis of multiple human cancer types, shares a structural ancestor with the four receptor tyrosine kinases that make up the ERBB family (ERBB1–ERBB4). 68% of HCC patients overexpress ERBB1 (also known as the epidermal growth factor receptor, or EGFR), 84% overexpress ERBB3, 21% overexpress ERBB2 (also known as HER2), and 61% overexpress ERBB4 (albeit at a lesser level), according to an analysis of these receptor tyrosine kinases. ERBB1 and ERBB3 expressions were linked to a more aggressive appearance, which included a high proliferation index, intrahepatic metastasis, dedifferentiation, and tumor size (Ito et al. 2001) (Sandgren et al. 1990).

According to Russell et al. (1996), hepatocarcinogen therapy causes smaller hepatic neoplasms in TGFα-deficient animals but speeds up the development of HCC in the TGFα transgenic strain. Compound TGFα and MYC transgenic mice exhibit elevated hepatocarcinogenesis linked to chromosomal losses and disruption of TGFβ1 signaling, some of which are syntenic with the RB tumor-suppressor locus found in human HCCs (Sargent et al. 1999). According to Santoni-Rugiu et al. (1996), TGFα can collaborate with HBV transgenic strains to successfully raise the incidence of HCC. Collectively, these investigations highlight the critical role that TGFα signaling plays in the development of HCC (Jakubczak et al. 1997).

3.5.2.3 Ras

The Ras family of proto-oncogenes, which consists of H-Ras, K-Ras, and N-Ras, convey signals related to muscle development to mitogen-activated protein kinases (MAPK1) MEK1 and MEK2 through the activity of serine/threonine kinases Raf1 (Merle and Trepo 2009). This process promotes cellular proliferation, differentiation, and programmed cell death. Aravalli et al. (2008) discovered that particular mutations occurring at codons 12, 13, 61, and 64 in the N-Ras, H-Ras, and K-Ras genes result in the activation of the Ras-family proto-oncogenes. A study found that Ras mutations are likely to be present in around 30% of HCCs (Kudo 2011), other previous studies found that the Ras family gene mutation rate in human HCC is rather low and uncommon (Merle and Trepo 2009; Aravalli et al. 2008).

3.5.2.4 c-myc

Most human hepatoma cell lines have overexpressed c-myc, while normal liver cells express very little to no c-myc. Its level increased gradually from a normal liver to chronic hepatitis, cirrhosis, and HCC. 40%–60% of HCC cases have either promoter hypomethylation or gene amplification leading to the overexpression of c-myc (Cha and DeMatteo 2005). Early human HCC has been observed to exhibit significant levels of c-myc expression. Furthermore, several studies suggest a strong association between the activation of c-myc and the progression of preneoplastic, high-grade dysplastic liver nodules into carcinogenic cells (Merle and Trepo 2009).

3.5.2.5 c-fos Activation

The c-fos proto-oncogene is a significant constituent of the activating protein-1 (AP-1) transcription factor. It is involved in cellular processes such as transformation, proliferation, differentiation, and apoptosis. The presence of c-fos is necessary during several stages of the cell cycle. HCC has been found to exhibit elevated levels of c-fos gene expression. The study conducted by Güller et al. (2008) found that hepatocytes that overexpress c-fos exhibit continuous proliferation, even in the absence of growth stimuli.

3.5.3 Telomerase Reactivation and Immortality in HCC

The ribonucleoprotein enzyme telomerase is essential for the replication of chromosomal termini in most eukaryotes. In many cancer cells, telomerase overexpression plays a crucial role in the transformation process (Delgado et al. 2015). Cells can divide because TERT stretches telomeres, and TERT mutations stimulate this activity. TERT mutations could be thought of as a tumor "gatekeeper" since they are among the first genetic abnormalities connected to malignant transformation in HCC (Nault and Villanueva 2015). An important process in the immortalization of hepatocellular cells is the reactivation of TERT, which prevents the shortening of telomeres throughout repeated cycles of cell division. Tahtouh et al. (2015) showed that inhibiting telomerase reduces the expression of alpha-fetoprotein (AFP) in people with (HCC and may hinder cell proliferation by weakening the repair of telomeres.

Telomere shortening has been described previously as a key feature of chronic hyperproliferative liver disease (Rudolph 2001), specifically occurring in the hepatocyte compartment (Wiemann et al. 2002). These findings have raised the possibility that hepatocyte turnover and telomere shortening linked to chronic liver illness are factors in the development of genomic instability that underlies human HCC. (Plentz et al. 2005).

A study conducted by Nault et al. (2013) confirmed that no mutations in the TERT gene were detected in cases of cirrhosis and hepatocellular adenoma. Nevertheless, the TERT mutation was the initial genetic alteration detected in cirrhotic macronodules, regardless of the presence or absence of dysplasia. In addition, cirrhosis is primarily characterized by the cessation of cell division in liver cells due to telomere-dependent senescence. However, the formation of HCC necessitates the activation of the TERT enzyme, which is absent in healthy liver cells. Hence, it is unsurprising that a significant telomerase activity was observed in 80–90% of HCCs (Nakayama et al. 1998). An additional study found that the frequencies of TERT mutations increased gradually with the development of hepatocellular carcinoma. Specifically, 6% of low-grade dysplastic nodules, 9% of high-grade dysplastic nodules, 61% of early hepatocellular carcinomas, and 42% of small and advanced hepatocellular carcinomas exhibited TERT mutations. Therefore, the presence of the TERT mutation is expected to indicate the initiation of a clearly cancerous condition, specifically early hepatocellular carcinoma, in the process of hepatocellular carcinogenesis (Nault et al. 2014).

Telomere shortening has been linked to increased chromosomal instability in human hepatomas, according to research (Plentz et al. 2004). Accordingly, telomere disruption has been linked to an increased risk of liver cancer in studies using a telomerase deletion mice model for HCC (Farazi and DePinho 2006). Strong telomerase activation, which is correlated with elevated TERT mRNA levels, is another feature of telomere biology shared by HCC that occurs in about 90% of human HCCs (Lee et al. 2004; Shimojima et al. 2004). Surprisingly, HBV has been demonstrated to integrate in the TERT locus in human HCCs, suggesting that TERT gene expression may be elevated by the close positioning of viral enhancers (Ferber et al. 2003). Amplification of the gene that encodes the telomerase RNA component (TERC) (Takeo et al. 2001) and the allelic loss of chromosome 10p (in a region that encodes a putative telomerase repressor) (Nishimoto et al. 2001) has been reported in HCCs.

Increased microvessel density (Piao et al. 2004) and HCC recurrence following resection (Youssef et al. 2001; Oh et al. 2003) have been linked to telomerase reactivation. Some research has linked telomerase to the onset of hepatocarcinogenesis (Ogami et al. 1999); Nevertheless, the presence of telomerase-positive invading lymphocytes and resident sinusoidal cells may account for the conflicting outcomes seen (Artandi et al. 2002). Moreover, the telomeres of HCCs have a shorter length compared to those of healthy livers, indicating that the activation of telomerase occurs at a later stage in the progression of HCCs. It is important to mention that telomerase may have carcinogenic features in addition to its role in maintaining telomeres (Artandi et al. 2002). Telomere shortening may contribute to the development of HCC by promoting the creation of a cirrhotic environment. When comparing mice with intact telomeres to telomerase knockout animals with short telomeres, it was observed that the latter group had increased liver fibrosis and cirrhosis after injury. This is likely due to the heightened apoptosis of hepatocytes as a result of the telomere checkpoint response, as stated by Rudolph (2001).

3.5.4 Epithelial to Mesenchymal Transition and HCC

EMT, or epithelial-mesenchymal transition, is an important process that occurs throughout embryogenesis. It is involved in various crucial stages, including neural crest delamination, heart valve creation, palatogenesis, and myogenesis (type I) (Thiery et al. 2009). EMT is also triggered during fibrosis and wound healing (type II) as well as cancer (type III) (Kalluri and Weinberg 2009). EMT often involves the reorganization of the cytoskeleton and the regulation of many genes, such as those responsible for cell adhesion. The EMT process involves various components, including cadherins, which are a group of glycoproteins located in the cell membrane that rely on calcium and are responsible for the adhesion between cells. They perform crucial roles in intercellular adhesion and are implicated in embryo development and the preservation of normal tissue. Cadherins are categorized into over ten subgroups, which include E-cadherin (found in epithelium), N-cadherin (found in nerve cells), P-cadherin (found in the placenta), and R-cadherin (found in the retina). E-cadherin expression alteration is a characteristic indicator of epithelial-mesenchymal transition (EMT). Tumor cells undergo a process called cadherin switching, where they decrease the expression of E-cadherin and transition from normal epithelial cells to mobile mesenchymal cancer cells. During this transition, they start expressing the adhesion protein N-cadherin, which gives them the ability to invade surrounding tissues (Stemmler 2008).

Hepatocyte growth factor (HGF) is a versatile cytokine that stimulates cell proliferation, cell motility, and the formation of multicellular tissue-like structures in epithelial cells (Nakamura et al. 2011). Prior research has shown that HGF plays a vital role in tissue regeneration, carcinogenesis, tumor invasion, and epithelial wound healing, due to its various roles (Imamura and Matsumoto 2017). The c-mesenchymal-epithelial transition receptor (c-MET) was first discovered as the fusion gene (tpr-met), which acts as the receptor for HGF and is encoded by the c-MET proto-oncogene (Cooper et al. 1984). The transmembrane receptor tyrosine kinase (RTK) was identified as such by Bottaro et al. in (1991). The activation of c-MET is pleiotropic because its cytoplasmic domain has the ability to interact with different proteins that are involved in diverse cellular signaling pathways. When HGF binds to c-MET, it activates c-MET and initiates a complicated biological process that promotes many activities such as cell proliferation, cell invasion, and protection against apoptosis. The movement and multiplication of cells are controlled by the HGF/MET axis. The physiologic regeneration of the liver is essential. c-MET has a crucial role in promoting the growth of placental tissue, liver, and brain precursors. It also regulates the migration and maturation of muscle tissue by controlling the process of epithelial-mesenchymal transition (EMT) in myogenic progenitor cells. This information is supported by studies conducted by Kim et al. (2016) and Szturz et al. (2017).

The activation of c-MET by HGF is tightly controlled. However, when the signaling pathway is abnormally activated, it results in enhanced cell motility, cell cycle progression, and various other signaling events that promote tumor growth. This aberrant activation has been observed in several types of cancer, including HCC (Meng and Chen 2021). The HGF/c-MET axis is a crucial signaling route in HCC and is closely linked to its highly aggressive characteristics. Cancer types, such as HCC, are facilitated in their onset, proliferation, invasion, and metastasis by the inappropriate activation of c-MET (Meng and Chen 2021). Activation of the MET pathway has been observed in 20–40% of HCC, mostly due to increased expression of both the receptor and its ligand. Genomic analysis identified the activation of this cascade in 40% of individuals with HCC using a gene signature created specifically for this purpose. Curiously, these patients had notably poorer prognoses (Sia and Villanueva 2011). In recent years, multiple studies have suggested that the HGF/c-MET signaling pathway holds great potential for guiding the therapy of HCC (Liu et al. 2016).

Multiple in vitro and in vivo analyzes have been conducted to elucidate the function of HGF/MET in HCC. The data obtained from experiments conducted outside of a living organism support the idea that HGF/MET has a tendency to promote invasion and this is linked to its capacity to initiate epithelial-mesenchymal transition (EMT) (Xie et al. 2010). Therefore, HCC cell lines that have elevated MET levels exhibit a mesenchymal character, as reported by Ogunwobi and Liu (2011). Various laboratories have examined the impacts of inactivating or overexpressing MET and/or HGF in in vivo experimental models of HCC, yielding inconsistent findings. For instance, in the case of HCC, the absence of MET in liver cells resulted in larger tumors that developed more quickly compared to the control group in the HCC model produced by DEN. In contrast, transgenic mouse models that have been genetically modified to have increased levels of MET expression in liver cells are known to develop liver tumors without any external intervention (Fan et al. 2017). Conversely, the absence of MET accelerates and intensifies the onset of HCC through pharmacological means, but has no impact on the development of HCC produced by phenobarbital (Takami et al. 2007). Hence, the situation is complex and implies that the context may be significant, and a delicate equilibrium of HGF/MET signaling is required to sustain liver homeostasis.

The HGF/MET signaling system is known to be excessively active in approximately 50% of individuals with HCC and virtually all cases of liver metastases. In addition, a comparative analysis of functional genomics revealed the presence of a MET-regulated signature in a specific subset of HCC characterized by an aggressive phenotype and unfavorable prognosis (Kaposi-Novak et al. 2006). Abnormal activation of MET signaling can occur through several mechanisms, including gene amplification, activating mutations, suppression of microRNAs that target MET, and autocrine signaling caused by excessive production of HGF or activation by other ligands (Yu et al. 2021). Nevertheless, both the expression of MET and the levels of HGF in the plasma are not suitable for use as diagnostic or prognostic indicators in HCC, due to conflicting findings in research investigations. Hence, it warrants additional scrutiny. One possible application is their usefulness in specific subgroups of patients, especially those with the MET-specific hallmark or pathological condition. An alternative approach would involve incorporating them among other factors that assess the risk of HCC (Arechederra et al. 2018; Wang et al. 2022).

Medical research has shown that the TME creates an environment that promotes the spread of tumors, and the process of epithelial-mesenchymal transition (EMT) triggered by many components in the TME is a crucial factor in the distant spread of HCC (He et al. 2017). HGF can induce metastatic alterations, such as EMT, increased mobility, and invasiveness in many types of cancer cells. Therefore, it can be described as a "metastatic growth factor." Hepatocyte growth factor (HGF) plays a crucial function in the progression of HCC among the variables that contribute to metastasis (Trusolino et al. 2010). Several studies have found that elevated levels of c-MET expression in hepatocellular carcinoma (HCC) can enhance cell motility and activate various signaling molecules through downstream signaling pathways, including vascular epidermal growth factor (VEGF) and Rac signaling molecules. This ultimately leads to the promotion of tumor neovascularization and metastasis of tumor cells (Menard et al. 2014). A study conducted by Bozkaya et al. (2012) has shown that the activation of c-MET by HGF can stimulate the invasion and migration of HCC cells.

In mice, the rapid formation of HCC is induced by the co-expression of c-Met and activated mutant versions of β-catenin; liver tumor development with a longer latency is also induced by the overexpression of c-Met and cyclin D1. However, Patil et al. (2009) demonstrated that cyclin D1 expression is not necessary for the formation of liver tumors caused by c-Met and activated mutant versions of β-catenin using Ccnd1-knockout mice. Mechanistically, the loss of cyclin D1 causes a compensatory upregulation of cyclin D2 expression in the liver.

3.6 Epigenetics, MicroRNA (miRNA), Long Non-coding RNA and HCC

Carcinogenesis is mostly influenced by aberrant epigenetic silencing of tumor suppressor genes caused by histone deacetylation and promoter DNA hypermethylation. According to Hellebrekers et al. (2007), treating these epigenetic aberrations with chromatin-modifying medicines is an appealing therapeutic approach because of their possible reversibility. Tischoff and Tannapfe (2008) has demonstrated that changes in epigenetics and miRNA are correlated with the development of hepatic carcinogenesis from precancerous lesions to HCC.

miRNAs are short non-coding RNAs of approximately 22 nucleotides that control the expression of many target genes (Saito et al. 2014). Histone modifications, including methylation of histone H3 lysine 9 (H3K9) and tri-methylation of H3K27, as well as DNA hypermethylation of CpG island promoters and histone deacetylation, may epigenetically silence tumor suppressor genes in HCC (Hellebrekers et al. 2007; Tischoff and Tannapfe 2008; Hodi et al. 2010; Brahmer et al. 2015). Furthermore, if a particular suppressor miRNA is epigenetically silenced, oncogenes that would typically be dormant due to that miRNA may become active (Saito et al. 2014). Therefore, a logical therapy strategy for HCC may use histone deacetylase and DNA methylation inhibitors to restore the production of tumor suppressor genes or tumor suppressor miRNA.

Long non-coding RNAs have been discovered to exhibit differential expressions in HCC and have been linked to the etiology of HCC. Non-coding RNAs were believed to constitute transcriptional "noise." Several researches, however, have demonstrated that these compounds have important regulatory functions. Endogenous cellular RNA molecules that are longer than 200 nucleotides are known as long non-coding RNAs, and they are unable to be translated into proteins. Since they alter gene expression through processes like chromatin modification and genomic imprinting, they play a vital role in epigenetic control. Long non-coding RNA has been associated with the onset, development, and metastasis of

HCC. However, understanding the chemicals in this illness and how to use them therapeutically is still a promising era of research (Liu et al. 2015).

3.6.1 miRNA Alteration in HCC

Epigenetic alterations through non-coding RNA have been described to impact the aberrant HCC (Wu et al. 2020). MicroRNAs (miRNAs) are conserved endogenous, nonprotein-coding RNAs composed of approximately 20–22 nucleotides in length (Chen et al. 2013). They are reported to regulate gene expression at the posttranslational level by suppressing target gene translation or by inducing the degradation of target mRNAs (Guo et al. 2015). The expression of several miRNAs has been observed to be altered in HCC, and these changes have an impact on the development and progression of HCC (Han et al. 2016). Some of miRNA functions to inhibit apoptosis (miR-221), promote cell invasion (miR-9) or inhibit migration and proliferation (miR23b) (Schütte et al. 2015). Additionally, some others appear to exhibit a TSG-like function (miR-101, 195, 122, 338) and are silenced in HCC (Lachenmayer et al. 2010). Mutant miR-1269a was reported to promote HCC progression (Min et al. 2017).

miR-128-2, miR-148a and miR-331-3p were identified to be upregulated in HCC tissues (Kanda et al. 2015). miR-34a was downregulated in metastatic HCC tissues (Kim et al. 2013). The miR-199a-5p is also downregulated in HCC tissues and is associated with the tumor size and prognosis of patient. (Guo et al. 2015). miR-29a, miR-425-5p, miR-487a, miR-219-5p and miR-1247-3p are metastasis-promoting miRNAs correlate with unfavorable clinical prognosis of HCC while miR-630, miR-503, miR-149, miR-137 and miR-129-3pare dysregulated in HCC and associated with a worse clinical prognosis (Weidle et al. 2020). Lower levels of miR-708 were related to aggressive progression of HCC (Sun et al. 2019).

It was demonstrated that miR-200b (Min et al. 2017) and miR-218 (Nie et al. 2018; Wu et al. 2018) were tumor suppressors for HCC by inhibiting BMI1 expression. miR-203 and miR-491-5p were reported to have suppressive effects in HCC tissues (Xu et al. 2023; Yang et al. 2015). Furthermore, miR-29c plays a role as a suppressor of *SIRT1* affects HCC (Bae et al. 2014). Whereas miR-34a and miR-142-3p target LDHA to suppress aerobic glycolysis and HCC progression (Li et al. 2016; Hua et al. 2018; Zhang et al. 2018). miR-100 and miR-125b were identified in HCC to act as suppressors of vessels that encapsulate the tumor cluster (VETC) formation and VETC-dependent metastasis (Zhou et al. 2016). By downregulating rho-kinase 2, miR-139 has been found to suppress metastasis and progression of HCC (Wong et al. 2011). miR-622 displays forceful tumor-suppressive functions in HCC (Linck-Paulus et al. 2020).

Several miRNAs were documented to affect HCC through different signaling pathways. miR-142-3p, miR-125a, and miR-7 were demonstrated to repress HCC progression through the PI3K/AKT/mTOR pathway (Fang et al. 2012; Tang et al. 2015; Zeng et al. 2022). miR-505, miR-342-3p, and miR-455-5p were all downregulated in HCC tissues through PI3K/AKT pathway or insulin growth factor receptor 1 (IGF-1R) (Liu et al. 2018; Hu et al. 2019; Ren et al. 2019a, b). miR-196 (a and b) could suppress cell proliferation and induce apoptosis in HCC cells through the interaction with the STAT3 pathway (Ren et al. 2019a, b; He and Tang 2020). miR-300 is a tumor-suppressive miRNA reported to inhibit the development of HCC through inhibition Wnt/β-catenin signaling (Wang et al. 2018a, b). miR-432, miR-610, miR-126a and miR-202 have been shown to inhibit the canonical pathway by targeting the LRP6 and suppress HCC proliferation and metastasis to angiogenesis (Du et al. 2014; Zeng et al. 2014; Zhang et al. 2014; Jiang et al. 2015). miR-199a miR-27a target FZD7 and inhibits HCC cells proliferation (Song et al. 2014) or increase response to chemotherapy (Chen et al. 2013). On the other hand, miR-522, an oncogenic miRNA, was reported as positive regulators of the Wnt pathway signaling antagonists DKK1 and SFRP2 regulating the proliferation of HCC cells (Zhang et al. 2016).

HIF-1α and c-Myc which participate in chemoresistance in HCC were inhibited by miR-199ab-5p and miR-3662 for HIF-1α (Li et al. 2017; Chen et al. 2018) and miR-129-5p and miR-23a for c-Myc (Reyes et al. 2014; Han et al. 2016). miR-331-3p induced the phosphorylation of *AKT* and the subsequent EMT on HCC cells (Kanda et al. 2015).

3.6.2 lncRNA Alteration in HCC

Approximately, 68% of non-coding RNAs in the human genome are long non-coding RNAs (lncRNAs) (DiStefano 2017). They are a class of functional RNAs of more than 200 nucleotides in length, do not have protein-coding ability and modulate target gene expression at the transcriptional and posttranscriptional levels (Li et al. 2018). Numerous studies investigate the role of lncRNAs in the initiation, progression, and metastasis of HCC (DiStefano 2017). LncRNA HOTTIP was reported to be associated with HCC progression and disease outcome (Huang et al. 2014; Parasramka et al. 2016). The CCAT1 informed to Promote HCC progression (DiStefano 2017).

Multiple long non-coding RNAs (lncRNAs), such as lncTCF7, lncβ-Catm, and lncRNA-LALR1, play a role in activating the Wnt/β-catenin pathway (He and Tang 2020). Furthermore, the study conducted by Yao et al. (2019) revealed that ASB16-AS1 plays a role in controlling the Wnt/β-catenin signaling pathway in hepatocellular carcinoma (HCC). In addition, a study by Liu et al. (2020a, b, c) found that the p38-inhibited cutaneous squamous cell carcinoma-associated lincRNA (PICSAR) activates the PI3K/AKT/mTOR signaling pathway in HCC. The study conducted by Li et al. (2018) revealed that the long non-coding RNA Ftx enhances the progression of HCC by activating the PPAR-γ pathway. In addition, the study conducted by Wei et al. (2017) revealed that Lnc-HOTAIR enhances glycolysis by activating the mTOR pathway.

Regarding the PI3K/AKT/mTOR signaling, a total of 67 signaling-related lncRNAs have been documented to play a prominent role in HCC (Wu et al. 2020). These lncRNA were divided into: 53 upregulated (lncARSR, PTTG3P, NR027113,

GAS6-AS2, AWPPH, FGFR3-AS1, HAGLROS, HULC, Linc00462, Myd88, CASC11, AK023948, CHRF, FOXP4-AS1, ANRIL, DLEU1, UCA1, ecCEBPA, LINC00963, LINC01133, CRNDE, H19, lncIHS, TP73-AS1, HOXA-AS2, DCST1-AS1, FOXD3-AS1, OR3A4, SNHG1, lncRNA PDPK2P, FOXD2-AS1, NEAT1, DUXAP10, CASC9, Linc-GALH, CDKN2B-AS1, AGAP2-AS1, LincRNAp21, LINC00707, TINCR, HOTAIR, MALAT1, LINC00152, HEIH, SNHG16, CUDR, SNHG20, GATA3-AS1, Linc01296, THOR, WEE2-AS1) and 14 downregulated (FER1L4, GAS5, MEG3, TCL6, OGFRP1, CADM1-AS1, uc002mbe.2, RP5-833A20.1, PTENP1, LINC01554, F11-AS1, LINC00657, linc-USP16, SEMA3B-AS1).

3.6.3 CircRNAs and Hepatocellular carcinoma

A newly acknowledged category of non-coding RNA is circular RNAs (circRNAs), which may influence cellular physiology, by interactions with binding proteins, regulation of gene expression, or sponging of microRNA. A variety of circRNA biological roles in HCC have been investigated throughout the past years (Yepmo et al. 2022). Several circRNAs have been displayed to have a role in the HCC tumorigenesis through various mechanisms, illuminating the complexity of HCC pathogenesis (Yao et al. 2019).

Numerous circ-RNA have been overexpressed on HCC samples including Circ-FOXP1 (Wang et al. 2020a). The interaction between hsa_circ_0088364 and hsa_circ_0090049 and mRNAs through miRNA sponges has been suggested to influence the course of HCC (Xiong et al. 2019). circ_KIAA1429 affects migration and invasion of HCC cells and facilitates EMT (Wang et al. 2020b). Moreover, Circ_0000502 and circ_0001955 have oncogenic effects and their silencing reduced the proliferation, invasion, and migration aptitude of HCC cells (Lei et al. 2019; Yao et al. 2019).

Several circRNAs have been found to promote HCC progression and invasion and could be used as biomarkers for the prognosis. circ_GFRA1 modulates the miR-498/NAP1L3 axis and promotes HCC progress (Lv et al. 2021). hsa_circRNA_104348 could promote HCC progression by upregulating the Wnt/β-catenin pathway and sponging miR-187-3p (Huang et al. 2020). Correlating with the severity of HCC, circTMEM45A promotes the progression of HCC by sponging miR-65 which activates the IGF2 pathway (Zhang et al. 2020). circ-CSPP1 Knocking down suppressed HCC development by miR-493-5p upregulation and HMGB1downregulation, intimating that circ-CSPP1 contributed to HCC pathogenesis (Yang et al. 2021).

On the other hand, functional studies have displayed the tumor suppressor role of circRNAs in HCC (Hussen et al. 2021). circ_0005986, has been suggested as a predictive biomarker and an inhibitor of carcinogenesis of HCC by inhibiting liver cell proliferation through sponging miR-129-5p and controlling Notch1 (Fu et al. 2017). circLIFR has been identified as a tumor suppressor in HCC, by blocking the β-catenin signaling pathway and sponging miR-624-5p and (Yang et al. 2022). CircRNA-5692 has reduced the malignant activities of HCC cells through interacting with miR-328-5p and subsequent upregulation of DAB2IP levels (Wu et al. 2019). Hsa_circ_0028502 and hsa_circ_0076251 were downregulated in HCC and their expression levels have been shown to be augmented from HCC to liver cirrhosis to chronic hepatitis (Jiang et al. 2019). Reduction in cSMARCA5 has been correlated with aggressive features of HCC. cSMARCA5 suppresses HCC proliferation and migration TIMP3 (Wang et al. 2018a, b).

3.6.4 Methylation of Cancer-Relevant Genes

Gene expression is epigenetically silenced when regulatory areas (especially promoters) of genes are abnormally methylated. Human HCC has been linked to aberrant DNA methylation patterns (Yu et al. 2003). According to Lee et al. (2003), methylation has been found at the outset of hepatocarcinogenesis and to a greater amount along the course of the tumor. Apoptosis-associated speck-like protein (ASC), COX2, p16(INK4a), E-cadherin, deleted in liver cancer 1 (DLC1), and others have all been the target of specific hypermethylation events in HCC (Murata et al. 2004; Maeta et al. 2005). In HCC cell lines, the biological importance of certain of these genes' hypermethylation in hepatocarcinogenesis has been assessed. P16(INK4a) and COX2 expression are increased when hepatoma cells are treated with a demethylating agent (Maeta et al. 2005). Hence, the process of suppressing the activity of crucial cancer-related genes through epigenetic mechanisms appears to be significant in the development of liver cancer and could potentially lead to the creation of a novel category of anti-cancer drugs.

In human HCC, an aberrant global hypomethylation background is complemented by an aberrant DNA hypermethylation pattern. Methylation usually happens during hepatocarcinogenesis's initiating and progressing phases (Li et al. 2005). In HCC, certain tumor suppressor genes, including p16INK4A, E-cadherin, BRCA1, IGFR-II/MP6, and COX-2, are silenced and their promoters are hypermethylated. (Feng et al. 2010).

3.7 Genetic and Epigenetic Factors in HCV-Induced HCC

HCC caused by HCV is linked to many genes. The first gene identified as being linked to the emergence of HCC was the tumor suppressor P53. A subset of genes is often mutated in HCV patients, according to recent investigations (Tornesello et al. 2016; Sghaier et al. 2017). A 30% mutation is present in the oncogene CTNNB1, which codes for the Wnt pathway's β-catenin protein. It has been noted that mutations in the Wnt pathway occur in HCC, stabilizing β-catenin. This β-catenin translocate to the nucleus, where it modulates genes involved in the survival and growth of cells. NS5A activates Akt and PI3K to indirectly control the Wnt pathway. HCV-infected cells have been shown to have elevated β-catenin. It is still unclear what role β-catenin plays in HCV-infected cells (Wang et al. 2017). Its level has, nevertheless, largely increased in HCC patients. In a similar vein, telomere shrinkage causes cellular senescence. Alongside other causes, HCC resulting from HCV infection has been linked to activating mutations in the telomerase reverse transcriptase (TERT) promoter gene (Chen et al. 2014; Nault et al. 2013, 2014). To inhibit the aging of liver cells, the HCV core protein reduces the level of CDKN2A expression. Primary human hepatocytes transfected with HCV core and exhibiting an immortalized phenotype demonstrated elevated telomerase activity, a characteristic commonly observed in cells that are prone to transformation or have already undergone transformation.

This finding is consistent with the finding that somatic mutations in the TERT promoter that increase TERT expression are among the most common and early neoplastic events linked to all major aetiologias, including HCV. An increased risk of HCC is also linked to host genetic variations (Dragani 2010). The PNPLA3 gene (patatin-like phospholipase domain-containing protein-2) shows a significant association with fatty liver disease in HCV patients who have a higher susceptibility to developing HCC (Valenti et al. 2010; Miura et al. 2012; Sato et al. 2014). Polymorphisms in a few other cytokine/receptor genes have also been linked to HCC in a similar manner. These include genes for vascular endothelial growth factor (VEGF), IL-10, TNF-α, and IL-23R, among other cytokines. The way a host reacts to variations in the viral genome varies. For instance, El-Shamy et al. (2013) revealed that HCV genotypes 1a and 1b are linked to HCC.

3.7.1 Molecular Mechanisms of HCV-Related HCC

The viral genome of HCV is 9.6 kb long and consists of a single-stranded RNA molecule. The molecule encodes a large polyprotein, known as the structural [core, envelope (E)1, and E2] proteins, and non-structural (NS) proteins, which include proteins p7, NS2, NS3, NS4A, NS4B, NS5A, and NS5B. Different epidemiologic studies from around the world have shown that HCC represents the major risk for HCV, or more generally, chronic liver diseases caused by this virus as well (Poduri 2003). However, historical research has found that chronic hepatitis C virus infection typically causes hepatic fibrosis, cirrhosis, and hepatocellular carcinoma later in life, often after many years. The pathogenesis of this disease was poorly understood until recently because there were no in vitro culture systems available for studying its development into chronic liver diseases, which was possible only through establishing cell lines harboring replicating genomes of HCV, but even then such models were not perfect, therefore researchers could only use transgenic animals expressing one or more viral proteins instead, according to Rusyn and Lemon (2014), who developed these models, though some scientists still doubt whether HCV alone can cause cancer as stated by Lerat et al. (2011).

After groundbreaking research on how viruses replicate in cell culture (Lindenbach et al. 2005), more research is being done on how HCV causes liver cancer. It is only in the cytoplasm of a host genome-free hepatocyte that HCV can replicate. When the host integrates viral elements into its genome, hepatocytes undergo direct oncogenic transformation. Numerous reports suggest that HCV is directly involved in the pathogenesis of HCC. Previous studies have already demonstrated the connection between HCC and the HCV core protein. The same protein turns on STAT3 through the IL-6 autocrine pathway (Tacke et al. 2011), which makes telomerase work harder (Zhu et al. 2010). This may cause liver cells to become cancerous. More ERK phosphorylation is caused by NS3/4A. This helps cells grow by decreasing p21 promoter activity and p53-mediated apoptosis suppression (He et al. 2007; Kwun et al. 2001). There are several ways that a long-term infection with the hepatitis C virus can lead to cancer. These include NF-kB causing strong, long-lasting inflammation (Yu et al. 2012); Choi and Hwang (2006) blocking the TGF-β signaling pathway through the T^2R-I/NS5A interaction; NS5A-directed changes to the wnt/β-catenin pathway; changes to tumor suppressor genes (Munakata et al. 2005); and oxidative stress-induced DNA mutagenesis (Korenaga et al. 2005). Furthermore, a recent study revealed that a lack of microRNA-122 causes high-frequency tumorigenesis in a mouse model, although its mechanism remains unknown (Tsai et al. 2012).

The reports show that people infected with HBV and HDV tend to have rapid and severe disease progression. It remains unclear how these two co-infections can accelerate hepatocarcinogenesis. One argument said that HDV replication makes liver cancer worse by causing noticeable inflammation, problems with nuclear signaling pathways, higher oxidative stress, and changes in epigenetics (Abbas et al. 2015).

Many studies have indicated that HCC is associated with abnormalities in genes responsible for regulating epigenetics (Ma et al. 2014).

For example, EZH2 is an enzyme that changes histone-lysine methylation in HCCs when it is expressed in a way that isn't normal (Sudo et al. 2005; Au et al. 2012). This causes miRNAs to stop the growth of the tumor. Li et al. (2005) observed a link between virus-induced tumors and changes in gene methylation levels. Tumor suppressor genes such as CDKN2A, GSTP1, GSTP1, RUNX3, APC, SOCSS-1, and RASSF1A exhibit heavy methylation in cases of HCV or HBV-induced HCCs (Feng et al. 2010). Non-coding RNAs and lncRNAs may act as mediators for miRNA-induced epigenetic changes during the hepatocellular carcinoma development stages. Numerous miRNAs have demonstrated a positive or negative influence on the replication process of the hepatitis C virus (Shrivastava et al. 2015).

3.8 Genetic and Epigenetic Factors in HBV-Related HCC

HBV is the primary causative agent that significantly raises the occurrence of HCC in East Asia and sub-Saharan Africa, making it the most prevalent risk factor for HCC. The HBV genome has four genes (C, S, X, and P) that encode the core protein, envelope protein, X protein, and a polymerase. One of these proteins, known as hepatitis B X protein (HBx), plays a crucial role in the development of HCC. Increasing evidence suggests that HBx has multiple functions, such as preventing cell death in liver cells (Liu et al. 2012) and influencing DNA repair processes by regulating the activity of p53 (Ferber et al. 2003). Additionally, HBx plays a role in facilitating cellular signal transmission, promoting cell cycle progression, and maintaining the stability of HBx by interacting with various host factors (Zhang and Ding 2015).

Chronic HBV infection allows the viral DNA to become part of the host genome, resulting in a cancer-causing change. A recent next-generation sequencing (NGS) study discovered that HBV integration was present in over 80% of Hepatitis B Virus-positive HCC cases. Furthermore, the integration was more prevalent in tumor tissue compared to the surrounding non-tumor tissue (Sung et al. 2012). Tumors that tested positive for HBV showed frequent integration of three genes associated with cancer: telomerase reverse transcriptase (TERT), mixed-lineage leukemia 4 (MLL4), and cyclin E1 (CCNE1). These data indicate a strong correlation between HBV integration and the development of liver cancer. Furthermore, TERT promoter mutations have been detected in over 50% of HCC tissue, as reported by Nault et al. (2013). While the exact process by which TERT is activated in cancer is not fully comprehended, a recent study discovered that the GA-binding protein transcription factor (GABP), which belongs to the E-twenty-six (ETS) transcription factor family, is specifically attracted to the mutated TERT promoter and triggers TERT expression (Bell et al. 2015).

Increasing data indicates that HBx plays a significant role in the development of liver cancer. HBx may operate through several methods at the molecular and cellular levels, including the following: The effects of the protein Yes-associated protein (YAP) include: (1) activating specific genes that contain the cAMP response element binding protein (CREB) response element (CRE) through transactivation (Zhang et al. 2012); (2) changing the DNA specificity of CREB and activating transcription factor 2 (ATF-2), leading to the binding and activation of the HBV enhancer (Maguire et al. 1991); (3) modifying the DNA-binding specificity of the p53 tumor suppressor, resulting in altered expression of its target genes (Chan et al. 2013); and (4) regulating various cellular signaling pathways, such as the Ras-Raf-MAPK pathway, Src-dependent pathway, PI3K-Akt pathway, inflammation-associated NF-kB/STAT-3 pathways, and wnt/β-catenin pathway (Yun et al. 2002). Furthermore, HBx influences changes in gene expression patterns by either increasing or decreasing the methylation levels of oncogenes and tumor suppressor genes. It also facilitates modifications in the acetylation status of histones and the expression of tumor-related genes, as well as modifications in the levels of certain microRNAs (Kong et al. 2011; Tian et al. 2013).

3.9 Studied Mutations Related to HCC in LMICs

Several reports documented mutations related to HCC risk/prognosis. The double mutations T1762/A1764 positions in HBV genotype C was related in most HCC patients in Bangladesh (Raihan et al. 2019). Moreover, HBV genotype C is the dominant genotype in Cambodia. Cambodian patients infected with HBV mutation in genotype C1 brings high possibility of HCC occurrence (Chuon et al. 2019).

Three studies reported associated mutations with hepatocarcinogenesis form Cameroon. The role of aflatoxin in HCC is commonly estimated through the prevalence of the 9S mutation of TP53, patients with TP53 mutations (R249S) displayed significantly increased circulating alpha-fetoprotein values, high HBV DNA loads in HCC patients from Cameroon and Central African Republic (Marchio et al. 2018). In addition, HBV viral genomes isolated for HCC patients are more heavily altered than those found in controls (Atsama Amougou et al. 2019). A case control study of HCV-related HCC demonstrated that infection with HCV-4 is strongly associated with HCC development and the risk of developing HCC increased significantly in case of infection with mutated HCV subtype 4f (Amougou-Atsama et al. 2020).

Several reports documented from Egypt. No association of TP53 mutations was observed in HCV genotype 4-associated **HCC** (Zekri et al. 2006). Furthermore, Mohamed et al. (2008) demonstrated that TP53 mutations are rather a late event in the carcinogenesis. Mutagenesis by aflatoxin could play a role in hepatocarcinogenesis in Egypt, TP53 mutations were demonstrated in 10% of HCC cases with underlying HCV with no mutations were found in CTNNB1 in HCC biopsies (Hosny et al. 2008). El-Kafrawy et al. (2005) verified about 41% of HCC samples had p53 mutations which previously reported to be associated with aflatoxin exposure. Moreover, the low frequency of Aflatoxin was documented to be associated with TP53 (c.747 G > T, p. R249S) mutation in HCC (Mosbeh et al. 2023). Mutations (H63D) in hemochromatosis gene (HFE) were studied and carriers of the D allele of H63D mutation were significantly more likely to develop HCC (Gharib et al. 2011). In a more recent study, this mutation did not associate with an increased risk of HCC in cirrhotic Egyptian patients (Dawood et al. 2021). No significant differences in the c-MET mutation frequency in HCC patients, although they found that the frequency of c-MET mutations was higher in ctDNA than in the gDNA samples from the same patient; thus, these mutations are somatic mutations, rather than germline mutations (Ahmed et al. 2023). The Lymphotoxin alpha (c.179 C > A; p. Thr60Asn; rs1041981) polymorphisms were autonomously associated with an increased risk for HCC in the Egyptian population (Alhelf et al. 2023). El-Mowafy et al. (2017) studied the mutational analysis in HBV viral genome (preS1/preS2 region) and detect no incidence of HCC development in patients infected with mutated HBV.

A number of research studies were carried out in India. The incidence of TP53 mutation in HBV-associated HCC samples was found to be very low, and it seems that the beta-catenin pathway does not play a substantial role in this process (Katiyar et al. 2000; Vivekanandan et al. 2011). Among primary HCC tissues that tested positive for HBV-DNA, the presence of a mutation in codon 12 of K-ras was found to be rare. Additionally, the levels of Ras expression in HCC were lower compared to those with normal liver and chronic liver disease. This suggests that the wild-type K-Ras may have a new role as a growth suppressor in the progression of hepatic cancer (Bose et al. 2011).

Mutations of the HBV genome were reported to be associated with HCC in many studies (Asim et al. 2010; Malik et al. 2012; Panigrahi et al. 2012; Gopalakrishnan et al. 2013; Tuteja et al. 2014; Malik et al. 2018; Shivlata et al. 2021; Kar et al. 2022).

From Iran, Abedi-Ardekani et al. (2011) reported no association between the TP53 R249S mutation and HBV genotypes D in Iranian HCC patients. The majority of HCC patients in Bahramali et al. (2008) study was infected with HBV mutant variants. The presence of a mutation in the activator protein-1 (AP2) binding site (−483 A to C) in the Astrocyte elevated gene-1 promoter is linked to an increased risk of hepatocellular carcinoma (HCC) in the Iranian population, according to a study by Motalleb et al. (2014).

In Mongolian-infected patients with HBV/D, the C1752 and/or V1753 mutation was associated with HCC (Elkady et al. 2008). The common driver mutations (TP53, CTNNB1) were found in pan-cancer analysis on Mongolian HCC patients in addition to exhibiting unique drivers (GTF2IRD2B, PNRC2, and SPTA1) which is associated with hepatitis D viral infection (Candia et al. 2020). Torrens et al. (2022) identified distinct genomic and transcriptomic footprints in Mongolian HCC, including a novel mutational signature, a higher number of mutations per tumor, and two molecular clusters not observed in Western HCC.

Two studies from Morocco, Akil et al. (2012) demonstrated that variants of the transcriptional coactivator genes (EP300 and PCAF) could influence HCC risk with low mutations or chromosomal instability rates. H63D mutation in hemochromatosis gene was reported to be conferred with an increased susceptibility to HCC while HFE C282Y and SERPINA1 mutations do not contribute to HCC development in Moroccan population (Ezzikouri et al. 2008).

From Nigeria, a case control study determines a significant association of p53 codon 249 mutation and HCC patients from South-Western Nigeria (Igetei et al. 2008). Moreover, mutations in the surface and polymerase genes of HBV genotype E associated with poor HCC prognosis in Nigerians (Olusola et al. 2021). Furthermore, mutations in the α-box of the enhancer II region of the HBx gene are associated with HCC prevalence in Pakistani HBV genotype D isolates (Khan et al. 2022). Multivariate analysis by Sakamoto et al. (2006) indicated that the core promoter gene mutations of HBV subtypes B and C were significant factors for HCC development in the Philippines. In Tajikistan, the T1762/A1764 mutation in the Basal Core Promoter region of HBV was associated with HCC (Khan et al. 2008). Concerning Vietnam, HBV PreS/S mutations are significantly associated with HCC in Vietnamese chronic hepatitis B-infected patients (Thi Cam Huong et al. 2022). The double mutation, namely A1762T-G1764A, exhibited the highest prevalence among HCC patients in Vietnam, as reported by Song et al. (2005), Truong et al. (2007), and Ho et al. (2022). Furthermore, Matsuo et al. (2017) discovered that there were genetic changes in the promoter region of HBV genotype B4 isolates, which were a combination of genotype C. This genetic combination was associated with an increased risk of HCC.

No data were reported from Angola, Algeria, Benin, Bhutan, Bolivia, Cabo Verde, Comoros, Congo, Rep., Côte d'Ivoire, Djibouti, Eswatini, Ghana, Guinea, Haiti, Honduras, Jordan, Kenya, Kiribati, Kyrgyz Republic, Lao PDR, Lebanon,

Lesotho, Mauritania, Micronesia, Fed. Sts., Nepal,Nicaragua, Papua New Guinea, Samoa, São Tomé and Principe, Senegal, Solomon Islands, Sri Lanka, Tanzania, Timor-Leste, Ukraine, Uzbekistan, Vanuatu, Zambia or Zimbabwe.

3.10 Conclusion

Research and therapies focusing on the molecular basis of HCC in LMICs are necessary. Understanding the various factors that increase the risk and the molecular properties of HCC in different situations will help in formulating targeted approaches for prevention, diagnosis, and treatment. This involves the application of genetic profiling tools and personalized therapeutics in resource-limited settings in LMICs.

References

Abbas Z, Abbas M, Abbas S, Shazi L. Hepatitis D and hepatocellular carcinoma. World J Hepatol. 2015;7(5):777–86. https://doi.org/10.4254/wjh.v7.i5.777.

Abdelhamed W, El-Kassas M. Hepatocellular carcinoma and hepatitis C virus treatments: The bold and the beautiful. J Viral Hepat. 2023;30(2):148–59. https://doi.org/10.1111/jvh.13778.

Abedi-Ardekani B, Gouas D, Villar S, Sotoudeh M, Hainaut P. TP53 mutations and HBX status analysis in Hepatocellular carcinomas from Iran: evidence for lack of association between HBV genotype D and TP53 R249S mutations. Hepat Res Treat. 2011;2011:475965. https://doi.org/10.1155/2011/475965.

Ahmed E, El-Dien AN, Sabet S, Khalifa M, El Hamshary M. Detection of MET gene somatic mutations in hepatocellular carcinoma of Egyptian patients using next-generation sequencing. Biomarkers. 2023;28(4):379–86. https://doi.org/10.1080/1354750X.2023.2184497.

Ahn SM, Jang SJ, Shim JH, et al. Genomic portrait of resectable hepatocellular carcinomas: implications of RB1 and FGF19 aberrations for patient stratification. Hepatology. 2014;60(6):1972–82. https://doi.org/10.1002/hep.27198.

Akil A, Ezzikouri S, El Feydi AE, et al. Associations of genetic variants in the transcriptional coactivators EP300 and PCAF with hepatocellular carcinoma. Cancer Epidemiol. 2012;36(5):e300–5. https://doi.org/10.1016/j.canep.2012.05.011.

Alhelf M, Shoaib RMS, Elsaid A, et al. Prognostic significance of the genetic variant of lymphotoxin alpha (p.Thr60Asn) in egyptian patients with advanced hepatocellular carcinoma. Mol Biol Rep. 2023;50(5):4317–27. https://doi.org/10.1007/s11033-023-08281-z.

Amougou-Atsama M, Jean Adrien Atangana P, Noah Noah D, Fewou Moundipa P, Pineau P, Njouom R. The role of hepatitis C virus genotypes and core mutations in hepatocellular carcinoma in Cameroon. J Viral Hepat. 2020;27(9):880–5. https://doi.org/10.1111/jvh.13303.

An FQ, Matsuda M, Fujii H, et al. Tumor heterogeneity in small hepatocellular carcinoma: analysis of tumor cell proliferation, expression and mutation of p53 AND beta-catenin. Int J Cancer. 2001;93(4):468–74. https://doi.org/10.1002/ijc.1367.

Angers S, Moon RT. Proximal events in Wnt signal transduction. Nat Rev Mol Cell Biol. 2009;10(7):468–77. https://doi.org/10.1038/nrm2717.

Aravalli RN, Steer CJ, Cressman EN. Molecular mechanisms of hepatocellular carcinoma. Hepatology. 2008;48(6):2047–63. https://doi.org/10.1002/hep.22580.

Arechederra M, Daian F, Yim A, et al. Hypermethylation of gene body CpG islands predicts high dosage of functional oncogenes in liver cancer [published correction appears in Nat Commun. 2018 Sep 25;9(1):3976]. Nat Commun. 2018;9(1):3164. https://doi.org/10.1038/s41467-018-05550-5.

Artandi SE, Alson S, Tietze MK, et al. Constitutive telomerase expression promotes mammary carcinomas in aging mice. Proc Natl Acad Sci USA. 2002;99(12):8191–6. https://doi.org/10.1073/pnas.112515399.

Asim M, Malik A, Sarma MP, et al. Hepatitis B virus BCP, Precore/core, X gene mutations/genotypes and the risk of hepatocellular carcinoma in India. J Med Virol. 2010;82(7):1115–25. https://doi.org/10.1002/jmv.21774.

Atsama Amougou M, Marchio A, Bivigou-Mboumba B, et al. Enrichment in selected genotypes, basal core and precore mutations of hepatitis B virus in patients with hepatocellular carcinoma in Cameroon. J Viral Hepat. 2019;26(9):1086–93. https://doi.org/10.1111/jvh.13131.

Attallah AM, Tabll AA, Salem SF, El-Sadany M, Ibrahim TA, Osman S, El-Dosoky IM. DNA ploidy of liver biopsies from patients with liver cirrhosis and hepatocellular carcinoma: a flow cytometric analysis. Cancer Lett. 1999;142(1):65–9.

Au SL, Wong CC, Lee JM, et al. Enhancer of zeste homolog 2 epigenetically silences multiple tumor suppressor microRNAs to promote liver cancer metastasis. Hepatology. 2012;56(2):622–31. https://doi.org/10.1002/hep.25679.

Audard V, Grimber G, Elie C, et al. Cholestasis is a marker for hepatocellular carcinomas displaying beta-catenin mutations. J Pathol. 2007;212(3):345–52. https://doi.org/10.1002/path.2169.

Bae HJ, Noh JH, Kim JK, et al. MicroRNA-29c functions as a tumor suppressor by direct targeting oncogenic SIRT1 in hepatocellular carcinoma. Oncogene. 2014;33(20):2557–67. https://doi.org/10.1038/onc.2013.216.

Bahramali G, Sadeghizadeh M, Amini-Bavil-Olyaee S, et al. Clinical, virologic and phylogenetic features of hepatitis B infection in Iranian patients. World J Gastroenterol. 2008;14(35):5448–53. https://doi.org/10.3748/wjg.14.5448.

Barbosa MC, Grosso RA, Fader CM. Hallmarks of aging: an autophagic perspective. Front Endocrinol (Lausanne). 2019;9:790.

Belinky F, Nativ N, Stelzer G, et al. PathCards: multi-source consolidation of human biological pathways. Database (Oxford). 2015;2015:bav006. https://doi.org/10.1093/database/bav006.

Bell RJ, Rube HT, Kreig A, et al. Cancer. The transcription factor GABP selectively binds and activates the mutant TERT promoter in cancer. Science. 2015;348(6238):1036–9. https://doi.org/10.1126/science.aab0015.

Benhamouche S, Decaens T, Godard C, et al. Apc tumor suppressor gene is the "zonation-keeper" of mouse liver. Dev Cell. 2006;10(6):759–70. https://doi.org/10.1016/j.devcel.2006.03.015.

Bhat M, Sonenberg N, Gores GJ. The mTOR pathway in hepatic malignancies. Hepatology. 2013;58(2):810–8. https://doi.org/10.1002/hep.26323.

Bose S, Sakhuja P, Bezawada L, et al. Hepatocellular carcinoma with persistent hepatitis B virus infection shows unusual downregulation of Ras expression and differential response to Ras mediated signaling. J Gastroenterol Hepatol. 2011;26(1):135–44. https://doi.org/10.1111/j.1440-1746.2010.06305.x.

Bottaro DP, Rubin JS, Faletto DL, et al. Identification of the hepatocyte growth factor receptor as the c-met proto-oncogene product. Science. 1991;251(4995):802–4. https://doi.org/10.1126/science.1846706.

Bozkaya G, Korhan P, Cokaklı M, et al. Cooperative interaction of MUC1 with the HGF/c-Met pathway during hepatocarcinogenesis. Mol Cancer. 2012;11:64. https://doi.org/10.1186/1476-4598-11-64.

Brahmer J, Reckamp KL, Baas P, et al. Nivolumab versus docetaxel in advanced squamous-cell non-small-cell lung Cancer. N Engl J Med. 2015;373(2):123–35. https://doi.org/10.1056/NEJMoa1504627.

Bruix J, Reig M, Sherman M. Evidence-based diagnosis, staging, and treatment of patients with hepatocellular carcinoma. Gastroenterology. 2016;150(4):835–53.

Bugter JM, Fenderico N, Maurice MM. Mutations and mechanisms of WNT pathway tumour suppressors in cancer [published correction appears in Nat Rev Cancer. 2020 Nov 4]. Nat Rev Cancer. 2021;21(1):5–21. https://doi.org/10.1038/s41568-020-00307-z.

Calvisi DF, Factor VM, Ladu S, Conner EA, Thorgeirsson SS. Disruption of beta-catenin pathway or genomic instability define two distinct categories of liver cancer in transgenic mice. Gastroenterology. 2004;126(5):1374–86. https://doi.org/10.1053/j.gastro.2004.02.014.
Candia J, Bayarsaikhan E, Tandon M, et al. The genomic landscape of Mongolian hepatocellular carcinoma. Nat Commun. 2020;11(1):4383. https://doi.org/10.1038/s41467-020-18186-1.
Cargill Z, Brown SE, Dusheiko G, Agarwal K. Risk stratification in chronic hepatitis B patients for hepatocellular carcinoma surveillance: management in migrant sub-Saharan African populations. Gut. 2021;70(3):629–30.
Cha C, Dematteo RP. Molecular mechanisms in hepatocellular carcinoma development. Best Pract Res Clin Gastroenterol. 2005;19(1):25–37. https://doi.org/10.1016/j.bpg.2004.11.005.
Chai ZT, Kong J, Zhu XD, Zhang YY, Lu L, Zhou JM, Wang LR, Zhang KZ, Zhang QB, Ao JY, Wang M, Wu WZ, Wang L, Tang ZY, Sun HC. MicroRNA-26a inhibits angiogenesis by down-regulating VEGFA through the PIK3C2α/Akt/HIF-1α pathway in hepatocellular carcinoma. PLoS One. 2013;8(10):e77957. https://doi.org/10.1371/journal.pone.0077957.
Chan C, Wang Y, Chow PK, Chung AY, Ooi LL, Lee CG. Altered binding site selection of p53 transcription cassettes by hepatitis B virus X protein. Mol Cell Biol. 2013;33(3):485–97. https://doi.org/10.1128/MCB.01189-12.
Chang PH, Sekine K, Chao HM, Hsu SH, Chern E. Chitosan promotes cancer progression and stem cell properties in association with Wnt signaling in colon and hepatocellular carcinoma cells. Sci Rep. 2017;8:45751. https://doi.org/10.1038/srep45751.
Chen C, Wang G. Mechanisms of hepatocellular carcinoma and challenges and opportunities for molecular targeted therapy. World J Hepatol. 2015;7(15):1964–70. https://doi.org/10.4254/wjh.v7.i15.1964.
Chen YL, Jeng YM, Chang CN, et al. TERT promoter mutation in resectable hepatocellular carcinomas: a strong association with hepatitis C infection and absence of hepatitis B infection. Int J Surg. 2014;12(7):659–65. https://doi.org/10.1016/j.ijsu.2014.05.066.
Chen Z, Ma T, Huang C, et al. MiR-27a modulates the MDR1/P-glycoprotein expression by inhibiting FZD7/β-catenin pathway in hepatocellular carcinoma cells. Cell Signal. 2013;25(12):2693–701. https://doi.org/10.1016/j.cellsig.2013.08.032.
Chen Z, Zuo X, Zhang Y, et al. MiR-3662 suppresses hepatocellular carcinoma growth through inhibition of HIF-1α-mediated Warburg effect. Cell Death Dis. 2018;9(5):549. https://doi.org/10.1038/s41419-018-0616-8.
Chidambaranathan-Reghupaty S, Fisher PB, Sarkar D. Hepatocellular carcinoma (HCC): Epidemiology, etiology and molecular classification. Adv Cancer Res. 2021;149:1–61.
Choi SH, Hwang SB. Modulation of the transforming growth factor-beta signal transduction pathway by hepatitis C virus nonstructural 5A protein. J Biol Chem. 2006;281(11):7468–78. https://doi.org/10.1074/jbc.M512438200.
Chuon C, Takahashi K, Matsuo J, et al. High possibility of hepatocarcinogenesis in HBV genotype C1 infected Cambodians is indicated by 340 HBV C1 full-genomes analysis from GenBank. Sci Rep. 2019;9(1):12186. https://doi.org/10.1038/s41598-019-48304-z.
Cieply B, Zeng G, Proverbs-Singh T, Geller DA, Monga SP. Unique phenotype of hepatocellular cancers with exon-3 mutations in beta-catenin gene. Hepatology. 2009;49(3):821–31. https://doi.org/10.1002/hep.22695.
Cooper CS, Park M, Blair DG, et al. Molecular cloning of a new transforming gene from a chemically transformed human cell line. Nature. 1984;311(5981):29–33. https://doi.org/10.1038/311029a0.
Cooray S. The pivotal role of phosphatidylinositol 3-kinase-Akt signal transduction in virus survival. J Gen Virol. 2004;85(Pt 5):1065–76. https://doi.org/10.1099/vir.0.19771-0.
Dakurah OB, Tamandjou CRT, Zunza M, Preiser W, Maponga TG. Viral hepatitis associated hepatocellular carcinoma on the African continent, the past, present, and future: a systematic review. BMC Cancer. 2021;21(1):715.
Dancey J. mTOR signaling and drug development in cancer. Nat Rev Clin Oncol. 2010;7(4):209–19. https://doi.org/10.1038/nrclinonc.2010.21.

Dawood RM, Abd El Meguid M, Elrobe W, et al. Significance of hereditary hemochromatosis gene (HFE) mutations in chronic hepatitis c and hepatocellular carcinoma patients in Egypt: a pilot study. Asian Pac J Cancer Prev. 2021;22(9):2837–45. https://doi.org/10.31557/APJCP.2021.22.9.2837.

Delgado E, Okabe H, Preziosi M, et al. Complete response of Ctnnb1-mutated tumours to β-catenin suppression by locked nucleic acid antisense in a mouse hepatocarcinogenesis model. J Hepatol. 2015;62(2):380–7. https://doi.org/10.1016/j.jhep.2014.10.021.

Dhanasekaran R, Venkatesh SK, Torbenson MS, Roberts LR. Clinical implications of basic research in hepatocellular carcinoma. J Hepatol. 2016;64(3):736–45.

Di Tommaso L, Spadaccini M, Donadon M, Personeni N, Elamin A, Aghemo A, Lleo A. Role of liver biopsy in hepatocellular carcinoma. World J Gastroenterol. 2019;25(40):6041–52.

DiStefano JK. Long noncoding RNAs in the initiation, progression, and metastasis of hepatocellular carcinoma. Noncoding RNA Res. 2017;2(3–4):129–36. https://doi.org/10.1016/j.ncrna.2017.11.001.

Dragani TA. Risk of HCC: genetic heterogeneity and complex genetics. J Hepatol. 2010;52(2):252–7. https://doi.org/10.1016/j.jhep.2009.11.015.

Du C, Lv Z, Cao L, et al. MiR-126-3p suppresses tumor metastasis and angiogenesis of hepatocellular carcinoma by targeting LRP6 and PIK3R2. J Transl Med. 2014;12:259. https://doi.org/10.1186/s12967-014-0259-1.

Edamoto Y, Hara A, Biernat W, et al. Alterations of RB1, p53 and Wnt pathways in hepatocellular carcinomas associated with hepatitis C, hepatitis B and alcoholic liver cirrhosis. Int J Cancer. 2003;106(3):334–41. https://doi.org/10.1002/ijc.11254.

Elderkin J, Al Hallak N, Azmi AS, Aoun H, Critchfield J, Tobon M, Beal EW. Hepatocellular carcinoma: surveillance, diagnosis. Evaluation and Management Cancers (Basel). 2023;15(21):5118.

Elkady A, Tanaka Y, Kurbanov F, Oynsuren T, Mizokami M. Virological and clinical implication of core promoter C1752/V1753 and T1764/G1766 mutations in hepatitis B virus genotype D infection in Mongolia. J Gastroenterol Hepatol. 2008;23(3):474–81. https://doi.org/10.1111/j.1440-1746.2008.05321.x.

El-Kafrawy SA, Abdel-Hamid M, El-Daly M, et al. P53 mutations in hepatocellular carcinoma patients in Egypt. Int J Hyg Environ Health. 2005;208(4):263–70. https://doi.org/10.1016/j.ijheh.2005.02.002.

El-Mowafy M, Elgaml A, El-Mesery M, Elegezy M. Molecular analysis of hepatitis B virus subgenotypes and incidence of preS1/preS2 region mutations in HBV-infected Egyptian patients from Mansoura. J Med Virol. 2017;89(9):1559–66. https://doi.org/10.1002/jmv.24828.

El-Sayed SS, El-Sadany M, Tabll AA, Soltan A, El-Dosoky I, Attallah AM. DNA ploidy and liver cell dysplasia in liver biopsies from patients with liver cirrhosis. Can J Gastroenterol. 2004;18(2):87–91.

El-Shamy A, Shindo M, Shoji I, Deng L, Okuno T, Hotta H. Polymorphisms of the core, NS3, and NS5A proteins of hepatitis C virus genotype 1b associate with development of hepatocellular carcinoma. Hepatology. 2013;58(2):555–63. https://doi.org/10.1002/hep.26205.

Ezzat R, Eltabbakh M, El Kassas M. Unique situation of hepatocellular carcinoma in Egypt: A review of epidemiology and control measures. World J Gastrointest Oncol. 2021;13(12):1919–38.

Ezzikouri S, El Feydi AE, El Kihal L, et al. Prevalence of common HFE and SERPINA1 mutations in patients with hepatocellular carcinoma in a Moroccan population. Arch Med Res. 2008;39(2):236–41. https://doi.org/10.1016/j.arcmed.2007.09.006.

Fan Q, Yang L, Zhang X, et al. Autophagy promotes metastasis and glycolysis by upregulating MCT1 expression and Wnt/β-catenin signaling pathway activation in hepatocellular carcinoma cells. J Exp Clin Cancer Res. 2018;37(1):9. https://doi.org/10.1186/s13046-018-0673-y.

Fan Y, Arechederra M, Richelme S, et al. A phosphokinome-based screen uncovers new drug synergies for cancer driven by liver-specific gain of nononcogenic receptor tyrosine kinases. Hepatology. 2017;66(5):1644–61. https://doi.org/10.1002/hep.29304.

Fang Y, Xue JL, Shen Q, Chen J, Tian L. MicroRNA-7 inhibits tumor growth and metastasis by targeting the phosphoinositide 3-kinase/Akt pathway in hepatocellular carcinoma [published correction appears in Hepatology. 2014 Mar;59(3):1216]. Hepatology. 2012;55(6):1852–62. https://doi.org/10.1002/hep.25576.

Farazi PA, DePinho RA. Hepatocellular carcinoma pathogenesis: from genes to environment. Nat Rev Cancer. 2006;6(9):674–87. https://doi.org/10.1038/nrc1934.

Feng Q, Stern JE, Hawes SE, Lu H, Jiang M, Kiviat NB. DNA methylation changes in normal liver tissues and hepatocellular carcinoma with different viral infection. Exp Mol Pathol. 2010;88(2):287–92. https://doi.org/10.1016/j.yexmp.2010.01.002.

Ferber MJ, Montoya DP, Yu C, et al. Integrations of the hepatitis B virus (HBV) and human papillomavirus (HPV) into the human telomerase reverse transcriptase (hTERT) gene in liver and cervical cancers. Oncogene. 2003;22(24):3813–20. https://doi.org/10.1038/sj.onc.1206528.

Franco-Juárez EX, González-Villasana V, Camacho-Moll ME, Rendón-Garlant L, Ramírez-Flores PN, Silva-Ramírez B, Peñuelas-Urquides K, Cabello-Ruiz ED, Castorena-Torres F, Bermúdez de León M. Mechanistic insights about sorafenib-, valproic acid- and metformin-induced cell death in hepatocellular carcinoma. Int J Mol Sci. 2024;25(3):1760.

Fruman DA, Chiu H, Hopkins BD, Bagrodia S, Cantley LC, Abraham RT. The PI3K pathway in human disease. Cell. 2017;170(4):605–35. https://doi.org/10.1016/j.cell.2017.07.029.

Fruman DA, Rommel C. PI3K and cancer: lessons, challenges and opportunities. Nat Rev Drug Discov. 2014;13(2):140–56. https://doi.org/10.1038/nrd4204.

Fu L, Chen Q, Yao T, et al. Hsa_circ_0005986 inhibits carcinogenesis by acting as a miR-129-5p sponge and is used as a novel biomarker for hepatocellular carcinoma. Oncotarget. 2017;8(27):43878–88. https://doi.org/10.18632/oncotarget.16709.

Galicia VA, He L, Dang H, et al. Expansion of hepatic tumor progenitor cells in Pten-null mice requires liver injury and is reversed by loss of AKT2. Gastroenterology. 2010;139(6):2170–82. https://doi.org/10.1053/j.gastro.2010.09.002.

Gharib AF, Karam RA, Pasha HF, Radwan MI, Elsawy WH. Polymorphisms of hemochromatosis, and alpha-1 antitrypsin genes in Egyptian HCV patients with and without hepatocellular carcinoma. Gene. 2011;489(2):98–102. https://doi.org/10.1016/j.gene.2011.08.010.

Gopalakrishnan D, Keyter M, Shenoy KT, et al. Hepatitis B virus subgenotype A1 predominates in liver disease patients from Kerala, India. World J Gastroenterol. 2013;19(48):9294–306. https://doi.org/10.3748/wjg.v19.i48.9294.

Gross-Goupil M, Riou P, Emile JF, et al. Analysis of chromosomal instability in pulmonary or liver metastases and matched primary hepatocellular carcinoma after orthotopic liver transplantation. Int J Cancer. 2003;104(6):745–51. https://doi.org/10.1002/ijc.11017.

Guichard C, Amaddeo G, Imbeaud S, et al. Integrated analysis of somatic mutations and focal copy-number changes identifies key genes and pathways in hepatocellular carcinoma. Nat Genet. 2012;44(6):694–8. https://doi.org/10.1038/ng.2256.

Gujral TS, Chan M, Peshkin L, Sorger PK, Kirschner MW, MacBeath G. A noncanonical Frizzled2 pathway regulates epithelial-mesenchymal transition and metastasis. Cell. 2014;159(4):844–56. https://doi.org/10.1016/j.cell.2014.10.032.

Güller M, Toualbi-Abed K, Legrand A, et al. C-Fos overexpression increases the proliferation of human hepatocytes by stabilizing nuclear cyclin D1. World J Gastroenterol. 2008;14(41):6339–46. https://doi.org/10.3748/wjg.14.6339.

Guo H, Zhou T, Jiang D, et al. Regulation of hepatitis B virus replication by the phosphatidylinositol 3-kinase-akt signal transduction pathway. J Virol. 2007;81(18):10072–80. https://doi.org/10.1128/JVI.00541-07.

Guo W, Qiu Z, Wang Z, et al. MiR-199a-5p is negatively associated with malignancies and regulates glycolysis and lactate production by targeting hexokinase 2 in liver cancer. Hepatology. 2015;62(4):1132–44. https://doi.org/10.1002/hep.27929.

Guri Y, Colombi M, Dazert E, et al. mTORC2 promotes tumorigenesis via lipid synthesis. Cancer Cell. 2017;32(6):807–823.e12. https://doi.org/10.1016/j.ccell.2017.11.011.

Guy J, Yee HF Jr. Health disparities in liver disease: Time to take notice and take action. Hepatology. 2009;50(1):309–13.

Han H, Li W, Shen H, Zhang J, Zhu Y, Li Y. microRNA-129-5p, a c-Myc negative target, affects hepatocellular carcinoma progression by blocking the Warburg effect. J Mol Cell Biol. 2016;8(5):400–10. https://doi.org/10.1093/jmcb/mjw010.

Hara K, Maruki Y, Long X, et al. Raptor, a binding partner of target of rapamycin (TOR), mediates TOR action. Cell. 2002;110(2):177–89. https://doi.org/10.1016/s0092-8674(02)00833-4].

He C, Zhou Z, Jiang H, et al. Epithelial-mesenchymal transition is superior to vessels-encapsulate tumor cluster in promoting metastasis of Hepatocellular carcinoma: a morphological evidence. J Cancer. 2017;8(1):39–47. https://doi.org/10.7150/jca.16736.

He Q, Cheng R, Chen Z, et al. Cell transformation and proteome alteration in QSG7701 cells transfected with hepatitis C virus non-structural protein 3. Acta Biochim Biophys Sin Shanghai. 2007;39(10):751–62. https://doi.org/10.1111/j.1745-7270.2007.00344.x.

He S, Tang S. WNT/β-catenin signaling in the development of liver cancers. Biomed Pharmacother. 2020;132:110851. https://doi.org/10.1016/j.biopha.2020.110851.

He TC, Sparks AB, Rago C, et al. Identification of c-MYC as a target of the APC pathway. Science. 1998;281(5382):1509–12. https://doi.org/10.1126/science.281.5382.1509.

He X, Hikiba Y, Suzuki Y, Nakamori Y, Kanemaru Y, Sugimori M, Sato T, Nozaki A, Chuma M, Maeda S. EGFR inhibition reverses resistance to lenvatinib in hepatocellular carcinoma cells. Sci Rep. 2022;12(1):8007.

Hellebrekers DM, Griffioen AW, van Engeland M. Dual targeting of epigenetic therapy in cancer. Biochim Biophys Acta. 2007;1775(1):76–91. https://doi.org/10.1016/j.bbcan.2006.07.003.

Higashitsuji H, Itoh K, Nagao T, et al. Reduced stability of retinoblastoma protein by gankyrin, an oncogenic ankyrin-repeat protein overexpressed in hepatomas. Nat Med. 2000;6(1):96–9. https://doi.org/10.1038/71600.

Ho PT, Balzanelli MG, Distratis P, et al. Characteristics of hepatitis B virus genotype and sub-genotype in Hepatocellular Cancer patients in Vietnam. Diagnostics (Basel). 2022;12(10):2393. https://doi.org/10.3390/diagnostics12102393.

Hodi FS, O'Day SJ, McDermott DF, et al. Improved survival with ipilimumab in patients with metastatic melanoma [published correction appears in N Engl J Med. 2010 Sep 23;363(13):1290]. N Engl J Med. 2010;363(8):711–23. https://doi.org/10.1056/NEJMoa1003466.

Horton S, Sullivan R, Flanigan J, Fleming KA, Kuti MA, Looi LM, Pai SA, Lawler M. Delivering modern, high-quality, affordable pathology and laboratory medicine to low-income and middle-income countries: a call to action. Lancet. 2018 May 12;391(10133): 1953–1964. J Hepatol. 2020;72(2):342–52.

Hosny G, Farahat N, Tayel H, Hainaut P. Ser-249 TP53 and CTNNB1 mutations in circulating free DNA of Egyptian patients with hepatocellular carcinoma versus chronic liver diseases. Cancer Lett. 2008;264(2):201–8. https://doi.org/10.1016/j.canlet.2008.01.031.

Hsieh AC, Liu Y, Edlind MP, et al. The translational landscape of mTOR signalling steers cancer initiation and metastasis. Nature. 2012;485(7396):55–61. https://doi.org/10.1038/nature10912.

Hsu HC, Jeng YM, Mao TL, Chu JS, Lai PL, Peng SY. Beta-catenin mutations are associated with a subset of low-stage hepatocellular carcinoma negative for hepatitis B virus and with favorable prognosis. Am J Pathol. 2000;157(3):763–70. https://doi.org/10.1016/s0002-9440(10)64590-7.

Hu Y, Yang Z, Bao D, Ni JS, Lou J. miR-455-5p suppresses hepatocellular carcinoma cell growth and invasion via IGF-1R/AKT/GLUT1 pathway by targeting IGF-1R. Pathol Res Pract. 2019;215(12):152674. https://doi.org/10.1016/j.prp.2019.152674.

Hua S, Liu C, Liu L, Wu D. miR-142-3p inhibits aerobic glycolysis and cell proliferation in hepatocellular carcinoma via targeting LDHA. Biochem Biophys Res Commun. 2018;496(3):947–54. https://doi.org/10.1016/j.bbrc.2018.01.112.

Huang F, Wang BR, Wang YG. Role of autophagy in tumorigenesis, metastasis, targeted therapy and drug resistance of hepatocellular carcinoma. World J Gastroenterol. 2018;24(41):4643–51.

Huang G, Liang M, Liu H, et al. CircRNA hsa_circRNA_104348 promotes hepatocellular carcinoma progression through modulating miR-187-3p/RTKN2 axis and activating Wnt/β-catenin pathway. Cell Death Dis. 2020;11(12):1065. https://doi.org/10.1038/s41419-020-03276-1.

Huang JL, Zheng L, Hu YW, Wang Q. Characteristics of long non-coding RNA and its relation to hepatocellular carcinoma. Carcinogenesis. 2014;35(3):507–14. https://doi.org/10.1093/carcin/bgt405.

Huang SM, Mishina YM, Liu S, et al. Tankyrase inhibition stabilizes axin and antagonizes Wnt signalling. Nature. 2009;461(7264):614–20. https://doi.org/10.1038/nature08356.

Hussen BM, Honarmand Tamizkar K, Hidayat HJ, Taheri M, Ghafouri-Fard S. The role of circular RNAs in the development of hepatocellular carcinoma. Pathol Res Pract. 2021;223:153495. https://doi.org/10.1016/j.prp.2021.153495.

Igetei R, Otegbayo JA, Ndububa DA, et al. Detection of p53 codon 249 mutation in Nigerian patients with hepatocellular carcinoma using a novel evaluation of cell-free DNA. Ann Hepatol. 2008;7(4):339–44. https://doi.org/10.1016/S1665-2681(19)31834-4.

Imamura R, Matsumoto K. Hepatocyte growth factor in physiology and infectious diseases. Cytokine. 2017;98:97–106. https://doi.org/10.1016/j.cyto.2016.12.025.

Ito Y, Takeda T, Sakon M, et al. Expression and clinical significance of erb-B receptor family in hepatocellular carcinoma. Br J Cancer. 2001;84(10):1377–83. https://doi.org/10.1054/bjoc.2000.1580.

Jakubczak JL, Chisari FV, Merlino G. Synergy between transforming growth factor alpha and hepatitis B virus surface antigen in hepatocellular proliferation and carcinogenesis. Cancer Res. 1997;57(16):3606–11.

Janku F, Kaseb AO, Tsimberidou AM, Wolff RA, Kurzrock R. Identification of novel therapeutic targets in the PI3K/AKT/mTOR pathway in hepatocellular carcinoma using targeted next generation sequencing. Oncotarget. 2014;5(10):3012–22. https://doi.org/10.18632/oncotarget.1687.

Jensen N, Kelly AH, Avendano M. Health equity and health system strengthening - Time for a WHO re-think. Glob Public Health. 2022;17(3):377–90.

Jiang N, Chen WJ, Zhang JW, et al. Downregulation of miR-432 activates Wnt/β-catenin signaling and promotes human hepatocellular carcinoma proliferation. Oncotarget. 2015;6(10):7866–79. https://doi.org/10.18632/oncotarget.3492.

Jiang Z, Shen L, Wang S, Wu S, Hu Y, Guo J, Fu L. Hsa_circ_0028502 and hsa_circ_0076251 are potential novel biomarkers for hepatocellular carcinoma. Cancer Med. 2019;8(17):7278–87. https://doi.org/10.1002/cam4.2584.

Kalluri R, Weinberg RA. The basics of epithelial-mesenchymal transition [published correction appears in J Clin Invest. 2010 May 3;120(5):1786]. J Clin Invest. 2009;119(6):1420–8. https://doi.org/10.1172/JCI39104.

Kanda M, Sugimoto H, Kodera Y. Genetic and epigenetic aspects of initiation and progression of hepatocellular carcinoma. World J Gastroenterol. 2015;21(37):10584–97. https://doi.org/10.3748/wjg.v21.i37.10584.

Kaposi-Novak P, Lee JS, Gòmez-Quiroz L, Coulouarn C, Factor VM, Thorgeirsson SS. Met-regulated expression signature defines a subset of human hepatocellular carcinomas with poor prognosis and aggressive phenotype. J Clin Invest. 2006;116(6):1582–95. https://doi.org/10.1172/JCI27236.

Kar P, Goswami B, Mahanta J, et al. Epidemiology, genotyping, mutational and phylogenetic analysis of hepatitis B virus infection in north-East India. J Clin Exp Hepatol. 2022;12(1):43–51. https://doi.org/10.1016/j.jceh.2021.04.002.

Katiyar S, Dash BC, Thakur V, Guptan RC, Sarin SK, Das BC. P53 tumor suppressor gene mutations in hepatocellular carcinoma patients in India. Cancer. 2000;88(7):1565–73. https://doi.org/10.1002/(sici)1097-0142(20000401)88:7<1565::aid-cncr10>3.0.co;2-9.

Kedar Mukthinuthalapati VVP, Sewram V, Ndlovu N, Kimani S, Abdelaziz AO, Chiao EY, Abou-Alfa GK. Hepatocellular carcinoma in Sub-Saharan Africa. JCO Glob Oncol. 2021;7:756–66.

Khan A, Kurbanov F, Tanaka Y, et al. Epidemiological and clinical evaluation of hepatitis B, hepatitis C, and delta hepatitis viruses in Tajikistan. J Med Virol. 2008;80(2):268–76. https://doi.org/10.1002/jmv.21057.

Khan M, Khan S, Gondal MF, et al. Genetic diversity in enhancer II region of HBV genotype D and its association with advanced liver diseases. PLoS One. 2022;17(1):e0261721. https://doi.org/10.1371/journal.pone.0261721.

Kim B, Jung N, Lee S, Sohng JK, Jung HJ. Apigenin inhibits Cancer stem cell-like phenotypes in human glioblastoma cells via suppression of c-met signaling. Phytother Res. 2016;30(11):1833–40. https://doi.org/10.1002/ptr.5689.

Kim HR, Roe JS, Lee JE, Cho EJ, Youn HD. p53 regulates glucose metabolism by miR-34a. Biochem Biophys Res Commun. 2013;437(2):225–31. https://doi.org/10.1016/j.bbrc.2013.06.043.

Kong G, Zhang J, Zhang S, Shan C, Ye L, Zhang X. Upregulated microRNA-29a by hepatitis B virus X protein enhances hepatoma cell migration by targeting PTEN in cell culture model. PLoS One. 2011;6(5):e19518. https://doi.org/10.1371/journal.pone.0019518.

Korenaga M, Wang T, Li Y, et al. Hepatitis C virus core protein inhibits mitochondrial electron transport and increases reactive oxygen species (ROS) production. J Biol Chem. 2005;280(45):37481–8. https://doi.org/10.1074/jbc.M506412200.

Kudo M. Signaling pathway and molecular-targeted therapy for hepatocellular carcinoma. Dig Dis. 2011;29(3):289–302. https://doi.org/10.1159/000327562.

Kwun HJ, Jung EY, Ahn JY, Lee MN, Jang KL. p53-dependent transcriptional repression of p21(waf1) by hepatitis C virus NS3. J Gen Virol. 2001;82(Pt 9):2235–41. https://doi.org/10.1099/0022-1317-82-9-2235.

Lachenmayer A, Alsinet C, Chang CY, Llovet JM. Molecular approaches to treatment of hepatocellular carcinoma. Dig Liver Dis. 2010;42(Suppl 3(0 3)):S264–72. https://doi.org/10.1016/S1590-8658(10)60515-4.

Lee CM, Hsu CY, Eng HL, et al. Telomerase activity and telomerase catalytic subunit in hepatocellular carcinoma. Hepato-Gastroenterology. 2004;51(57):796–800.

Lee S, Lee HJ, Kim JH, Lee HS, Jang JJ, Kang GH. Aberrant CpG island hypermethylation along multistep hepatocarcinogenesis. Am J Pathol. 2003;163(4):1371–8. https://doi.org/10.1016/S0002-9440(10)63495-5.

Lei B, Zhou J, Xuan X, Tian Z, Zhang M, Gao W, Lin Y, Ni B, Pang H, Fan W. Circular RNA expression profiles of peripheral blood mononuclear cells in hepatocellular carcinoma patients by sequence analysis. Cancer Med. 2019;8(4):1423–33. https://doi.org/10.1002/cam4.2010.

Lerat H, Higgs M, Pawlotsky JM. Animal models in the study of hepatitis C virus-associated liver pathologies. Expert Rev Gastroenterol Hepatol. 2011;5(3):341–52. https://doi.org/10.1586/egh.11.14.

Levine AJ, Oren M. The first 30 years of p53: growing ever more complex. Nat Rev Cancer. 2009;9(10):749–58. https://doi.org/10.1038/nrc2723.

Li B, He L, Zuo D, He W, Wang Y, Zhang Y, Liu W, Yuan Y. Mutual regulation of MiR-199a-5p and HIF-1α modulates the Warburg effect in Hepatocellular carcinoma. J Cancer. 2017;8(6):940–9. https://doi.org/10.7150/jca.17496.

Li HP, Leu YW, Chang YS. Epigenetic changes in virus-associated human cancers. Cell Res. 2005;15(4):262–71. https://doi.org/10.1038/sj.cr.7290295.

Li J, Quan H, Liu Q, Si Z, He Z, Qi H. Alterations of axis inhibition protein 1 (AXIN1) in hepatitis B virus-related hepatocellular carcinoma and overexpression of AXIN1 induces apoptosis in hepatocellular cancer cells. Oncol Res. 2013;20(7):281–8. https://doi.org/10.3727/096504013x13639794277608.

Li W, He P, Huang Y, Li YF, Lu J, Li M, Kurihara H, Luo Z, Meng T, Onishi M, Ma C, Jiang L, Hu Y, Gong Q, Zhu D, Xu Y, Liu R, Liu L, Yi C, Zhu Y, Ma N, Okamoto K, Xie Z, Liu J, He RR, Feng D. Selective autophagy of intracellular organelles: recent research advances. Theranostics. 2021;11(1):222–56.

Li X, Lu P, Li B, et al. Sensitization of hepatocellular carcinoma cells to irradiation by miR-34a through targeting lactate dehydrogenase-a. Mol Med Rep. 2016;13(4):3661–7. https://doi.org/10.3892/mmr.2016.4974.

Li X, Zhao Q, Qi J, et al. lncRNA Ftx promotes aerobic glycolysis and tumor progression through the PPARγ pathway in hepatocellular carcinoma. Int J Oncol. 2018;53(2):551–66. https://doi.org/10.3892/ijo.2018.4418.

Liew CT, Li HM, Lo KW, et al. High frequency of p16INK4A gene alterations in hepatocellular carcinoma. Oncogene. 1999;18(3):789–95. https://doi.org/10.1038/sj.onc.1202359.

Linck-Paulus L, Hellerbrand C, Bosserhoff AK, Dietrich P. Dissimilar appearances are deceptive-common microRNAs and therapeutic strategies in liver cancer and melanoma. Cells. 2020;9(1):114. https://doi.org/10.3390/cells9010114.

Lindenbach BD, Evans MJ, Syder AJ, et al. Complete replication of hepatitis C virus in cell culture. Science. 2005;309(5734):623–6. https://doi.org/10.1126/science.1114016.

Liu F, Wu X, Qian Y, Jiang X, Wang Y, Gao J. PIK3C3 regulates the expansion of liver CSCs and PIK3C3 inhibition counteracts liver cancer stem cell activity induced by PI3K inhibitor. Cell Death Dis. 2020a;11(6):427. https://doi.org/10.1038/s41419-020-2631-9.

Liu L, Liao JZ, He XX, Li PY. The role of autophagy in hepatocellular carcinoma: friend or foe. Oncotarget. 2017;8(34):57707–22.

Liu M, Jiang L, Guan XY. The genetic and epigenetic alterations in human hepatocellular carcinoma: a recent update. Protein Cell. 2014;5(9):673–91. https://doi.org/10.1007/s13238-014-0065-9.

Liu P, Liang B, Liu M, et al. Oncogenic mutations in armadillo repeats 5 and 6 of β-catenin reduce binding to APC, increasing signaling and transcription of target genes. Gastroenterology. 2020b;158(4):1029–1043.e10. https://doi.org/10.1053/j.gastro.2019.11.302.

Liu W, Kang L, Han J, Wang Y, Shen C, Yan Z, Tai Y, Zhao C. miR-342-3p suppresses hepatocellular carcinoma proliferation through inhibition of IGF-1R-mediated Warburg effect. Onco Targets Ther. 2018;11:1643–53. https://doi.org/10.2147/OTT.S161586.

Liu W, Zheng L, Zhang R, et al. Circ-ZEB1 promotes PIK3CA expression by silencing miR-199a-3p and affects the proliferation and apoptosis of hepatocellular carcinoma. Mol Cancer. 2022;21(1):72. https://doi.org/10.1186/s12943-022-01529-5.

Liu WT, Jing YY, Yu GF, et al. Hepatic stellate cell promoted hepatoma cell invasion via the HGF/c-met signaling pathway regulated by p53. Cell Cycle. 2016;15(7):886–94. https://doi.org/10.1080/15384101.2016.1152428.

Liu Y, Chang CC, Marsh GM, Wu F. Population attributable risk of aflatoxin-related liver cancer: systematic review and meta-analysis. Eur J Cancer. 2012;48(14):2125–36. https://doi.org/10.1016/j.ejca.2012.02.009.

Liu YR, Tang RX, Huang WT, et al. Long noncoding RNAs in hepatocellular carcinoma: novel insights into their mechanism. World J Hepatol. 2015;7(28):2781–91. https://doi.org/10.4254/wjh.v7.i28.2781.

Liu Z, Mo H, Sun L, et al. Long noncoding RNA PICSAR/miR-588/EIF6 axis regulates tumorigenesis of hepatocellular carcinoma by activating PI3K/AKT/mTOR signaling pathway. Cancer Sci. 2020c;111(11):4118–28. https://doi.org/10.1111/cas.14631.

Llovet JM, Montal R, Sia D, Finn RS. Molecular therapies and precision medicine for hepatocellular carcinoma. Nat Rev Clin Oncol. 2018;15(10):599–616.

Llovet JM, Villanueva A, Lachenmayer A, Finn RS. Advances in targeted therapies for hepatocellular carcinoma in the genomic era [published correction appears in Nat Rev Clin Oncol. 2015 Aug;12(8):436]. Nat Rev Clin Oncol. 2015;12(7):408–24. https://doi.org/10.1038/nrclinonc.2015.103.

Llovet JM, Zucman-Rossi J, Pikarsky E, et al. Hepatocellular carcinoma. Nat Rev Dis Primers. 2016;2:16018. https://doi.org/10.1038/nrdp.2016.18.

Lu LC, Shao YY, Lee YH, et al. β-catenin (CTNNB1) mutations are not associated with prognosis in advanced hepatocellular carcinoma. Oncology. 2014;87(3):159–66. https://doi.org/10.1159/000362821.

Lv S, Li Y, Ning H, Zhang M, Jia Q, Wang X. CircRNA GFRA1 promotes hepatocellular carcinoma progression by modulating the miR-498/NAP1L3 axis. Sci Rep. 2021;11(1):386. https://doi.org/10.1038/s41598-020-79321-y.

Ma L, Chua MS, Andrisani O, So S. Epigenetics in hepatocellular carcinoma: an update and future therapy perspectives. World J Gastroenterol. 2014;20(2):333–45. https://doi.org/10.3748/wjg.v20.i2.333.

Maehama T, Fukasawa M, Date T, Wakita T, Hanada K. A class II phosphoinositide 3-kinase plays an indispensable role in hepatitis C virus replication. Biochem Biophys Res Commun. 2013;440(1):150–6. https://doi.org/10.1016/j.bbrc.2013.09.048.

Maeta Y, Shiota G, Okano J, Murawaki Y. Effect of promoter methylation of the p16 gene on phosphorylation of retinoblastoma gene product and growth of hepatocellular carcinoma cells. Tumour Biol. 2005;26(6):300–5. https://doi.org/10.1159/000089288.
Maguire HF, Hoeffler JP, Siddiqui A. HBV X protein alters the DNA binding specificity of CREB and ATF-2 by protein-protein interactions. Science. 1991;252(5007):842–4. https://doi.org/10.1126/science.1827531.
Malik A, Kumar D, Khan AA, et al. Hepatitis B virus precore G1896A mutation in chronic liver disease patients with HBeAg negative serology from North India. Saudi J Biol Sci. 2018;25(7):1257–62. https://doi.org/10.1016/j.sjbs.2016.05.004.
Malik A, Singhal DK, Albanyan A, Husain SA, Kar P. Hepatitis B virus gene mutations in liver diseases: a report from New Delhi. PLoS One. 2012;7(6):e39028. https://doi.org/10.1371/journal.pone.0039028.
Maloberti T, De Leo A, Sanza V, Gruppioni E, Altimari A, Riefolo M, Visani M, Malvi D, D'Errico A, Tallini G, Vasuri F, de Biase D. Correlation of molecular alterations with pathological features in hepatocellular carcinoma: Literature review and experience of an Italian center. World J Gastroenterol. 2022;28(25):2854–66.
Mao J, Wang D, Wang Z, et al. Combretastatin A-1 phosphate, a microtubule inhibitor, acts on both hepatocellular carcinoma cells and tumor-associated macrophages by inhibiting the Wnt/β-catenin pathway. Cancer Lett. 2016;380(1):134–43. https://doi.org/10.1016/j.canlet.2016.06.020.
Marchio A, Amougou Atsama M, Béré A, et al. Droplet digital PCR detects high rate of TP53 R249S mutants in cell-free DNA of middle African patients with hepatocellular carcinoma. Clin Exp Med. 2018;18(3):421–31. https://doi.org/10.1007/s10238-018-0502-9.
Matsuo J, Do SH, Yamamoto C, et al. Clustering infection of hepatitis B virus genotype B4 among residents in Vietnam, and its genomic characters both intra- and extra-family. PLoS One. 2017;12(7):e0177248. https://doi.org/10.1371/journal.pone.0177248.
Menard L, Parker PJ, Kermorgant S. Receptor tyrosine kinase c-met controls the cytoskeleton from different endosomes via different pathways. Nat Commun. 2014;5:3907.
Meng W, Chen T. Association between the HGF/c-MET signaling pathway and tumorigenesis, progression and prognosis of hepatocellular carcinoma (Review). Oncol Rep. 2021;46(3):191.
Merle P, Trepo C. Molecular mechanisms underlying hepatocellular carcinoma. Viruses. 2009;1(3):852–72. https://doi.org/10.3390/v1030852.
Michelotti A, de Scordilli M, Palmero L, Guardascione M, Masala M, Roncato R, Foltran L, Ongaro E, Puglisi F. NAFLD-related hepatocarcinoma: the malignant side of metabolic syndrome. Cells. 2021;10(8):2034.
Min P, Li W, Zeng D, et al. A single nucleotide variant in microRNA-1269a promotes the occurrence and process of hepatocellular carcinoma by targeting to oncogenes SPATS2L and LRP6. Bull Cancer. 2017;104(4):311–20. https://doi.org/10.1016/j.bulcan.2016.11.021.
Minouchi K, Kaneko S, Kobayashi K. Mutation of p53 gene in regenerative nodules in cirrhotic liver. J Hepatol. 2002;37(2):231–9. https://doi.org/10.1016/s0168-8278(02)00144-7.
Miura M, Maekawa S, Kadokura M, et al. Analysis of viral amino acids sequences and the IL28B SNP influencing the development of hepatocellular carcinoma in chronic hepatitis C. Hepatol Int. 2012;6(1):386–96. https://doi.org/10.1007/s12072-011-9307-6.
Mohamed WS, Omar MM, Khayri TM, Fakhr IM. Assessment of the proliferative marker Ki-67 and p53 protein expression in HBV- and HCV-related Hepatocellular carcinoma cases in Egypt. Int J Health Sci (Qassim). 2008;2(1):27–34.
Monga SP. B-Catenin signaling and roles in liver homeostasis, injury, and tumorigenesis. Gastroenterology. 2015;148(7):1294–310. https://doi.org/10.1053/j.gastro.2015.02.056.
Mosbeh A, Abdelmaguid W, Ezzat S, Kohla M, Sultan MM, Abdel-Rahman MH. Low frequency of aflatoxin induced TP53 gene codon 249 mutation in hepatocellular carcinoma from Egyptian patients living in the Nile delta region. Asian Pac J Cancer Prev. 2023;24(9):3165–8. https://doi.org/10.31557/APJCP.2023.24.9.3165.

Motalleb G, Gholipour N, Samaei NM. Association of the human astrocyte elevated gene-1 promoter variants with susceptibility to hepatocellular carcinoma. Med Oncol. 2014;31(4):916. https://doi.org/10.1007/s12032-014-0916-5.

Motta BM, Masarone M, Torre P, Persico M. From non-alcoholic steatohepatitis (NASH) to hepatocellular carcinoma (HCC): epidemiology, incidence, predictions, risk factors, and prevention. Cancers (Basel). 2023;15(22):5458.

Munakata T, Nakamura M, Liang Y, Li K, Lemon SM. Down-regulation of the retinoblastoma tumor suppressor by the hepatitis C virus NS5B RNA-dependent RNA polymerase. Proc Natl Acad Sci USA. 2005;102(50):18159–64. https://doi.org/10.1073/pnas.0505605102.

Murata H, Tsuji S, Tsujii M, et al. Promoter hypermethylation silences cyclooxygenase-2 (cox-2) and regulates growth of human hepatocellular carcinoma cells. Lab Investig. 2004;84(8):1050–9. https://doi.org/10.1038/labinvest.3700118.

Nakamura T, Sakai K, Nakamura T, Matsumoto K. Hepatocyte growth factor twenty years on: much more than a growth factor. J Gastroenterol Hepatol. 2011;26(Suppl 1):188–202. https://doi.org/10.1111/j.1440-1746.2010.06549.x.

Nakayama J, Tahara H, Tahara E, et al. Telomerase activation by hTRT in human normal fibroblasts and hepatocellular carcinomas. Nat Genet. 1998;18(1):65–8. https://doi.org/10.1038/ng0198-65.

Nault JC, Calderaro J, Di Tommaso L, et al. Telomerase reverse transcriptase promoter mutation is an early somatic genetic alteration in the transformation of premalignant nodules in hepatocellular carcinoma on cirrhosis. Hepatology. 2014;60(6):1983–92. https://doi.org/10.1002/hep.27372.

Nault JC, Mallet M, Pilati C, et al. High frequency of telomerase reverse-transcriptase promoter somatic mutations in hepatocellular carcinoma and preneoplastic lesions [published correction appears in Nat Commun. 2013;4:2577. Zucman Rossi, Jessica [corrected to Zucman-Rossi, Jessica]]. Nat Commun. 2013;4:2218. https://doi.org/10.1038/ncomms3218.

Nault JC, Villanueva A. Intratumor molecular and phenotypic diversity in hepatocellular carcinoma. Clin Cancer Res. 2015;21(8):1786–8. https://doi.org/10.1158/1078-0432.CCR-14-2602.

Neuveut C, Wei Y, Buendia MA. Mechanisms of HBV-related hepatocarcinogenesis. J Hepatol. 2010;52(4):594–604. https://doi.org/10.1016/j.jhep.2009.10.033.

Nie X, Liu Y, Chen WD, Wang YD. Interplay of miRNAs and canonical Wnt signaling pathway in hepatocellular carcinoma. Front Pharmacol. 2018;9:657. https://doi.org/10.3389/fphar.2018.00657.

Nishimoto A, Miura N, Horikawa I, et al. Functional evidence for a telomerase repressor gene on human chromosome 10p15.1. Oncogene. 2001;20(7):828–35. https://doi.org/10.1038/sj.onc.1204165.

Ogami M, Ikura Y, Nishiguchi S, Kuroki T, Ueda M, Sakurai M. Quantitative analysis and in situ localization of human telomerase RNA in chronic liver disease and hepatocellular carcinoma. Lab Investig. 1999;79(1):15–26.

Ogunwobi OO, Liu C. Hepatocyte growth factor upregulation promotes carcinogenesis and epithelial-mesenchymal transition in hepatocellular carcinoma via Akt and COX-2 pathways. Clin Exp Metastasis. 2011;28(8):721–31. https://doi.org/10.1007/s10585-011-9404-x.

Oh BK, Jo Chae K, Park C, et al. Telomere shortening and telomerase reactivation in dysplastic nodules of human hepatocarcinogenesis. J Hepatol. 2003;39(5):786–92. https://doi.org/10.1016/s0168-8278(03)00395-7.

Okeke E, Davwar PM, Roberts L, Sartorius K, Spearman W, Malu A, Duguru M. Epidemiology of liver cancer in Africa: current and future trends. Semin Liver Dis. 2020;40(2):111–23.

Olusola BA, Faneye AO, Oluwasemowo OO, et al. Profiles of mutations in hepatitis B virus surface and polymerase genes isolated from treatment-naïve Nigerians infected with genotype E. J Med Microbiol. 2021;70(3) https://doi.org/10.1099/jmm.0.001338.

Omar MA, Omran MM, Farid K, Tabll AA, Shahein YE, Emran TM, Petrovic A, Lucic NR, Smolic R, Kovac T, Smolic M. Biomarkers for hepatocellular carcinoma: from origin to clinical diagnosis. Biomedicines. 2023;11(7):1852.

Panigrahi R, Biswas A, Banerjee A, et al. Subgenotype D5, BCP and MHR mutations in hepatic complications among hepatitis B virus infected patients from Orissa. India Infect Genet Evol. 2012;12(8):1622–9. https://doi.org/10.1016/j.meegid.2012.06.015.

Parasramka MA, Maji S, Matsuda A, Yan IK, Patel T. Long non-coding RNAs as novel targets for therapy in hepatocellular carcinoma. Pharmacol Ther. 2016;161:67–78. https://doi.org/10.1016/j.pharmthera.2016.03.004.

Pate KT, Stringari C, Sprowl-Tanio S, et al. Wnt signaling directs a metabolic program of glycolysis and angiogenesis in colon cancer. EMBO J. 2014;33(13):1454–73. https://doi.org/10.15252/embj.201488598.

Patil MA, Lee SA, Macias E, et al. Role of cyclin D1 as a mediator of c-met- and beta-catenin-induced hepatocarcinogenesis. Cancer Res. 2009;69(1):253–61. https://doi.org/10.1158/0008-5472.CAN-08-2514.

Peng SY, Chen WJ, Lai PL, Jeng YM, Sheu JC, Hsu HC. High alpha-fetoprotein level correlates with high stage, early recurrence and poor prognosis of hepatocellular carcinoma: significance of hepatitis virus infection, age, p53 and beta-catenin mutations. Int J Cancer. 2004;112(1):44–50. https://doi.org/10.1002/ijc.20279.

Peng YY, He YH, Chen C, et al. NLRC5 regulates cell proliferation, migration and invasion in hepatocellular carcinoma by targeting the Wnt/β-catenin signaling pathway. Cancer Lett. 2016;376(1):10–21. https://doi.org/10.1016/j.canlet.2016.03.006.

Perugorria MJ, Olaizola P, Labiano I, et al. Wnt-β-catenin signalling in liver development, health and disease. Nat Rev Gastroenterol Hepatol. 2019;16(2):121–36. https://doi.org/10.1038/s41575-018-0075-9.

Petrowsky H, Fritsch R, Guckenberger M, De Oliveira ML, Dutkowski P, Clavien PA. Modern therapeutic approaches for the treatment of malignant liver tumours. Nat Rev Gastroenterol Hepatol. 2020;17(12):755–72.

Piao YF, He M, Shi Y, Tang TY. Relationship between microvessel density and telomerase activity in hepatocellular carcinoma. World J Gastroenterol. 2004;10(14):2147–9. https://doi.org/10.3748/wjg.v10.i14.2147.

Piñero F, Mauro E, Casciato P, Forner A. From evidence to clinical practice: Bridging the gap of new liver cancer therapies in Latin America. Ann Hepatol. 2023;1:101185.

Plentz RR, Caselitz M, Bleck JS, et al. Hepatocellular telomere shortening correlates with chromosomal instability and the development of human hepatoma. Hepatology. 2004;40(1):80–6. https://doi.org/10.1002/hep.20271.

Plentz RR, Schlegelberger B, Flemming P, et al. Telomere shortening correlates with increasing aneuploidy of chromosome 8 in human hepatocellular carcinoma. Hepatology. 2005;42(3):522–6. https://doi.org/10.1002/hep.20847.

Poduri CD. Hepatitis C virus (HCV)--a review molecular biology of the virus, immunodiagnostics, genomic heterogeneity and the role of virus in hepatocellular carcinoma. Indian J Exp Biol. 2003;41(6):549–62.

Poillet-Perez L, Sarry JE, Joffre C. Autophagy is a major metabolic regulator involved in cancer therapy resistance. Cell Rep. 2021;36(7):109528.

Poillet-Perez L, White E. Role of tumor and host autophagy in cancer metabolism. Genes Dev. 2019;33(11–12):610–9.

Pourbagheri-Sigaroodi A, Fallah F, Bashash D, Karimi A. Unleashing the potential of gene signatures as prognostic and predictive tools: A step closer to personalized medicine in hepatocellular carcinoma (HCC). Cell Biochem Funct. 2024;42(1):e3913.

Raihan R, Akbar SMF, Al Mahtab M, et al. Genomic analysis of hepatitis B virus and its association with disease manifestations in Bangladesh. PLoS One. 2019;14(6):e0218744. https://doi.org/10.1371/journal.pone.0218744.

Raj R, Aykun N, Wehrle CJ, Maspero M, Krishnamurthi S, Estfan B, Kamath S, Aucejo F. Immunotherapy for advanced hepatocellular carcinoma-a large tertiary center experience. J Gastrointest Surg. 2023;27(10):2126–34.

Ramakrishna G, Rastogi A, Trehanpati N, Sen B, Khosla R, Sarin SK. From cirrhosis to hepatocellular carcinoma: new molecular insights on inflammation and cellular senescence. Liver Cancer. 2013;2(3–4):367–83. https://doi.org/10.1159/000343852.
Rashed WM, Kandeil MAM, Mahmoud MO, Ezzat S. Hepatocellular Carcinoma (HCC) in Egypt: a comprehensive overview. J Egypt Natl Canc Inst. 2020;32(1):5.
Ren L, Yao Y, Wang Y, Wang S. MiR-505 suppressed the growth of hepatocellular carcinoma cells via targeting IGF-1R. Biosci Rep. 2019a;39(7):BSR20182442. https://doi.org/10.1042/BSR20182442.
Ren W, Wu S, Wu Y, Liu T, Zhao X, Li Y. MicroRNA-196a/−196b regulate the progression of hepatocellular carcinoma through modulating the JAK/STAT pathway via targeting SOCS2. Cell Death Dis. 2019b;10(5):333. https://doi.org/10.1038/s41419-019-1530-4.
Reyes RK, Motiwala T, Jacob ST. Regulation of glucose metabolism in hepatocarcinogenesis by microRNAs. Gene Expr. 2014;16(2):85–92. https://doi.org/10.3727/105221614X13919976902093.
Rich NE. Changing epidemiology of hepatocellular carcinoma within the united states and worldwide. Surg Oncol Clin N Am. 2024;33(1):1–12.
Roberts LO, Jopling CL, Jackson RJ, Willis AE. Viral strategies to subvert the mammalian translation machinery. Prog Mol Biol Transl Sci. 2009;90(C):313–67. https://doi.org/10.1016/S1877-1173(09)90009-6.
Romualdo GR, Heidor R, Bacil GP, Moreno FS, Barbisan LF. Past, present, and future of chemically induced hepatocarcinogenesis rodent models: Perspectives concerning classic and new cancer hallmarks. Life Sci. 2023;330:121994.
Ronan B, Flamand O, Vescovi L, et al. A highly potent and selective Vps34 inhibitor alters vesicle trafficking and autophagy. Nat Chem Biol. 2014;10(12):1013–9. https://doi.org/10.1038/nchembio.1681.
Rosenberg L, Rosenberg D. Human genes and genomes. 1st ed. Lawrenceville, NJ: Scientific Publishing Consultant; 2012.
Rudolph KL. DrPinho RA. In: Arias I, Fausto N, Boyer J, Chisari F, Shafritz D, editors. The liver biology and pathobiology. Philadelphia: Lippincott Williams and Wilkins; 2001. p. 1001–11.
Russell JO, Monga SP. Wnt/β-catenin signaling in liver development, homeostasis, and pathobiology. Annu Rev Pathol. 2018;13:351–78. https://doi.org/10.1146/annurev-pathol-020117-044010.
Russell WE, Kaufmann WK, Sitaric S, Luetteke NC, Lee DC. Liver regeneration and hepatocarcinogenesis in transforming growth factor-alpha-targeted mice. Mol Carcinog. 1996;15(3):183–9. https://doi.org/10.1002/(SICI)1098-2744(199603)15:3<183::AID-MC4>3.0.CO;2-J.
Rusyn I, Lemon SM. Mechanisms of HCV-induced liver cancer: what did we learn from in vitro and animal studies? Cancer Lett. 2014;345(2):210–5. https://doi.org/10.1016/j.canlet.2013.06.028.
Sahin F, Kannangai R, Adegbola O, Wang J, Su G, Torbenson M. mTOR and P70 S6 kinase expression in primary liver neoplasms. Clin Cancer Res. 2004;10(24):8421–5. https://doi.org/10.1158/1078-0432.CCR-04-0941.
Saito Y, Hibino S, Saito H. Alterations of epigenetics and microRNA in hepatocellular carcinoma. Hepatol Res. 2014;44(1):31–42. https://doi.org/10.1111/hepr.12147.
Sakamoto T, Tanaka Y, Orito E, et al. Novel subtypes (subgenotypes) of hepatitis B virus genotypes B and C among chronic liver disease patients in The Philippines. J Gen Virol. 2006;87(Pt 7):1873–82. https://doi.org/10.1099/vir.0.81714-0.
Sandgren EP, Luetteke NC, Palmiter RD, Brinster RL, Lee DC. Overexpression of TGF alpha in transgenic mice: induction of epithelial hyperplasia, pancreatic metaplasia, and carcinoma of the breast. Cell. 1990;61(6):1121–35. https://doi.org/10.1016/0092-8674(90)90075-p.
Santoni-Rugiu E, Nagy P, Jensen MR, Factor VM, Thorgeirsson SS. Evolution of neoplastic development in the liver of transgenic mice co-expressing c-myc and transforming growth factor-alpha. Am J Pathol. 1996;149(2):407–28.
Sargent LM, Zhou X, Keck CL, et al. Nonrandom cytogenetic alterations in hepatocellular carcinoma from transgenic mice overexpressing c-Myc and transforming growth factor-alpha in the liver. Am J Pathol. 1999;154(4):1047–55. https://doi.org/10.1016/s0002-9440(10)65357-6.

Sato M, Kato N, Tateishi R, et al. Impact of PNPLA3 polymorphisms on the development of hepatocellular carcinoma in patients with chronic hepatitis C virus infection. Hepatol Res. 2014;44(10):E137–44. https://doi.org/10.1111/hepr.12258.

Satoh S, Daigo Y, Furukawa Y, et al. AXIN1 mutations in hepatocellular carcinomas, and growth suppression in cancer cells by virus-mediated transfer of AXIN1. Nat Genet. 2000;24(3):245–50. https://doi.org/10.1038/73448.

Schütte K, Schulz C, Link A, Malfertheiner P. Current biomarkers for hepatocellular carcinoma: surveillance, diagnosis and prediction of prognosis. World J Hepatol. 2015;7(2):139–49. https://doi.org/10.4254/wjh.v7.i2.139.

Schwaederlé M, Lazar V, Validire P, et al. VEGF-A expression correlates with TP53 mutations in non-small cell lung Cancer: implications for Antiangiogenesis therapy. Cancer Res. 2015;75(7):1187–90. https://doi.org/10.1158/0008-5472.CAN-14-2305.

Sghaier I, Mouelhi L, Rabia NA, et al. Genetic variants in IL-6 and IL-10 genes and susceptibility to hepatocellular carcinoma in HCV infected patients. Cytokine. 2017;89:62–7. https://doi.org/10.1016/j.cyto.2016.10.004.

Shadi Y, Heshmati B, Poorolajal J. Interaction between hepatitis B, hepatitis C and smoking in the development of hepatocellular carcinoma: a systematic review and meta-analysis. J Public Health (Oxf). 2024;46(1):51–60.

Shi YZ, Hui AM, Takayama T, Li X, Cui X, Makuuchi M. Reduced p21(WAF1/CIP1) protein expression is predominantly related to altered p53 in hepatocellular carcinomas. Br J Cancer. 2000;83(1):50–5. https://doi.org/10.1054/bjoc.2000.1310.

Shimojima M, Komine F, Hisatomi H, Shimizu T, Moriyama M, Arakawa Y. Detection of telomerase activity, telomerase RNA component, and telomerase reverse transcriptase in human hepatocellular carcinoma. Hepatol Res. 2004;29(1):31–8. https://doi.org/10.1016/j.hepres.2004.02.005.

Shivlata L, Pacholi S, Chouksey VK, Barde PV. Molecular characterization of hepatitis B virus reveals circulation of multiple subgenotypes of genotype D with clinically important mutations in central India. Indian J Med Microbiol. 2021;39(1):67–72. https://doi.org/10.1016/j.ijmmb.2021.01.002.

Shrivastava S, Steele R, Ray R, Ray RB. MicroRNAs: role in hepatitis C virus pathogenesis. Genes Dis. 2015;2(1):35–45. https://doi.org/10.1016/j.gendis.2015.01.001.

Shtutman M, Zhurinsky J, Simcha I, et al. The cyclin D1 gene is a target of the beta-catenin/LEF-1 pathway. Proc Natl Acad Sci USA. 1999;96(10):5522–7. https://doi.org/10.1073/pnas.96.10.5522.

Sia D, Villanueva A. Signaling pathways in hepatocellular carcinoma. Oncology. 2011;81(Suppl 1):18–23. https://doi.org/10.1159/000333254.

Singal AG, Kanwal F, Llovet JM. Global trends in hepatocellular carcinoma epidemiology: implications for screening, prevention and therapy. Nat Rev Clin Oncol. 2023;20(12):864–84.

Song J, Gao L, Yang G, Tang S, Xie H, Wang Y, Wang J, Zhang Y, Jin J, Gou Y, Yang Z, Chen Z, Wu K, Liu J, Fan D. MiR-199a regulates cell proliferation and survival by targeting FZD7. PLoS One. 2014;9(10):e110074. https://doi.org/10.1371/journal.pone.0110074.

Song J, Xie C, Jiang L, et al. Transcription factor AP-4 promotes tumorigenic capability and activates the Wnt/β-catenin pathway in hepatocellular carcinoma. Theranostics. 2018;8(13):3571–83. https://doi.org/10.7150/thno.25194.

Song LH, Duy DN, Binh VQ, Luty AJ, Kremsner PG, Bock CT. Low frequency of mutations in the X gene, core promoter and precore region of hepatitis B virus infected Vietnamese. J Viral Hepat. 2005;12(2):160–7. https://doi.org/10.1111/j.1365-2893.2005.00560.x.

Soussi T. p53 alterations in human cancer: more questions than answers. Oncogene. 2007;26(15):2145–56. https://doi.org/10.1038/sj.onc.1210280.

Stemmler MP. Cadherins in development and cancer. Mol BioSyst. 2008;4(8):835–50. https://doi.org/10.1039/b719215k.

Street A, Macdonald A, McCormick C, Harris M. Hepatitis C virus NS5A-mediated activation of phosphoinositide 3-kinase results in stabilization of cellular beta-catenin and stimulation of beta-catenin-responsive transcription. J Virol. 2005;79(8):5006–16. https://doi.org/10.1128/JVI.79.8.5006-5016.2005.

Sudo T, Utsunomiya T, Mimori K, et al. Clinicopathological significance of EZH2 mRNA expression in patients with hepatocellular carcinoma. Br J Cancer. 2005;92(9):1754–8. https://doi.org/10.1038/sj.bjc.6602531.

Sun SN, Hu S, Shang YP, et al. Relevance function of microRNA-708 in the pathogenesis of cancer. Cell Signal. 2019;63:109390. https://doi.org/10.1016/j.cellsig.2019.109390.

Sung WK, Zheng H, Li S, et al. Genome-wide survey of recurrent HBV integration in hepatocellular carcinoma. Nat Genet. 2012;44(7):765–9. https://doi.org/10.1038/ng.2295.

Szturz P, Raymond E, Abitbol C, Albert S, de Gramont A, Faivre S. Understanding c-MET signalling in squamous cell carcinoma of the head & neck. Crit Rev Oncol Hematol. 2017;111:39–51. https://doi.org/10.1016/j.critrevonc.2017.01.004.

Tacke RS, Tosello-Trampont A, Nguyen V, Mullins DW, Hahn YS. Extracellular hepatitis C virus core protein activates STAT3 in human monocytes/macrophages/dendritic cells via an IL-6 autocrine pathway. J Biol Chem. 2011;286(12):10847–55. https://doi.org/10.1074/jbc.M110.217653.

Tahtouh R, Azzi AS, Alaaeddine N, et al. Telomerase inhibition decreases alpha-fetoprotein expression and secretion by hepatocellular carcinoma cell lines: in vitro and in vivo study. PLoS One. 2015;10(3):e0119512. https://doi.org/10.1371/journal.pone.0119512.

Takai A, Dang HT, Wang XW. Identification of drivers from cancer genome diversity in hepatocellular carcinoma. Int J Mol Sci. 2014;15(6):11142–60. https://doi.org/10.3390/ijms150611142.

Takami T, Kaposi-Novak P, Uchida K, et al. Loss of hepatocyte growth factor/c-met signaling pathway accelerates early stages of N-nitrosodiethylamine induced hepatocarcinogenesis. Cancer Res. 2007;67(20):9844–51. https://doi.org/10.1158/0008-5472.CAN-07-1905.

Takeo S, Arai H, Kusano N, et al. Examination of oncogene amplification by genomic DNA microarray in hepatocellular carcinomas: comparison with comparative genomic hybridization analysis. Cancer Genet Cytogenet. 2001;130(2):127–32. https://doi.org/10.1016/s0165-4608(01)00479-4.

Tang H, Li RP, Liang P, Zhou YL, Wang GW. miR-125a inhibits the migration and invasion of liver cancer cells via suppression of the PI3K/AKT/mTOR signaling pathway. Oncol Lett. 2015;10(2):681–6. https://doi.org/10.3892/ol.2015.3264.

Tannapfel A, Buss C, Weinans L, et al. INK 4A-ARF alterations and p53 mutations in hepatocellular carcinomas. Oncogene. 2001;20:7104–9.

Thi Cam Huong N, Trung NQ, Luong BA, et al. Mutations in the HBV PreS/S gene related to hepatocellular carcinoma in Vietnamese chronic HBV-infected patients. PLoS One. 2022;17(4):e0266134. https://doi.org/10.1371/journal.pone.0266134.

Thiery JP, Acloque H, Huang RY, Nieto MA. Epithelial-mesenchymal transitions in development and disease. Cell. 2009;139(5):871–90. https://doi.org/10.1016/j.cell.2009.11.007.

Thorgeirsson SS, Grisham JW. Molecular pathogenesis of human hepatocellular carcinoma. Nat Genet. 2002;31(4):339–46. https://doi.org/10.1038/ng0802-339.

Thorpe LM, Yuzugullu H, Zhao JJ. PI3K in cancer: divergent roles of isoforms, modes of activation and therapeutic targeting. Nat Rev Cancer. 2015;15(1):7–24. https://doi.org/10.1038/nrc3860.

Tian Y, Yang W, Song J, Wu Y, Ni B. Hepatitis B virus X protein-induced aberrant epigenetic modifications contributing to human hepatocellular carcinoma pathogenesis. Mol Cell Biol. 2013;33(15):2810–6. https://doi.org/10.1128/MCB.00205-13.

Tischoff I, Tannapfe A. DNA methylation in hepatocellular carcinoma. World J Gastroenterol. 2008;14(11):1741–8. https://doi.org/10.3748/wjg.14.1741.

Tornesello ML, Buonaguro L, Izzo F, Buonaguro FM. Molecular alterations in hepatocellular carcinoma associated with hepatitis B and hepatitis C infections. Oncotarget. 2016;7(18):25087–102. https://doi.org/10.18632/oncotarget.7837.

Torrens L, Puigvehí M, Torres-Martín M, et al. Hepatocellular carcinoma in Mongolia delineates unique molecular traits and a mutational signature associated with environmental agents. Clin Cancer Res. 2022;28(20):4509–20. https://doi.org/10.1158/1078-0432.CCR-22-0632.

Toyama T, Lee HC, Koga H, Wands JR, Kim M. Noncanonical Wnt11 inhibits hepatocellular carcinoma cell proliferation and migration. Mol Cancer Res. 2010;8(2):254–65. https://doi.org/10.1158/1541-7786.MCR-09-0238.

Truong BX, Seo Y, Yano Y, et al. Genotype and variations in core promoter and pre-core regions are related to progression of disease in HBV-infected patients from Northern Vietnam. Int J Mol Med. 2007;19(2):293–9.

Trusolino L, Bertotti A, Comoglio PM. MET signalling: principles and functions in development, organ regeneration and cancer. Nat Rev Mol Cell Biol. 2010;11(12):834–48. https://doi.org/10.1038/nrm3012.

Tsai WC, Hsu SD, Hsu CS, et al. MicroRNA-122 plays a critical role in liver homeostasis and hepatocarcinogenesis. J Clin Invest. 2012;122(8):2884–97. https://doi.org/10.1172/JCI63455.

Tuteja A, Siddiqui AB, Madan K, et al. Mutation profiling of the hepatitis B virus strains circulating in North Indian population. PLoS One. 2014;9(3):e91150. https://doi.org/10.1371/journal.pone.0091150.

Uma Devi P. Basics of carcinogenesis. Health Adm. 1989;17:16–24.

Umemura A, Park EJ, Taniguchi K, et al. Liver damage, inflammation, and enhanced tumorigenesis after persistent mTORC1 inhibition. Cell Metab. 2014;20(1):133–44. https://doi.org/10.1016/j.cmet.2014.05.001.

Valenti L, Al-Serri A, Daly AK, et al. Homozygosity for the patatin-like phospholipase-3/adiponutrin I148M polymorphism influences liver fibrosis in patients with nonalcoholic fatty liver disease. Hepatology. 2010;51(4):1209–17. https://doi.org/10.1002/hep.23622.

Vanhaesebroeck B, Guillermet-Guibert J, Graupera M, Bilanges B. The emerging mechanisms of isoform-specific PI3K signalling. Nat Rev Mol Cell Biol. 2010;11(5):329–41. https://doi.org/10.1038/nrm2882.

Vasudevan KM, Barbie DA, Davies MA, et al. AKT-independent signaling downstream of oncogenic PIK3CA mutations in human cancer. Cancer Cell. 2009;16(1):21–32. https://doi.org/10.1016/j.ccr.2009.04.012.

Vivekanandan P, Torbenson M, Ramakrishna B. Hepatitis B virus-associated hepatocellular carcinoma from India: role of viral genotype and mutations in CTNNB1 (beta-catenin) and TP53 genes. J Gastrointest Cancer. 2011;42(1):20–5. https://doi.org/10.1007/s12029-010-9222-4.

Waly Raphael S, Yangde Z, Yuxiang C. Hepatocellular carcinoma: focus on different aspects of management. ISRN Oncol. 2012;2012:421673. https://doi.org/10.5402/2012/421673.

Wang B, Chen H, Zhang C, et al. Effects of hsa_circRBM23 on Hepatocellular carcinoma cell viability and migration as produced by regulating miR-138 expression. Cancer Biother Radiopharm. 2018a;33(5):194–202. https://doi.org/10.1089/cbr.2017.2424.

Wang M, Yang Y, Yang J, Yang J, Han S. circ_KIAA1429 accelerates hepatocellular carcinoma advancement through the mechanism of m6A-YTHDF3-Zeb1. Life Sci. 2020a;257:118082. https://doi.org/10.1016/j.lfs.2020.118082.

Wang P, Guo QS, Wang ZW, Qian HX. HBx induces HepG-2 cells autophagy through PI3K/Akt-mTOR pathway. Mol Cell Biochem. 2013;372(1–2):161–8. https://doi.org/10.1007/s11010-012-1457-x.

Wang Q, Xu L, Wu Q, Zhang M, Zhang J. Association between the risk of hepatitis virus-related hepatocellular carcinoma and EGF polymorphism: a PRISMA-compliant updated meta-analysis. Medicine (Baltimore). 2022;101(42):e31280. https://doi.org/10.1097/MD.0000000000031280.

Wang Q, Yu WN, Chen X, et al. Spontaneous Hepatocellular carcinoma after the combined deletion of Akt isoforms. Cancer Cell. 2016;29(4):523–35. https://doi.org/10.1016/j.ccell.2016.02.008.

Wang R, Yu Z, Chen F, et al. miR-300 regulates the epithelial-mesenchymal transition and invasion of hepatocellular carcinoma by targeting the FAK/PI3K/AKT signaling pathway. Biomed Pharmacother. 2018b;103:1632–42. https://doi.org/10.1016/j.biopha.2018.03.005.

Wang W, Li Y, Li X, et al. Circular RNA circ-FOXP1 induced by SOX9 promotes hepatocellular carcinoma progression via sponging miR-875-3p and miR-421. Biomed Pharmacother. 2020b;121:109517. https://doi.org/10.1016/j.biopha.2019.109517.

Wang W, Pan Q, Fuhler GM, Smits R, Peppelenbosch MP. Action and function of Wnt/β-catenin signaling in the progression from chronic hepatitis C to hepatocellular carcinoma [published correction appears in J Gastroenterol. 2017 Oct 11]. J Gastroenterol. 2017;52(4):419–31. https://doi.org/10.1007/s00535-016-1299-5.

Wei S, Fan Q, Yang L, et al. Promotion of glycolysis by HOTAIR through GLUT1 upregulation via mTOR signaling. Oncol Rep. 2017;38(3):1902–8. https://doi.org/10.3892/or.2017.5840.
Weidle UH, Schmid D, Birzele F, Brinkmann U. MicroRNAs involved in metastasis of Hepatocellular carcinoma: target candidates, functionality and efficacy in animal models and prognostic relevance. Cancer Genomics Proteomics. 2020;17(1):1–21. https://doi.org/10.21873/cgp.20163.
Wheler JJ, Janku F, Naing A, et al. TP53 alterations correlate with response to VEGF/VEGFR inhibitors: implications for targeted therapeutics. Mol Cancer Ther. 2016;15(10):2475–85. https://doi.org/10.1158/1535-7163.MCT-16-0196.
Wiemann SU, Satyanarayana A, Tsahuridu M, et al. Hepatocyte telomere shortening and senescence are general markers of human liver cirrhosis. FASEB J. 2002;16(9):935–42. https://doi.org/10.1096/fj.01-0977com.
Wogan GN, Kensler TW, Groopman JD. Present and future directions of translational research on aflatoxin and hepatocellular carcinoma. A review. Food Addit Contam Part A Chem Anal Control Expo Risk Assess. 2012;29(2):249–57.
Wong CC, Wong CM, Tung EK, et al. The microRNA miR-139 suppresses metastasis and progression of hepatocellular carcinoma by down-regulating Rho-kinase 2. Gastroenterology. 2011;140(1):322–31. https://doi.org/10.1053/j.gastro.2010.10.006.
Wu J, Jiang ZM, Xie Y, et al. miR-218 suppresses the growth of hepatocellular carcinoma by inhibiting the expression of proto-oncogene Bmi-1. J BUON. 2018;23(3):604–10.
Wu J, Liu C, Wang F. Disparities in hepatocellular carcinoma survival by insurance status: a population-based study in China. Front Public Health. 2021;9:742355.
Wu J, Liu S, Xiang Y, Qu X, Xie Y, Zhang X. Bioinformatic analysis of circular RNA-associated ceRNA network associated with hepatocellular carcinoma. Biomed Res Int. 2019;2019:8308694. https://doi.org/10.1155/2019/8308694.
Wu Y, Zhang Y, Qin X, Geng H, Zuo D, Zhao Q. PI3K/AKT/mTOR pathway-related long non-coding RNAs: roles and mechanisms in hepatocellular carcinoma. Pharmacol Res. 2020;160:105195. https://doi.org/10.1016/j.phrs.2020.105195.
Xie B, Xing R, Chen P, et al. Down-regulation of c-Met expression inhibits human HCC cells growth and invasion by RNA interference. J Surg Res. 2010;162(2):231–8. https://doi.org/10.1016/j.jss.2009.04.030.
Xiong DD, Feng ZB, Lai ZF, Qin Y, Liu LM, Fu HX, He RQ, Wu HY, Dang YW, Chen G, Luo DZ. High throughput circRNA sequencing analysis reveals novel insights into the mechanism of nitidine chloride against hepatocellular carcinoma. Cell Death Dis. 2019;10(9):658. https://doi.org/10.1038/s41419-019-1890-9.
Xu Q, Dou C, Liu X, et al. Corrigendum to "Oviductus ranae protein hydrolysate (ORPH) inhibits the growth, metastasis and glycolysis of HCC by targeting miR-491-5p/PKM2 axis" [Biomed. Pharmacother. 107 (2018) 1692–1704]. Biomed Pharmacother. 2023;157:113979. https://doi.org/10.1016/j.biopha.2022.113979.
Xu X, Sakon M, Nagano H, et al. Akt2 expression correlates with prognosis of human hepatocellular carcinoma. Oncol Rep. 2004;11(1):25–32.
Xu Z, Xu M, Liu P, et al. The mTORC2-Akt1 Cascade is crucial for c-Myc to promote hepatocarcinogenesis in mice and humans. Hepatology. 2019;70(5):1600–13. https://doi.org/10.1002/hep.30697.
Xue J, Ni H, Wang F, Xu K, Niu M. Advances in locoregional therapy for hepatocellular carcinoma combined with immunotherapy and targeted therapy. J Interv Med. 2021;4(3):105–13.
Yang F, Lv LZ, Cai QC, Jiang Y. Potential roles of EZH2, Bmi-1 and miR-203 in cell proliferation and invasion in hepatocellular carcinoma cell line Hep3B. World J Gastroenterol. 2015;21(47):13268–76. https://doi.org/10.3748/wjg.v21.i47.13268.
Yang G, Xu Q, Wan Y, Zhang L, Wang L, Meng F. Circ-CSPP1 knockdown suppresses hepatocellular carcinoma progression through miR-493-5p releasing-mediated HMGB1 downregulation. Cell Signal. 2021;86:110065. https://doi.org/10.1016/j.cellsig.2021.110065.

Yang JD, Hainaut P, Gores GJ, Amadou A, Plymoth A, Roberts LR. A global view of hepatocellular carcinoma: trends, risk, prevention and management. Nat Rev Gastroenterol Hepatol. 2019;16(10):589–604.

Yang L, Tan W, Wei Y, et al. CircLIFR suppresses hepatocellular carcinoma progression by sponging miR-624-5p and inactivating the GSK-3β/β-catenin signaling pathway. Cell Death Dis. 2022;13(5):464. https://doi.org/10.1038/s41419-022-04887-6.

Yao Z, Xu R, Yuan L, Xu M, Zhuang H, Li Y, Zhang Y, Lin N. Circ_0001955 facilitates hepatocellular carcinoma (HCC) tumorigenesis by sponging miR-516a-5p to release TRAF6 and MAPK11. Cell Death Dis. 2019;10(12):945. https://doi.org/10.1038/s41419-019-2176-y.

Yepmo M, Potier JB, Pinget M, Grabarz A, Bouzakri K, Dumond BA. Discussing the role of circular RNA in the pathogenesis of non-alcoholic fatty liver disease and its complications. Front Endocrinol (Lausanne). 2022;13:1035159. https://doi.org/10.3389/fendo.2022.1035159.

Youssef N, Paradis V, Ferlicot S, Bedossa P. In situ detection of telomerase enzymatic activity in human hepatocellular carcinogenesis. J Pathol. 2001;194(4):459–65. https://doi.org/10.1002/path.901.

Yu GY, He G, Li CY, et al. Hepatic expression of HCV RNA-dependent RNA polymerase triggers innate immune signaling and cytokine production. Mol Cell. 2012;48(2):313–21. https://doi.org/10.1016/j.molcel.2012.07.032.

Yu J, Chen GG, Lai PBS. Targeting hepatocyte growth factor/c-mesenchymal-epithelial transition factor axis in hepatocellular carcinoma: rationale and therapeutic strategies. Med Res Rev. 2021;41(1):507–24. https://doi.org/10.1002/med.21738.

Yu J, Zhang HY, Ma ZZ, Lu W, Wang YF, Zhu JD. Methylation profiling of twenty four genes and the concordant methylation behaviours of nineteen genes that may contribute to hepatocellular carcinogenesis. Cell Res. 2003;13(5):319–33. https://doi.org/10.1038/sj.cr.7290177.

Yun C, Um HR, Jin YH, et al. NF-kappaB activation by hepatitis B virus X (HBx) protein shifts the cellular fate toward survival. Cancer Lett. 2002;184(1):97–104. https://doi.org/10.1016/s0304-3835(02)00187-8.

Yuzugullu H, Benhaj K, Ozturk N, et al. Canonical Wnt signaling is antagonized by noncanonical Wnt5a in hepatocellular carcinoma cells. Mol Cancer. 2009;8:90. https://doi.org/10.1186/1476-4598-8-90.

Zekri AR, Bahnassy AA, Madbouly MS, Asaad NY, El-Shehaby AM, Alam El Din HM. p53 mutation in HCV-genotype-4 associated hepatocellular carcinoma in Egyptian patients. J Egypt Natl Canc Inst. 2006;18(1):17–29.

Zeng C, Yuan G, Hu Y, et al. Repressing phosphatidylinositol-4,5-bisphosphate 3-kinase catalytic subunit gamma by microRNA-142-3p restrains the progression of hepatocellular carcinoma. Bioengineered. 2022;13(1):1491–506. https://doi.org/10.1080/21655979.2021.2020549.

Zeng XC, Liu FQ, Yan R, et al. Downregulation of miR-610 promotes proliferation and tumorigenicity and activates Wnt/β-catenin signaling in human hepatocellular carcinoma. Mol Cancer. 2014;13:261. https://doi.org/10.1186/1476-4598-13-261.

Zhang H, Yu C, Chen M, et al. miR-522 contributes to cell proliferation of hepatocellular carcinoma by targeting DKK1 and SFRP2. Tumour Biol. 2016;37(8):11321–9. https://doi.org/10.1007/s13277-016-4995-0.

Zhang HF, Wang YC, Han YD. MicroRNA-34a inhibits liver cancer cell growth by reprogramming glucose metabolism. Mol Med Rep. 2018;17(3):4483–9. https://doi.org/10.3892/mmr.2018.8399.

Zhang T, Jing B, Bai Y, Zhang Y, Yu H. Circular RNA circTMEM45A acts as the sponge of MicroRNA-665 to promote Hepatocellular carcinoma progression. Mol Ther Nucleic Acids. 2020;22:285–97. https://doi.org/10.1016/j.omtn.2020.08.011.

Zhang X, Ding HG. Key role of hepatitis B virus mutation in chronic hepatitis B development to hepatocellular carcinoma. World J Hepatol. 2015;7(9):1282–6. https://doi.org/10.4254/wjh.v7.i9.1282.

Zhang T, Zhang J, You X, et al. Hepatitis B virus X protein modulates oncogene yes-associated protein by CREB to promote growth of hepatoma cells. Hepatology. 2012;56(6):2051–9. https://doi.org/10.1002/hep.25899.

Zhang Y, Zheng D, Xiong Y, et al. miR-202 suppresses cell proliferation in human hepatocellular carcinoma by downregulating LRP6 post-transcriptionally. FEBS Lett. 2014;588(10):1913–20. https://doi.org/10.1016/j.febslet.2014.03.030.

Zhou HC, Fang JH, Shang LR, et al. MicroRNAs miR-125b and miR-100 suppress metastasis of hepatocellular carcinoma by disrupting the formation of vessels that encapsulate tumour clusters. J Pathol. 2016;240(4):450–60. https://doi.org/10.1002/path.4804.

Zhu Z, Wilson AT, Gopalakrishna K, Brown KE, Luxon BA, Schmidt WN. Hepatitis C virus core protein enhances Telomerase activity in Huh7 cells. J Med Virol. 2010;82(2):239–48. https://doi.org/10.1002/jmv.21644.

Zucman-Rossi J, Villanueva A, Nault JC, Llovet JM. Genetic landscape and biomarkers of hepatocellular carcinoma. Gastroenterology. 2015;149(5):1226–1239.e4.

Environmental Carcinogens for Development of Hepatocellular Carcinoma

4

Amal Saad-Hussein and Haidi Karam-AllahRamadan

Abstract

Hepatocellular carcinoma (HCC) is one of the common cancers causing death worldwide, especially in low/middle-income countries. There are many environmental exposures to chemical and biological risky factors to increase the risk for the development of HCC. Environmental and occupational exposures to carcinogenic chemical pollutants in the workplaces and during unhealthy domestic life are traging factors for increasing the risk of HCC development. Also, exposure to biological factors; such as infection with viral hepatitis B or C, exposure to the carcinogenic fungal metabolites, and other biological toxins are well documented to cause increase the risk of development of HCC.

This chapter discusses the chemical and biological carcinogens risky for increasing HCC cases, and the impacts of ecological factors in low/middle-income countries that may increase the risk of HCC development.

Keywords

Hepatocellular carcinoma · Liver cirrhosis · Environmental chemical pollutants · Biological carcinogens · Hepatoma · Hepatocellular carcinoma · Carcinogenic agents · Low/middle-income countries · Climate changes

A. Saad-Hussein (✉)
Department of Environmental and Occupational Medicine, Environment and Climate Change Research Institute, National Research Centre, Giza, Egypt
e-mail: al.hussein@nrc.sci.eg

H. Karam-AllahRamadan
Department of Tropical Medicine and Gastroenterology, Faculty of Medicine, Assiut University, Asyut, Egypt
e-mail: haidikaram@aun.edu.eg

R. Elwakil et al. (eds.), *Approach to Hepatocellular Carcinoma (HCC) Management in Low/Middle-Income Countries*,
https://doi.org/10.1007/978-981-96-3894-9_4

Abbreviations

A. flavus	*Aspergillus flavus*
A. niger	*Aspergillus niger*
AF-alb	Aflatoxin-albumin adducts
AFB1	Aflatoxin B1
AFB1-FABY	AFB1-formamidopyrimidine adduct
AFB1-N7-Gua	AFB1-8,9 dihydro8-(N7 guanyl)-9-hydroxy
AFM1	Aflatoxin M1
AFP	Alpha-fetoprotein
AFs	Aflatoxins
AFU	Alpha-L-fucosidase
As	Arsenic
BaP	benzo(a)pyrene
BPA	Bisphenol A
BPDE	benzo(a)pyrene -diol epoxide
CCE	Cactus cladode extract
Cd	Cadmium
CSC	Cancer stem cell
Cu	Copper
CYN	cyanotoxin
EB	electron beam
EPA	Environmental Protective Agency
EU	European Union
FDA	Food and Drug Administration
G	guanine
GR	Glutathione reductase
GRAS	Generally Recognized As Safe
GSTP	Glutathione-S-transferase Pi
HABs	harmful algal blooms
HBV	Hepatitis B virus
HCC	Hepatocellular carcinoma
HCHO	Formaldehyde
HCV	Hepatitis C virus
hCYP1A2	human cytochrome-P450 1A2
IARC	International Agency for Research on Cancer
L	leucine
LD50	Lethal dose 50
MC	Microcystins
MDA	Malondialdehyde
MENA	Middle East and North Africa region
NAFLD	Nonalcoholic fatty liver disease
Ni	Nickel

NODS	nodularins
PAHs	Polycyclic aromatic hydrocarbons
PL	pulsed light
PP	protein phosphatase
ppb	Parts per billion
PSII	Photosystem II
PVC	Polymer polyvinyl chloride
R	arginine
RNS	Reactive nitrogen species
ROS	Reactive oxygen species
Se	selenium
SOD	superoxide dismutase
STXs	saxitoxins
T	thymine
TDP	Total Dissolved Phosphorus
TNFAIP8	TNF-α-Induced Protein 8
TNFα	Tumor necrosis factor alpha
UHT	Ultra-high temperature
UV	ultraviolet
VCM	Vinyl chloride monomer
WHO	World health organization
WSP	water safety plans
Y	tyrosine
Zn	Zinc

4.1 Introduction

Primary liver cancer; mainly hepatocellular carcinoma (HCC), is the third cancer causing death in the world (Cicalese et al. 2017a). There are many risky exposures that increase the risk for the development of HCC. Occupational exposure to environmental carcinogenic toxins in the workplaces is still remarkable risk factor for HCC worldwide, especially in developing countries due to unavailability of expensive controlling exposure programs (Uccello et al. 2012). Environmental exposure to carcinogenic pollutants during the domestic life, such as tobacco smoking, alcohol consumption, pesticides, un-complete combustion of fuels, daily usage of microplastics sources, and so on, are increasing the risk of development of HCC.

There are also many biological risk factors for induction of HCC, including infections with hepatic viruses (hepatitis B or hepatitis C), exposure to biological metabolites of fungi; such as aflatoxin, are well-documented risk factors that increase the incidence of hepatic cancers (Su et al. 2007).

This chapter discusses the chemical and biological carcinogens risk for increasing HCC cases, and the impacts of ecological factors in low/middle-income countries that may increase the risk of HCC development.

4.2 Environmental Chemical Pollutants Causing HCC

The liver is the main organ involved in metabolism and in toxicokinetics of chemicals. For that, it is considered to be a target organ of the toxicity of these chemicals. Adverse effects of chemical exposure may lead to hepatotoxicity, cholestatic liver injury, fatty liver, cirrhosis, and cancers, including HCC (Rapisarda et al. 2016).

There are great evidences about the association between environmental exposure to hazardous air pollutants and the increase in HCC cases in certain counties (Cicalese et al. 2017a). Occupational exposure to chemicals is another risk factor for HCC, even if this relationship is not always clear (Rapisarda et al. 2016), because HCC is a multifactorial disease (Cicalese et al. 2017a).

4.2.1 Mechanism of Action

Liver plays an essential role in the metabolism of chemical pollutants, being rich in high blood supply and handling many metabolic and excretory processes, this makes the liver sensitive to hepatotoxic chemicals.

Environmental chemical pollutants; such as pesticides, may cause HCC through several mechanisms; as pesticides are metabolized in the liver, causing ultrastructural, metabolic, and mitochondrial damage in liver (VoPham et al. 2017). Experimentally, Ji et al. (2016) demonstrated that oral gavage and intraperitoneal injection with benzo(a)pyrene (BaP) resulted in dose-dependent manner of the depletion of antioxidants and Krebs cycle's enzymes, and enhancement of the lipid peroxidation in the mitochondria of different organs; including the liver. Mitochondrial damage is crucial in the mechanism of cytotoxicity (Ji et al. 2016). Telomeres are DNA–protein structures that protect chromosome ends from degradation and fusion, shortened telomere length caused mainly by oxidative stress, and was found to be significantly dose-response on cumulative exposure to pollutants; such as Coke Oven Emissions, and was associate with development of cancers (Wang et al. 2019).

Occupational exposure to pesticides was found to be a cause of significant DNA damage, this may be an initiator to the process of chemical carcinogenesis (Kapka-Skrzypczak et al. 2011). This could be through cell adhesion alterations, genotoxicity, cytotoxicity, tumor promotion, immunotoxicity, and hormonal actions (VoPham et al. 2017). Moreover, exposure to environmental chemical pollutants can lead to damage of the mitochondrial, in addition to oxidative stress and endoplasmic reticulum stress, that will lead to cellular dysfunction (Li et al. 2023).

Formaldehyde (HCHO) proved to be associated with DNA reactivity, gene mutation, chromosomal breakages, aneuploidy, epigenetic effects, glutathione depletion, oxidative stress, and cytotoxicity-induced cellular proliferation (Lu et al. 2008).

The role of multidrug resistance-associated protein 2 (ABCC2) and ATP-binding cassette transporters breast cancer resistance protein (ABCG2) in hepatobiliary elimination of toxins and their metabolites is well proved. These transporters may have a protective function against carcinogenic chemical pollutants; such as BaP in human, due to its important role for the hepatobiliary elimination of BaP via bile (Kranz et al. 2014). The detoxification gene Glutathione-S-transferase Pi (*GSTP*) found to have an important detoxification role in BaP, therefore, *GSTP* will has a potential protective role against induction of HCC due to BaP exposures (Tian et al. 2016).

Reduction of excretion of chemical pollutants increases the susceptibility to these pollutants to induce carcinogenesis. Therefore, bioaccumulation of heavy metals in the human body due to the long biological half-life of it could increase its hazardous effects, e.g., Cd has biological half-life between 10 and 33 years (Clemens et al. 2013). That biological half-life will lead to an increase in the burden of heavy time over time. After Cd; as an example, will be absorbed, it will be bind with albumin, and then distributed through blood to the whole body (Vacchi-Suzzi et al. 2016).

Niture and his colleagues (2023) proved that even low concentration of Cd can play a significant role in the development of nonalcoholic fatty liver disease (NAFLD), that may promote liver disease or HCC through induction of reactive oxygen species (ROS) and cell proliferation in HCC cells. They found that exposure to low concentrations of Cd modulates AKT/mTOR signaling, in addition to the increase in phosphorylation of AKT-S473 and mTOR-S4448 in HCC cells and increased notch ligand Jagged1 expression, NTM of cleaved Notch1, Notch2, and Notch3, and Notch downstream Hes1 protein expression on exposure to Cd for 24–72 hours or for 50 days (Niture et al. 2023). AKT/mTOR is known to be involved in HCC proliferation (Ferrín et al. 2020), and Notch signaling is constitutively active in HCC (Huang et al. 2019).

Niture et al. (2023) also found that acute and chronic exposure to low concentration of Cd can modulate tumor signaling in HCC. They also found that Cd induced expression of the pro-inflammatory cytokine TNFα and the TNFα downstream oncogene TNFAIP8 as well as cancer stem cells (CSC) marker Nanog (Niture et al. 2023). The expression of TNFAIP8 increases HCC cell proliferation, survival, and drug resistance (Niture et al. 2020), and therefore Niture et al. (2023) suggested that even a low concentration of Cd can trigger oncogenic signaling in HCC.

The incidence of development of HCC proved to be increased due to occupational exposure to hepatocellular carcinogenic chemical pollutants if the workers have predisposing liver viral affection. Saad et al. (2004) found that there are synergistic effects of hepatitis C (HCV) and smoking with the occupational exposure to thermal degradation of polyurethane. They found that alpha-fetoprotein (AFP), tumor biomarker of hepatic cancers, was found to significantly higher among the smoker workers with positive HCV compared to the negative HCV workers (Saad et al. 2004).

4.2.2 Types

4.2.2.1 Pesticides

Exposure to excess amounts of pesticides is considered a risk for developing HCC. There are significant associations between occupational exposures to organophosphate and carbamate pesticides and the development of HCC (Ezzat et al. 2005). Saad-Hussein et al. (2019) found that, however, the tumor biomarkers; P53 protein, AFP, and Alpha-L-fucosidase (AFU), were within the normal range, there was prominent increase in the DNA damage, with shortening of telomere length and variation in telomerase enzyme activity in organophosphate sprayers, and that changes were related to the elevated levels of Butyrylcholinesterase (a marker indicating the level of exposure). Therefore, the authors recommended using telomere relative length and comets assay as predictors for liver cancer among workers exposed to pesticide (Saad-Hussein et al. 2019).

4.2.2.2 Heavy Metals

Cadmium (Cd)

Cadmium (Cd) is a hepatotoxic environmental pollutant. According to the International Agency for Research on Cancer (IARC), Cd is considered to be among Group1 carcinogenic heavy metal (IARC 2012a). Several epidemiological studies proved the strong connection between Cd accumulation in the human body and the development of various cancers; including liver cancer (Satarug 2012; Barsouk et al. 2021).

Occupational exposure to Cd may cause HCC to the exposed workers in Cd mining. Also, workers in the manufacture of Cd-containing ores, Ni-Cd battery manufacturing, and Cd alloy, are occupationally exposed to high concentration of Cd. The non-occupational exposures to Cd can occur through consumption of Cd-contaminated drinking water, food, and cigarettes (Luevano and Damodaran 2014).

Arsenic (As)

Arsenic (As) is an essential trace element for healthy life, the total human body content of As must be between 3 and 4 mg (WHO 1983), and its lethal dose is 125 mg (Bates et al. 1994). IARC (2012a, b) considered to be among Group 1 carcinogenic heavy metals (IARC 2012a). Occupational exposure to As are mainly in As extraction industry, lead processing, some pharmaceutical industries, glass industry, leather preservatives and antifouling paints, agrochemical production such as pesticides, microelectronics, and optical industries (Rapisarda et al. 2016).

The non-occupational exposures to As are mainly smoking and high consumption of fish and animal protein, that was found to be the principal cause of As accumulation in the general Egyptian population (Saad and Hassanien 2001).

4.2.2.3 Formaldehyde (HCHO)

Environmental Protective Agency (EPA) considers HCHO to be among Group B1 (carcinogenic for animal and probable human carcinogen), the inhalation of HCHO was found to cause DNA single-strand breaks in the liver of male rats (Im et al. 2006). Moreover, an association was detected between occupational exposure to HCHO and the increase of chromosomal aberrations in pathology lab workers, and these aberrations was significantly increasing with the duration of exposure, but, there was no significant elevation of the tumor biomarker P53 (Saad et al. 2006).

Therefore, the authors concluded that the increase in chromosomal aberrations cannot be neglected as predictors for its carcinogenic effect, and they recommended that regular follow-up of the workers is essential.

4.2.2.4 Bisphenol A (BPA)

The chemical structure of BPA is [(CH3)2C(C6H4OH)2], it is a synthetic precursor chemical in the manufacture of plastics and resins. BPA is an endocrine-disrupting, and it may be probable human carcinogenic doses less than the oral reference dose sated by EPA (Khan et al. 2021).

BPA can enter human body orally, or through inhalation or dermal during manufacturing, or as a result of leaching from plastic-lined food and drink containers contain acidic liquids, or during repeating heating or washing with detergents (Tsai 2006). The unconjugated BPA concentrations will be elevated in human body, if there are any abnormalities in the liver enzyme UDP-glucuronosyltransferases 2B15. This enzyme is responsible for formation of BPA-glucuronide to be excreted from the body either through bile or urine (Thongkorn et al. 2019). Accumulation of unconjugated BPA in human body may cause epigenome-wide changes, mitochondrial damage, oxidative stress, and reduction in the antioxidant activities of glutathione, catalase, and others enzymes, which may lead to liver injuries and development of hepatic cancers with chronic exposures (Khan et al. 2021).

4.2.2.5 Polycyclic Aromatic Hydrocarbons (PAHs)

PAHs are compounds released from incomplete combustion of coal, oil, gas, wood, or other carbon-containing organic substances. Also, PAHs are emitted in gas-burning motor vehicle, wood-burning furnaces, cigarette smoke, industrial smoke or soot, and charcoal-broiled foods (ATSDR 1995). IARC (2010a, b) recorded it as human carcinogens compounds (IARC 2010b).

4.2.2.6 Vinyl Chloride Monomer (VCM)

IARC considered VCM to be among Group 1 carcinogens (IARC 2012b). Cicalese et al. (2017a, b) found that vinyl chloride is a significant contributor to the increase in the incidence of HCC in Texas in both the year 2002 and 2005, that association with HCC rate was proved through using logistic regression, and with HCC magnitude through using gamma regression. The two statistical models were used to assess the nonlinear relationship between HCC and environmental vinyl chloride to provide more insight into the tested associations by reinforcement of the finding (Cicalese et al. 2017b).

VCM occurs in cigarette smoke and is mainly used in the production of polymer polyvinyl chloride (PVC), and in the manufacture of plastics, plumbing, cabling, house framing, waterproof clothing, medical devices, and food packaging industry (Rapisarda et al. 2016). VCM enters the human body through inhalation, and metabolized primarily in the liver, to be excreted in human urine as a thiodiglycolic acid (Rapisarda et al. 2016). Exposure to high environmental concentrations of VCM may lead to the development of angiosarcoma of the liver (Sherman 2009), and HCC due to specific gene mutations in the liver (Fedeli and Mastrangelo 2011).

4.2.2.7 Organic Solvents

Many organic solvents, such as aromatic, chlorinated, aliphatic, or alicyclic hydrocarbons, are commonly used in different industries and causes increase the risk of HCC (Uccello et al. 2012).

Building and chemical workers, painters, persons exposed to solvents, and textile industry workers are reported to be at high risk for HCC (Chen and Seaton 1996; Steenland and Palu 1999). Occupational exposure to organic solvents found to have hazardous effects on the liver that leaded to significant elevation of liver enzymes, the hepatic tumor biomarker alpha-fetoprotein (AFP), and oxidative stress biomarker MDA, and the significant decline in the antioxidant enzymes superoxide dismutase (SOD) and glutathione reductase (GR) and some trace elements such as selenium (Se), zinc (Zn) and copper (Cu) (Hussein et al. 2008). However, the authors could not detect protective roles of antioxidants and trace elements were not proved, as there were no significant relations between these antioxidants and oxidative stress, AFP, and liver enzymes.

4.2.2.8 Benzo(a)pyrene (BaP)

Incomplete combustion of organic materials from various anthropogenic activity will result in increasing the delivery of BaP as an environmental contaminant. The highly reactive metabolite of BaP is BaP diol epoxide (BPDE), that is binding to DNA forming BPDE-DNA adducts, this adducts increases the risk of developing HCC (Su et al. 2014).

4.2.3 Prevention and Control of Chemical Pollutants

Prolonged exposure to environmental pollutants either indoor or outdoor proved to have significant impacts on the liver of the exposed persons that were range from hepatotoxicity to the development of hepatic malignancy. For that, health surveillance is essential and reasonable for workers heavily exposed to hepatotoxic chemicals, especially in the presence of other risk factors; such as smoking habits, viral hepatitis, or gene susceptibility.

Liver function must be monitored regularly; particularly for highly exposed workers for early detection of any abnormalities in liver enzymes, especially alanine aminotransferase (ALT), aspartate aminotransferase (AST), gamma glutamyl transpeptidase (GGT), alkaline phosphatase, and bilirubin levels. Hepatic tumor biomarkers; such as alpha-fetoprotein (AFP), must be done even if there was no alterations in the liver enzymes, and no cirrhosis or fatty liver or any hepatic lesion detected by ultrasonography. Therefore, surveillance must be performed to facilitate early detection of hepatic diseases, including malignancies in the workers exposed to high chemical concentrations (Uccello et al. 2012).

The well controlling of hepato-carcinogens environmental pollutants; especially in closed ill ventilated places, quitting of cigarette smoking, reduction of alcohol drinking, and universal hepatitis B virus (HBV) vaccination of all newborn infants, proved to be the important clues for the prevention of HCC (Su et al. 2014).

Routine examination of the polymorphism of susceptible genes implemented in detoxification of environmental chemical pollutants will be of high value to minimize the rate of development of HCC among exposed workers. Examples about that are the polymorphisms of *GSTT1* and *GSTP1* gene among pesticide exposed persons (Saad-Hussein et al. 2017, 2022), and *GSTP* promoter DNA methylation regulates among persons exposed to BaP (Tian et al. 2016). These gene's expressions will have potential protective role against induction of HCC due to environmental exposures to chemical pollutants, and these genes are placing role in the detoxification of these pollutants. So, it will be cost benefit for workers with deficiency of detoxification, must be replaced their working place to minimize the dose of exposure to decrease the hazardous impacts of these exposures.

4.3 Biological Carcinogens

4.3.1 Types and Mechanism of Actions

Biological carcinogens include viral hepatitis, mycotoxins mainly aflatoxin and cyantotoxins particularly microcystins.

Mechanism of viral hepatic carcinogenesis was discussed in detail in Chap. 2.

4.3.1.1 Mechanism of Carcinogenesis by Mycotoxins

Mycotoxins are found in many food sources such as cereals, spices, dried fruits, coffee beans, and nuts. They are heat stable so they can survive high temperature during baking and roasting. Subsequently, contamination of processed food can contaminate animal products such as milk, eggs, and meat (Chain et al. 2020). Aflatoxin represents one of these mycotoxins which is produced by *Aspergillus flavus* and *Aspergillus paraciticus* fungi (Kew 2013).

The four main types of aflatoxins (AFB1, AFB2, AFG1, and AFG2) are potentially carcinogenic. Epidemiological evidence by IARC classifies aflatoxins as a human carcinogen (IARC 2012b). It could have synergistic effect on HCC occurrence with concomitant chronic HBV or HCV infections (Jin et al. 2023).

The optimum conditions for the growth of these fungi are the warm and moist environmental conditions. Therefore, *A. flavus* growth can occur at any time in the pre- or postharvest stage, so food contamination will be difficult to control. During storage, a large amount of AFB1 contamination can occur, because of the lack of the ability to store food in dry, temperature-controlled conditions (Liu and Wu 2010). The acceptable level of aflatoxin exposure for human consumption in food ranges from 0 to 40 parts per billion (ppb), while levels in animal feed could reach up to 300 ppb (Dohlman 2003).

Chronic HBV infection and aflatoxin increase the risk of HCC up to 30 times greater than exposure to aflatoxin alone (Liu et al. 2010). Genetic characteristics of hepatitis virus, and the age and sex of the infected patient may play a role in increasing the risk of aflatoxin-induced HCC (Kirk et al. 2006).

The parent molecule of aflatoxin is harmless, but it becomes carcinogenic when it is metabolized by members of the cytochrome p450 superfamily into mutagenic electrophilic intermediates (Kensler et al. 2003).

The main site of aflatoxin metabolism is in the liver where cytochrome p450 enzymes convert it into anafatoxin-8,9-exo-epoxide and, to a lesser extent, an aflatoxin8,9-endo-epoxide. Exo-epoxide is highly reactive and form derivatives with DNA, RNA, and proteins and reacts with the p53 tumor suppressor gene (Bressac et al. 1991). Following binding to DNA, there will be formation of the promutagenic 8,9 dihydro8-(N7 guanyl)-9-hydroxy AFB1 adduct (AFB1-N7-Gua) (Wild and Turner 2002).

4.3.1.2 Mechanism of Hepatic Carcinogenesis by Cyanotoxins

Cyanotoxins are naturally occurring secondary metabolites produced by cyanobacterial harmful algal blooms (HABs), present in nearly all global terrestrial and aquatic environments. Cyanotoxins are classified according to the affected organ as hepatotoxins (such as anatoxin, saxitoxin (STXs), and microcystin), neurotoxins (such as nodularins (NODs) and cylindrospermopsin), and dermatotoxins (such as aplysiatoxin and lyngbyatoxin-A) (Carmichael and Boyer 2016).

Human exposure to cyanotoxins occurs through ingestion of the drinking water and food such as fish, mussels, and crustaceans or through inhalation and dermal contacts during water activity (Massey et al. 2018; Nielsen and Jiang 2020).

Microcystins (MC) are cyclic peptides produced by numerous cyanobacteria, including the genera *Aphanizomenon, Dolichospermum, Fischerella, Microcystis, Nostoc, Oscillatoria, Planktothrix, Synechococcus, and Trichodesmium* (Du et al. 2019). More than 279 variants of microcystin have been identified (Bouaïcha et al. 2019). The most common three microcystin variants are originating from tyrosine (Y), leucine (L), or arginine (R) forming MC-YR, MC-LR, and MC-RR (Díez-Quijada et al. 2019b).

The highly toxic, MC-LR, is the most common and best characterized. MC-LR are classified as human carcinogens (IARC 2010a) through inhibition of protein serine/threonine phosphatases PP1 and PP2A (Du et al. 2019). In a study in China, serum MCs levels were found to be an independent risk factor for hepatocellular carcinoma (YU 1995).

The liver is the primary site of MCs distribution (Ito et al. 2000). MCs are stable and can be accumulated in the liver causing severe health hazards. However, there are variations in the absorption and distribution of MCs in different species, and these species-specific differences could contribute to different types of toxicities. For example, the LD50 of MC-LR in mammals is 100 times lower than in fishes. In the liver, cyanotoxin has been shown to be cytotoxic, genotoxic, and potentially carcinogenic and inhibits the synthesis of endogenous antioxidants such as protein and glutathione, leading to oxidative stress and DNA damage (Humpage et al. 2005; Yang et al. 2021).

Among cyanotoxins, MCs have strong hepatotoxic and genotoxic properties. MCs bind to the catalytic subunit of protein phosphatase (PP1 and PP2A) and inhibit its activity (Díez-Quijada et al. 2019a). These abnormal phosphorylation of the protein substrates of PP1 and PP2A were found to cause increased inflammation, cellular apoptosis, cytoskeletal destabilization, the disruption of DNA repair, and tumor formation (Liu and Sun 2015). Moreover, MCs were found to cause direct interaction with mitochondrial proteins, triggering oxidative stress and apoptosis (Ding and Nam Ong 2003). In addition, the levels of cyanotoxin were found to be significantly correlated with tumor expression of genes functioning in PPAR pathway and lipid metabolism (Hernandez et al. 2023).

4.3.1.3 Viral Carcinogens

HBV and HCV infections represent the most common and important hepatic carcinogens. Difference in the geographical distribution of both viruses determines the variation in HCC incidence among different countries. Global incidence of HBV in cirrhosis is high particularly in Western pacific and Africa, intermediate incidence in most Mediterranean countries and in eastern Europe, and low incidence in most countries of South and North America and western-Europe (Alberts et al. 2022).

HBV represents the liver carcinogen in about half of cases of HCC. At least one-quarter of infected patients will develop the tumor (Parkin 2006) with 15–20 times greater risk among HBV infected as compared to uninfected population (Shi et al. 2005), and incidence of 3.7 person years in patients with compensated cirrhosis (Fattovich et al. 2008). Development of HCC at younger age among those infected by HBV and HCV in some African countries suggests that specific environmental, biological, or genetic factors might determine the likelihood of development of HCC at a younger age in these countries (Gong et al. 2003).

4.3.2 Biological Pollutants as Risk Factors for HCC

N.B. Details on the HBV and HCV as risk factors are discussed in Chap. 2.

4.3.2.1 Mycotoxins

Aflatoxins in Low/Middle-Income Countries

These warm conditions and humidity are common during storage of many agricultural commodities in many marketplaces particularly in the low- and middle-income countries such as Pakistan, India, and Bangladesh, especially in the months following the monsoon (Nisa et al. 2014). Many studies from low-income countries estimated that about 4.5 billion persons had chronic exposure to high amount of aflatoxin in their environment such as Sub-Saharan Africa and Southeast Asia (Williams et al. 2004).

In countries like Kenya and India, severe outbreaks of AFB1 contamination in food resulted in large number of deaths due to acute exposures (Probst et al. 2007; Azziz-Baumgartner et al. 2005). Samples of maize from Kenya, showed that 35% had aflatoxin levels more than 100 μg/kg and 7% has level more than 1000 μg/kg (Lewis et al. 2005).

In The Gambia and Guinea, more than 90% of children at the age of 3 years had similar exposure to that observed in adult (Wild et al. 1993; Turner et al. 2000).

Early weaning of these children using aflatoxin contaminated food such as maize could be the reason in these regions. Aflatoxin-albumin adducts (AF-alb) as a biomarker of acute aflatoxin exposure was detected in the sera of Beninese children younger than 1 year of age (Gong et al. 2003).

Official monitoring of maize in developing countries particularly in sub-Saharan Africa is rare. High levels of aflatoxins have been found in both pre- and postharvest maize in Bénin (Hell et al. 2000).Other cereals such as wheat, barely, oat, and sorghum were less likely to be contaminated at preharvest stage (Wagacha and Muthomi 2008). In Egypt, aflatoxin level was high both in urine and serum of cirrhotic patients particularly from Upper Egypt as compared to Delta Egypt (Mokhles et al. 2007).

Raw milk also represents a source of aflatoxin contamination in low–/middle-income countries. In the Middle East, the highest concentration of aflatoxin in raw milk was reported in Syria. Meanwhile, the highest concentration of aflatoxin in ultra-high temperature processing (UHT) milk was recorded in Iran and Saudi Arabia. Studies on the contamination of pasteurized milk were conducted in Turkey and Iran. The highest carcinogenic risk in both adults and children due to consuming aflatoxin contaminated raw milk was observed in Syria; pasteurized milk in Turkey and UHT milk in Iran (Rahmani et al. 2018).

The Food and Drug Administration (FDA) sets an action level for AFM1 in milk is 500 ng/L (FDA 2005). In MENA region (Middle East and North Africa), 80% of the dry bread was highly contaminated by aflatoxins. In Algeria; the most contaminated country, 87% of animal feed was contaminated by aflatoxins and Fusarium. Fusarium was the highest mycotoxins detected in animal feed (1240.01 μg/kg) (Jalilzadeh-Amin et al. 2023).

Contamination by *A. flavus* and aflatoxins was reported in the diet formulated for feeding dairy cows and in the dairy food chain in Mexican Highland Plateau (Álvarez-Días et al. 2022). Silva et al. reported that isolated fungi from coffee of a farm located in Brazil were predominantly *A. flavus* and *A. nige*r, which increased during storage (Silva et al. 2008).

4.3.2.2 Cyanotoxins

MCs if detected in rivers, streams, lakes, and lagoons; which are the main global sources of irrigation and drinking water, will increase the risk of toxin transport into crops and drinking water systems (De Figueiredo et al. 2004). The World Health Organization (WHO) provisional guideline level of microcystin-LR is set at a dose of 1 μg/L as a safe level in the drinking water (Falconer et al. 1999).

Cyanotoxins in soil can be released and infiltrate to deeper layers and potentially contaminate groundwater (Bouaïcha and Corbel 2016). High levels of MCs in groundwater have been reported in different regions in China (Chaohu) and Saudi Arabia (Mutoti et al. 2023).

Microcystin (MCs) in Crops

MCs contamination of crops could occur through contamination of irrigation water either ground or surface water (Mohamed et al. 2022) or the use of cyanobacterial biomass as a fertilizer in agriculture (Xiang et al. 2020). MCs contamination in ground and surface water is increasing with increased eutrophication in freshwater systems and agricultural soils. This will pose threats to aquatic and terrestrial plants and other crop production. Owing to high chemical stability and low molecular weight of microcystin, it can survive in high quantities in the leaves, stems, and roots of the exposed plants. Studies have indicated potential health risks associated with consumption of fruits and vegetables contaminated by MCs from polluted irrigated water (Melaram et al. 2022).

Following the irrigation with toxin-contaminated water, agricultural plants become contaminated (Machado et al. 2017; Zhang et al. 2021). These plants include lettuce, ryegrass, clover, and rape (Crush et al. 2008). Cyanotoxins was found to be accumulated in different parts of rice, including grains. Dermal exposures may cause allergic dermatitis or even systemic toxic effects, that could occur during water activities, such as fishing or recreational sporting (Giannuzzi et al. 2011).

Irrigation of plants with MC contaminated water increases the possibility of accumulation and translocation of MC in different plant parts, including the edible parts (Llana-Ruiz-Cabello et al. 2019). For example, in Guatemala tomato and peppers irrigated with contaminated water from Lake Amatitlán, MC was found to be accumulated in different parts, including fruit and seed parts (Romero-Oliva et al. 2014).

A meta-analysis reported that MCs bio-accumulate in the leafy vegetables were three times higher than in other plants. MCs were found in durum wheat, corn, white mustard, and garden cress (Zhang et al. 2021). Moreover, elimination of MCs may take between 29 and 37 days (Cordeiro-Araújo et al. 2016).

Cyanotoxins in Low/Middle-Income Countries

Research conducted in China and Brazil during 2000–2021 found that seafood contaminated by cyanotoxins were more frequent comparing with that in the other developing countries in Africa, Asia, and Latin America. In Latin America, data on cyanotoxin occurrence in seafood have been reported in Brazil followed by Mexico, Argentina, and Guatemala (Abdallah et al. 2021).

WHO mentioned that 19% of samples from fish, carb, and shrimps collected from Sepetiba Bay in Brazil showed low levels of MCs, but, it was higher than the provisional tolerable daily intake (0.04 μg/kg of body weight per day) (Magalhaes et al. 2003). Low levels of MCs were also detected in Nile tilapia collected from Lake Zumpango in Mexico City, but MCs' level was two times above the recommended levels in cases consuming contaminated mesa silverside (Zamora-Barrios et al. 2019).

Numerous cities in Brazil and other South American countries use surface reservoirs, including lakes and rivers, as a main source of drinking water. These water bodies became eutrophicated ecosystems with recurrent cyanobacterial outbreaks making this an emerging concern to public health authorities (Frias et al. 2006; Echenique et al. 2006).

In Asia, cyanotoxin was detected in muscles of three edible fish species collected in Turkey for the first time in 2013 (Akcaalan et al. 2014; Gurbuz et al. 2016). Later, both MCs and cyanotoxins were detected by a survey in different water sources (Koker et al. 2017). MCs contamination in muscles of Iranian fish was reported in the Anzali wetland which exceeded the permissible levels for human consumption (Rezaitabar et al. 2017).

In Thailand, studies conducted to evaluate of MCs accumulation in cultured Nile tilapia and freshwater prawns showed higher levels of MCs in prawn in comparison to the levels detected in Nile tilapia fish. However, it was unclear whether the water green system as well as the feeding system in these studies contributed significantly to MCs accumulation in the selected species (Ruangrit et al. 2013).

In Vietnam, MCs were detected in high concentrations in the locally consumed *Corbicula* and *Ensidens* sp. (Pham et al. 2017). Another study from Vietnam, sampled and analyzed Apple snails' samples for eight MCs variants and NODs. MCs variant was detected in three samples of the muscular part of Apple snails, and its concentrations were ten times higher in the viscera of these snails. Meanwhile, NODs were not detected in the examined snails (Trung et al. 2018).

In Singapore, a study conducted on water reservoirs from January 2012 to February 2019, showed that CYN was the most commonly detected cyanotoxin, occurring in more than half of all samples. In addition, MC-RR was the next most commonly detected toxin, occurring in 37.6% of samples (Lim et al. 2020).

In Indian markets, MCs were detected at variable concentrations in the muscles of two commercially cultivated fish species, carp and catfish, which indicates a species variation in MCs adsorption and accumulation (Singh and Asthana 2014).

In Africa, most of the studies conducted on cyanotoxins have focused on MCs. Almost all the published surveys were mainly targeting total MCs in the seafood (Modley et al. 2019). The published data were mainly from few African countries, in the north; such as Algeria and Egypt, in the east; such as Ethiopia, Kenya, Uganda, and Tanzania, and in the south; such as South Africa and Mozambique. Nevertheless, the data about cyanobacteria and their toxins in food are lacking in the rest of the African countries, and there are no available data on cyanotoxin contamination in the edible aquatic organisms.

Most of the available data were obtained from the analysis of blooms occurred in lakes, reservoirs, rivers, and dams in large number of African countries. Humpage and Falconer (2003) detected MCs in *O. niloticus* muscles in fishponds blooms located in the southern part of Egypt, and they detected MCs 1.3 to 14 times higher concentrations than the recommended permissible guidelines levels during summer and fall seasons due to the growth of bacterial bloom. They also noticed the high resistance of the investigated *O. niloticus* sp. to the impacts of MCs, as there was no increase in the mortality rates observed.

Moreover, a total of 19 species of cyanobacteria were isolated from mats on the Nile River and irrigation canal sediments in Egypt. Five species showed hepatotoxic effects to mice within 6 h after injection (Mohamed et al. 2006). Common carp muscles in Algeria were the main source for MCs exposure, as the concentrations of

MCs for 1-year survey were above the provisional tolerable daily intake (Amrani et al. 2014).

In Ethiopia, MCs contamination was reported to be of high concentrations in the muscles and liver of Nile tilapia, carps, and African sharp tooth catfish (Zewde et al. 2018). MCs contamination was also found in 25% of the samples from the popular food for the Kenyan population, the small fish (*Rastrineobola argentea* sp.) collected from Victoria Lake, therefore, drying these fish under sunlight was found to be useful to reduce MCs contents (Simiyu et al. 2018). Moreover, anatoxin was detected almost 20 years ago in two freshwater lakes in Kenya during cyanobacterial bloom, but there are no reports on its contamination to the sea foods (Kotut et al. 2006).

Recently, a meta-analysis found that in various water bodies MCs have been detected in concentrations 1.4–2803 times higher than the WHO provisional guideline for human lifetime exposure via drinking water (1 μg/L) in 12 of 15 African countries where data were available (Zhao et al. 2023).

A survey done in Uganda detected high levels of MCs contaminating fish muscles in two different lakes (Nyakairu et al. 2010). However, in the same year, another survey detected MCs with lower concentrations in the same species (Semyalo et al. 2010). Three tropical lakes and four smaller lakes in Uganda showed MCs contamination in 19 different fish species with significant variations due to diet, species, and the season (Poste et al. 2011). In Tanzania, multiple cyanotoxins were detected in the serum of Tanzanians living in the Ukerewe district in Mwanza at variable concentrations (Mchau et al. 2021).

These data from Mozambique and from surrounding countries (South Africa, Lesotho, Botswana, Malawi, Zambia, and Tanzania) provide an evidence for the need conduct an operational monitoring program of MCs to avoid the possible cases of intoxications since the drinking water quality control tests recommended by the Ministry of Health do not include an MC test (Tamele and Vasconcelos 2020).

4.3.3 Prevention and Control of Biological Hepatic Carcinogens

4.3.3.1 Prevention and Control of Viral Carcinogens

Proper adequate screening for viral infection in blood or its products as well as reduction of promiscuous unprotected sexual activities are the major prevention and control methods against hepatitis viral transmission. Long-term health educational programs to reduce the sharing of needles and equipment used in dental, surgical, or intravenous implication between the users is also an important recommendation, particularly in countries with low HBV endemicity. Meanwhile, newborns' HBV vaccination is an essential preventive measure in countries with high and medium HBV endemicity, because HBV is more frequently acquired at birth or in early childhood. Similarly, prevention of HCV requires careful blood and its products screening, as well as educational programs for the healthcare personnel and all other categories at risk of infection (Sagnelli et al. 2020).

4.3.3.2 Intervention to Control Aflatoxins and Prevent Aflatoxin-Induced HCC (Fig. 4.1)

This can be achieved by maintaining food safety or ensuring hepatoprotection to the host against the carcinogenic effect of aflatoxin and creating aflatoxin awareness.

Food Safety

Strategies to control aflatoxin contamination can be either at an individual level or community level. At the individual level, a change in dietary practice to avoid food contamination or chemo-prevention approaches could be used. At the community level, these include preharvest or postharvest interventions. Preharvest methods include irrigation practices, use of pesticides or fungicides, biocontrol, or crops genetic modification to improve crop resistance, and timely harvest (Wild 2007).

Methods to control fungal contamination in the preharvest phase can be achieved through the following:

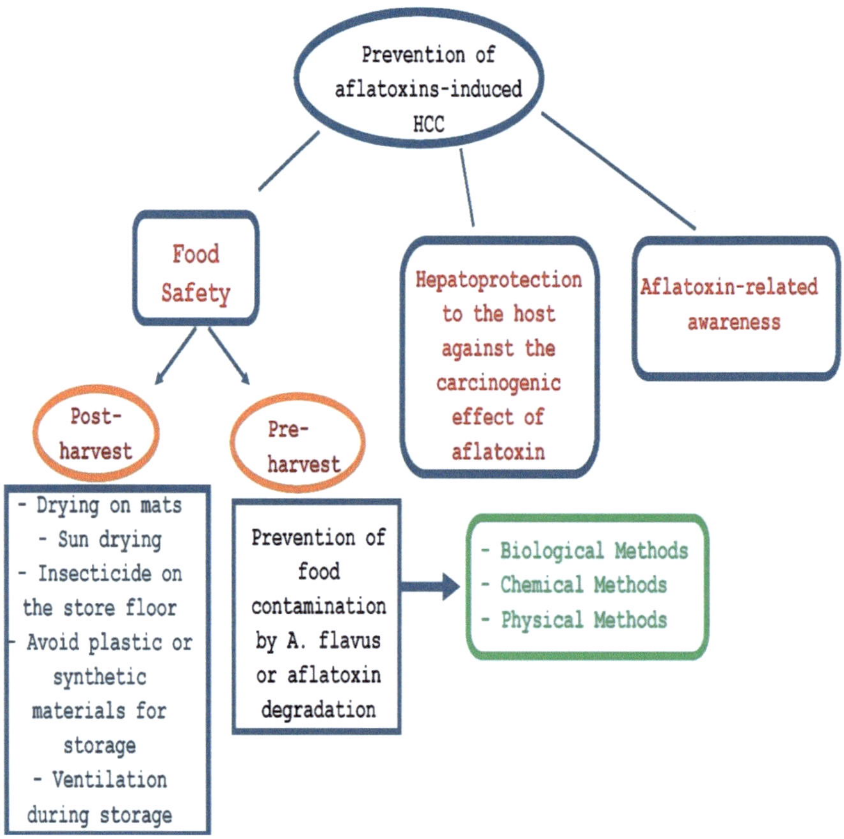

Fig. 4.1 Intervention to control aflatoxins and prevent aflatoxin-induced HCC

I. **Biological Methods**

Variable methods using natural substances can suppress the formation of aflatoxigenic producing fungi that may cause aflatoxin contamination of food products. Therefore, these natural substances were found to prevent production of aflatoxins and degrading aflatoxins. These inhibitors were found to have potential effects and can replace or supplement the existing ways of combatting aflatoxin contamination in food (Ahmad et al. 2022). This can be achieved by:

(a) **Microbial degradation of aflatoxins**: Many strains of *Pseudomonas, Rhodococcus, Bacillus* species, *Escherichia coli,* and *Streptomyces* were found to be capable of degrading aflatoxins (Guo et al. 2021). The white-rot fungi from the genus *Pleurotus* were suggested to have detoxification capability to aflatoxins (Jackson and Pryor 2017).
(b) **Enzymatic degradation of aflatoxins:** This can be achieved by isolation and identification of aflatoxin-degrading enzymes from microbes. The on-toxigenic *A. niger* can be used in the food industry by production of important enzymes; such as amyloglucosidase, amylase, cellulases, lactase, invertase, pectinases, and acid proteases (Sun et al. 2016). Peroxidases, laccases, and oxidases also have aflatoxins degradation effects. Novel aflatoxin-degrading enzymes are being explored such as extracellular enzyme MADE from *Myxococcus fulvus*, purified enzyme BADE from *Bacillus shackletonii*, enzyme PADE from *Pantoea* sp. However, up till now, there has been a lack of scientific standardized methods to investigate the activity of mycotoxin degrading enzymes in the digestive systems of animals (Guo et al. 2021).

II. **Chemical Methods**

a. **Aflatoxins degradation with ozone:** Ozone is a powerful oxidizing agent capable of detoxifying a wide range of emerging food contaminants, such as mycotoxins. Generally Recognized As Safe (GRAS) status granted mycotoxins degradation by ozone for use in food and water (FDA 1982). Application of ozone has already been successfully employed for the removal of aflatoxins in laboratory scale trials in food, such as corn, red pepper, wheat, and peanuts with reduction of hepatotoxicity and nephrotoxicity of aflatoxins (Diao et al. 2013).
b. **Aflatoxins degradation with electrolyzed oxidizing water:** Electrolyzed oxidizing water is a novel safe broad-spectrum disinfectant. It is formed through the passage of solution with diluted salt; 1% NaCl, in the electrolytic chamber, where the anode and cathode are separated by a membrane (Guo et al. 2021).
c. **Aflatoxins degradation with organic acids:** Global food safety control authorities consider organic acids as food-grade additives. The degradation of aflatoxins in the agriculture products; such as pepper, rice, and soybeans, by soaking in organic acids has been proved to be effective in laboratory

studies (Lee et al. 2015). Fruit juice contains high level of organic acids could be used as natural and readily available sources for the degradation of aflatoxins in the contaminated food.

d. **Aflatoxins degradation with plant extracts:** Natural plant extracts have anti-microbial, anti-inflammatory, antioxidant, and immune boosting activities. Potential use of natural plant extracts for mycotoxin detoxification has become of increasing importance. The leaf extract of *Adhatoda vasica* Nees, aqueous leave extracts of *Rosmarinus officinalis*, aqueous extract of *Ocimum tenuiflorum*, aqueous extracts of *Corymbia citriodora* and *Trachyspermum ammi* were also evaluated (Guo et al. 2021).Addition of garlic, ginger, cardamom, and black cumin to detoxify AFB1 on spice mix red pepper powder (*berbere*) and sauté resulted in an AFB1 level below the detection limit(Medalcho et al. 2023).

III. **Physical Methods**

These methods depend on aflatoxin degradation by irradiation. In general, irradiation used for aflatoxin degradation is classified into two forms: ionizing and non-ionizing irradiation.

Ionizing Irradiation

a. **Degradation by gamma irradiation:** Because of their high reactivity and penetrability, gamma rays are preferred as a source of irradiation for food processing, as irradiation of food contents up to 10 kGy has no hazardous effects or nutritional problems (Organization 1999). However, for fatty foods or foods with high vitamin content, gamma irradiation seemed not to be suitable, as it increases the formation of oxidative rancidity in these foods (Caulfeld et al. 2008).
b. **Degradation by electron beam irradiation** (EB): The equipment for this technology is of low cost with control of the emitted dosages, and the technology itself has short processing time. The use of EB-irradiation technology leads to significant decrease in the mutagenicity and cytotoxicity effects of aflatoxins (Liu et al. 2016).
c. **Degradation by ultraviolet irradiation (UV):** UV irradiation has effective physical effects on aflatoxins, as it can cause photosensitive destruction of aflatoxins without toxic effects or waste generation (Gayán et al. 2014). Nevertheless, penetration capacity of UV light into solid materials is limited, and can result in production of high suspended solids contents and low decontamination efficiency in food products (Fan et al. 2017).
d. **Degradation by photocatalysis:** UV–visible irradiation is using combination of UV with semiconducting photocatalysts that can increase aflatoxins degradation efficiency in liquid matrix (Sun et al. 2019). The most widely used photocatalyst is TiO2, that is active under UV irradiation. This technology is non-toxic, highly efficient, and has long-term photostability as studied on Sudanese peanut oil

(Magzoub et al. 2019). However, very little information exists on the stability and safety of this technology.

e. **Degradation by pulsed light (PL):** PL is a non-thermal technology implemented for inactivation of the cytotoxicity and mutagenicity of aflatoxins; particularly AFB1 and AFB2 (Wang et al., 2016). PL is rapid and efficient surface decontamination technology of food products with an upper limit influence of 12 J cm−2 (FDA, 1996). Despite the progress made in PL studies, the breakdown products of aflatoxins after PL treatment are still under investigation.

Non-ionizing Irradiation

a. **Degradation by microwave heating:** Microwave heating mechanism if through transforming the electromagnetic field energy to thermal energy by polarization effects of the electromagnetic radiation (Soni et al. 2020). Microwave heating results in degrading aflatoxins in various food substances (Guo et al. 2021). During microwave heating, there is difference in the distribution of the temperature, which may result in the formation of cold and hot spots in the treated food (Menon et al. 2020), which leads to variation in the effect on aflatoxins. In cold spots, aflatoxin cannot be effectively detoxified, while in hot spots, the quality of nutritional components may be lost or deteriorated.
b. **Degradation by cold plasma:** Plasma can be loosely categorized into thermal and cold plasma. It is highly energized ionized gas, and consists of electrons, ions, UV irradiation and reactive neutral species such as reactive oxygen species (ROS) and reactive nitrogen species (RNS) (Kogelschatz 2004). Further research is required to study the impact of plasma process conditions on the different food substances.

Hepatoprotection to the Host Against the Carcinogenic Effect of Aflatoxin

Natural products; such as the cactus cladode extract (CCE) from *cactus Opuntia ficus indica*, were found to have potential chemo-preventive effects in counteracting aflatoxin induction of hepatic carcinogenic or aflatoxicosis (Brahmi et al. 2011). Fruits and vegetables contain anti-carcinogenic compounds that act through antioxidant mechanism, for examples:

- Apiaceous vegetables were found to have an inhibitory action on human cytochrome-P450 1A2 (hCYP1A2); a liver enzyme known to activate several procarcinogens including aflatoxins (Peterson et al. 2006). Carrots, parsnips, celery and parsley are common examples of apiaceous vegetables.
- Grapefruits have a protective effect against aflatoxin induced liver DNA damage through a reduction in hepatic CYP3A activity (Miyata et al. 2004).
- Coffee may also provide protection against both genotoxicity and cytotoxicity of aflatoxin B1, as coffee induces enzymes involved in xenobiotic detoxification processes detected in the rat liver and primary hepatocytes (Cavin et al. 2008).

Postharvest approaches are generally simple and less expensive compared with preharvest strategies. Approach to postharvest fungal prevention can be done through improved drying, sorting prior to storage in a ventilated storage, use of insecticides, and sorting prior to consumption (Wild 2007).

Avoiding unseasonal rain damage prior to storage also plays a vital role. Removal of obviously damaged kernels or pods can reduce the quantity of aflatoxins (Dickens and Whitaker 1975). Avoiding contact with earth during storage can avoid high humidity. This can be done by raising on wooden pallets or a concrete floor and ensure adequate ventilation in the storage facility.

The development of affordable and acceptable intervention strategies, such as those demonstrated for groundnuts in Guinea, must be prioritized to prevent aflatoxin food contamination. There is little emphasis on combatting aflatoxin and few regulatory controls in developing countries. In addition, the climate conditions, the agricultural practice, and the economic factors, make aflatoxin exposure is a major problem in these countries.

Aflatoxin-Related Awareness

Creating awareness among stakeholders such as farmers, consumers, or policymakers does not receive much attention compared to other aflatoxins control strategies. Non-educated and socially unexposed farmers in Tanzania were found to have deficient aflatoxin awareness (Ayo et al. 2018). Similar low awareness levels were reported from Ethiopia, Uganda (Guchi 2015; Nakavuma et al. 2020), Nigeria and Vietnam (Adekoya et al. 2017; Lee et al. 2017).

However, misleading aflatoxin-related news headlines in Ghana and Ethiopia resulted in panic among consumers, necessitating interventions by governments and the scientific community (Stepman 2018). Therefore, the right information regarding aflatoxin should be adequately delivered to stakeholders.

4.3.3.3 Prevention and Control of Cyanotoxins

Few studies have been conducted in the developing countries regarding strategies for elimination of cyanotoxins. The selected treatment strategy should be able to remove both the cyanobacteria and its toxins, in addition to other water pollutants. Application of multiple strategies will be more effective than depending on single strategy. The following methods represent different methods that could be used to minimize accumulation of cyanotoxins in aquatic ecosystems:

Management of Nutrients

Control of the amounts of phosphorus, nitrogen, and carbon, are important long-term approaches to prevent the occurrence of cyanobacterial blooms enhanced under eutrophication. This can be achieved through the implementation of improved wastewater treatment programs that will lower the organic compounds, the main nutrients contents for cyanobacteria. In addition to the usage of special clay type; such as lanthanum modified bentonite, to bind with phosphorus to reduce eutrophication. But this technique is not always economically feasible, in addition, the ability of this type of clay is hindered by competing oxyanions (Copetti et al. 2016).

Moreover, controlling the usage of fertilizer and manure in agriculture with the reduction of the anthropogenic activities are important approaches to decrease the nutrient loads.

Biological Approach

Biological control is considered to be environmentally safe approach; as no chemicals will be used which avoids the risk of potential harmful effects of the used chemical on environmental and human health. However, its application is limited compared to chemical and physical approaches to remove cyanotoxins. For example, the usage of certain fish species, such as silver carp and bighead carp can be applied to decrease the formation of bloom by grazing it (Chen et al. 2006, 2007).

Other studies focused on the bacterial degradation of cyanotoxins; particularly MCs, that could be implemented using various species, such as *Bacillus* sp., *Sphingomonas* sp., *Sphingopyxis* sp., *Bordetella* sp., *Lactobacillus rhamnosus* sp., *Pseudomonas* sp., *Rahnella aquatilis* sp., and *Rhodococcus* sp. (He et al. 2016). Moreover, critical factors affecting water quality, such as water temperature, pH, type, and concentration of toxins, and the availability of nutrients will affect the efficacy and the process of bacterial degradation in controlling MCs concentrations (Li et al. 2017). More studies are needed to evaluate the ability of the used bacterial strains to degrade the different cyanotoxins.

Chemical Approach

The chemical and physical properties of MCs molecule, such as water-solubility, stability under sunlight, cyclic structure, and neutral pH, makes the conventional water treatment processes using flocculation, coagulation, sedimentation or dissolved air flotation, rapid sand filtration, or disinfection provide limited removal of the MCs contaminants (D'Anglada et al. 2015). The increase of the dissolved MCs concentrations requires additional processes such as chemical oxidation, adsorption, membrane filtration, or biodegradation (USEPA 2015).

The recommendation of WHO to adopt water safety plans (WSP) are mainly included modeling of risk analysis, assessment and management by water suppliers, preferably to be applied to all water supply components (WHO 2009). However, there is a gap of data regarding cyanotoxins potential health risks associated with oral exposure due to the insufficient capacity of water treatment technologies to reach acceptable limits in water in the developing countries.

Using chemical algicides to destroy the bloom has been considered to be an urgent intervention (Wu et al. 2017). However, several disadvantages exist for this method as these compounds mixture could lead to cell lysis and the liberation of cyanotoxins in water (Li et al. 2020), and its persistence in the environment can harm the ecosystem.

Hydrogen peroxide in low concentrations has good efficacy against cyanobacteria, and it has less destructive effect on the environment (Matthijs et al. 2012). However, the possibility of bloom reformation could occur.

The oxidation processes, such as application of ozone and chlorine, have been shown complete MCs removal at the laboratory scale (Lawton and Robertson 1999).

The oxidant dose is mainly depending on the MCs concentrations in addition to the water quality factors; like pH, natural organic matter, and presence of other contaminants in the water (Ma et al. 2012).

Ozone gas was reported to have high efficacy against *M. aeruginosa* but the cell lysis rate was high, which may result in increase the risk of toxin liberation (Roegner et al. 2014; Zamyadi et al. 2020).

The application of adsorbent materials has been widely used for the removal of trace contaminants from the water, such as activated carbon and iron-based adsorbents. Mesoporous activated carbon has more effective adsorption effect of MCs than micro- or macro-sized ones. Furthermore, wood-based activated carbon has the highest removal rate of various materials against cyanotoxins (Park et al. 2018). Iron-based adsorbents, e.g., magnetic bentonite material, have good affinity for adsorption of MCs in river water samples, especially at pH 2.1 (Lian et al. 2014). At low pH with high ionic strength, iron-based adsorbents, such as iron oxides, are more efficient with better results against MCs (Lee and Walker 2011).

Physical Approach

Bank filtration is an effective method for the removal of cyanobacterial cells and their associated toxins (Rose et al. 2018). Romero-Oliva et al. (2014) have focused on the physicochemical parameters involved in filtration, for the effectiveness of bank filtration for the removal of cyanobacteria (Romero-Oliva et al. 2014). Harvey et al. focused on the importance of colmation layer in the removal of cells (Harvey et al. 2015). However, it was demonstrated that cyanobacteria can be found in water filtered through bank filtration, as these cyanobacterial cells are capable of penetrating the bank filter (Rose et al. 2018).

In contrast, successful bio-sand filter operation was reported for the MC-LR removal using bioaugmentation (Kumar et al. 2020b). Most of these studies were performed at the bench-scale only. Moreover, bioaugmentation involves at least 2–3 weeks for a mature biofilm layer formation and can represent an obstacle when the filter adsorbent is used in a filter for household applications such as drinking and cooking.

The sand filter is not an energy-intensive treatment process, without chemical additives and is economical too. However, non-bioaugmented sand-based filters have resulted in poor MC-LR adsorption (<20% adsorption capacity) (Kumar et al. 2020a).

In Egypt, MCs in outflow tank water were detected in high concentrations (1.1–3.6 μg L^{-1}), exceeding WHO provisional guideline value of 1 μg L^{-1} for MC-LR in drinking water. During treatment processes, cyanobacterial cells were incompletely removed by coagulation/flocculation/sedimentation or sand filtration. However, coagulation/flocculation induced the release of MCs into the ambient water, and the toxins were not completely removed or degraded during further treatment stages by filtration and chlorination. (Mohamed et al. 2015).

The application of germicidal UV at a wavelength of 254 nm generates highly reactive hydroxyl radicals that causes limited photolysis of the extracellular cyanotoxins in water (He et al. 2015). Meanwhile, UV light irradiation followed by ozone were found to produce highly reactive hydroxyl radicals, that have better degradation rate for MCs in water (Chang et al. 2015). More studies are still required to confirm the efficacy of these approaches against other MCs contamination (Xie et al. 2021).

Another strategy is ultrasonication on cyanobacterial and algal cell growth which works through deteriorating gas vacuoles and cell walls and decreasing photosynthetic activities. The effect of ultrasonication on the development rate of algal cells and cyanobacteria depends on the sonication period, its frequency, and power (Dehghani 2016).

Increase of Public Awareness

Public awareness can have significant effect in reduction of human exposures to cyanotoxins either during recreational activities, consuming seafood, or drinking contaminated water. Improving social practices and avoiding throwing waste materials into the water sources are important approaches to limit bacterial bloom formation. Therefore, the media should highlight the effect of climate change on food safety, especially in developing countries. The categorical classification of cyanotoxins into low, medium, and high risks will be helpful in selection of the proper actions. Therefore, governments should issue laws to ensure that undesirable industrial waste is properly managed before reaching water bodies (Abdallah et al. 2021).

4.3.4 Role of Climate Change

4.3.4.1 Impact of Climate Changes on Chemical Pollutants

Global climate change proved to have an increase effect of chemical pollutants on the liver health in general. Changes in the temperature could increase the degradation of chemical pollutants in the environment and release these degradations with aggravation in its toxicity and carcinogenicity. Also, the change in wind speeds and directions can lead to the mobilization of chemical pollutants and transport it to other locations. Moreover, wind speeds may also cause dispersion of chemical pollutants and its degradations to be deposited in another location not well prepared to these pollutants. In addition, wind stagnation may cause increase the exposure time to high concentrations of these chemical pollutants (Saad-Hussein and Ramadan 2023).

4.3.4.2 Impact of Climate Changes on Aflatoxin

The increase level of CO_2 in the atmosphere resulted in global warming of 2–5 °C (Medina et al. 2015). This global warming with the subsequent increase in droughts, precipitation and floods will result in deterioration of crop quality with change in harvesting, drying and storage practices (Daou et al. 2021). Environmental conditions such as adequate temperature, relative humidity, oxygen, pH, water activity, and nutrients are all considered essential for the growth of fungi in feed on the crops (Alshannaq and Yu 2017).

The variation of temperature and humidity from country to another and within the same country affects the mycotoxin contamination. Regions of dry conditions are less susceptible as compared to tropical and sub-tropical areas (Prandini et al. 2009). Meanwhile, in Upper Egypt, an area of high temperature and low precipitation, a higher incidence of Aflatoxin M1 (AFM1) was detected in 85.5% of winter buffalo milk samples than in 78.5% of summer milk samples (AHMED et al. 2023).

Aflatoxin contamination can occur at two phases, first phase is infection of the developing crop (preharvest), and the second phase is after crop maturation (postharvest). Climate change affects both phases in a different manner. Fungal contamination can occur in the preharvest phase by wounding of the developing crop by birds, mammals, insects, or the hot dry conditions. The developing crops are usually resistant to the fungal contamination by *A. flavus*. However, aflatoxin contamination of the developing crops occurs when the environmental conditions favor both fungal growth and crop susceptibility. In the warm semi-arid regions like the valleys and mesas of the Sonoran Desert, most of the organic matter in soils is contaminated by *A. flavus* (Boyd and Cotty 2001).

The second phase of aflatoxin contamination may occur between crop maturation and consumption. During this phase, toxin increases in both components infected during the first phase and those infected after maturation. Contamination of the mature crop occurs when exposed to warm moist conditions either in the field or during transportation or storage (Cotty 1991). Fungal compositions set up during the first phase influence the second phase to a great extent. Indeterminate crops, like cotton, usually are not economic to harvest as they mature. Thus, early maturing components are exposed to weather in the field while late components mature.

The impact of climate changes over aflatoxin is evident in maize. It has become stable for years in warm regions of Africa, Asia, and the Americas. It became vulnerable to change in climate as occurred in Kenya (Lewis et al. 2005).

Moreover, the quality of aflatoxin producing fungi varies with climate. The quantity of *A. flavus* in cool areas is low compared to warmer areas where fungi become more common in soils, air, and on crop surfaces (Shearer et al. 1992). Although *A. flavus* is present on crops in almost all areas examined, *A. parasiticus, A. nomius,* and several unnamed taxa, which produce both B and G aflatoxins, are frequently absent or uncommon in certain regions (Cotty and Cardwell 1999).

Reports on the impact of climate changes on aflatoxin in low- middle- income countries:

In MENA region, 46% of animal feed was contaminated with mycotoxins. Algeria, Egypt, Libya, Morocco, and Tunisia are highly suffering from mycotoxin contamination, mainly aflatoxins, ochratoxin A, fumonisin, and zearalenone mycotoxin. Mycotoxins were detected in raw milk and cereals; mainly wheat, barley, maize, and cereal-based products (Jalilzadeh-Amin et al. 2023).

In Africa, milk purchased in Nairobi was found to contain a high level of aflatoxin above the recommended level with a seasonal variation (Lindahl et al. 2018).

In Asia, high temperatures and humidity favor Aspergillus growth in grains. Therefore, 95% of the samples in South Asia and three-quarters of the samples in China and the South East Asia and Pacific region (Indonesia, Philippines, Vietnam) showed aflatoxin contamination (Nutrition 2022). The warm and humid climate in Malaysia provides optimal growth conditions for *A flavus* in food (Shuib et al. 2017).

The highest mean of AFM1 in Ecuador occurs in the dry season and the tropical climatic region, assuming that food under these conditions is more contaminated by AFB1 (Puga-Torres et al. 2020).

In eastern Jordan, the climate has changed, and it became hotter and more humid favoring the production of more mycotoxins. Moreover, shortage in dairy feeds during dry seasons has forced farmers to store feeds during the rainy season for long periods in poor conditions (Bani Ismail et al. 2020). In Yemen, fresh samples of poultry rations (ground maize) from different regions were found to contain high level of aflatoxins and fumonisin (Algabr et al. 2018).

4.3.4.3 Impact of Climate Changes on Microcystin

Eutrophication is an environmental problem characterized by excessive algal and plant growth in aquatic ecosystems. Climate change was found to worsen these excessive growths, in addition to the effects of human population growth and increase industrialization (Withers et al. 2014). Eutrophication results in increasing hypoxia, poor water quality, and harmful algal blooms, such as cyanobacterial blooms (Padedda et al. 2017).

Global climate change can potentially promote the increase in the frequency and duration of harmful algal blooms and can lead to geographical extension of cyanobacteria in water (Paerl and Paul 2012). Optimal environmental factors associated with this climate change can enhance cyanobacterial bloom formation and cyanotoxin production including increased atmospheric carbon dioxide, environmental pollutants, nutrients, light intensity, increase pH, temperature, trace metals, water salinity, and ultraviolet radiation (Neilan et al. 2013; Paerl and Paul 2012).

Water temperature could be used to forecast harmful algal bloom severity**.** The mean of global water temperature is expected to increase by 0.8–1.6 °C in 2071–2100 compared to that was in 1971–2000 (van Vliet et al. 2013). Cyanobacteria exhibit optimal growth at high temperatures (20–25 °C) (Coles and Jones 2000).

Long periods of warm temperature were found to strengthen and increase the duration of the vertical stratification of marine and freshwater systems (Peeters et al. 2007). Cyanobacterial strains can use vertical stratification via the formation of intracellular gas vesicles (Walsby et al. 2006). Increased irradiation of the surface water is efficiently absorbed by cyanobacteria with minimal photosynthetic damage due to the composition of photoprotective accessory pigments and light-induced changes in photosystem II (PSII) (Ohad et al. 2010). Furthermore, cyanobacteria can prevent sunlight penetration to deeper layers of the water system, which can prevent the normal growth of eukaryotic phytoplankton (Amorim and do Nascimento Moura 2021).

Due to climate change, there is increase in salt concentrations of the estuaries due to sea level rise and frequent droughts that leads to vertical density stratification

(Paerl and Paul 2012). Cyanobacteria can tolerate temporary increase in salt concentration up to 7.5 g/L, but, may lead to increase leakage of toxins into the surrounding environment to prevent the osmotic damage (Georges des Aulnois et al. 2019). This is usually detected in brackish waters, where the salt concentration is higher due to the proximity to sea water (Kanoshina et al. 2003). Moreover, periods of intense rainfall followed by periods of severe drought increase nutrient runoff from agricultural land and industries into bodies of water causing water eutrophication (Chen et al. 2003). A strong correlation between the NO3–N and MCs in groundwater exists. High concentrations of NO3–N influence toxin production in groundwater.

Countries around the Mediterranean have the most favorable climate conditions for the development of cyanobacteria. However, studies of toxicology of cyanobacteria in the Mediterranean region are scarce, particularly in North Africa (Mohamed et al. 1999; Oudra et al. 2001).

Scarcity of water resources in arid and semi-arid regions is linked with global changes, and it is associated with the expansion of MC-producing cyanoblooms. For example, in the semi-arid regions of Morocco, microcystis aeruginosa has been dominant during the summer and autumn seasons in the eutrophic reservoir (El Khalloufi et al. 2013).

In Egypt, one study showed that cyanobacterial cell density and intracellular MCs in the water increased with the increase in temperature and nutrients, with maximum values obtained in August (Mohamed et al. 2015).

A study reported the presence of MCs in Saudi Arabia groundwater. High temperature and conductivity, a high concentration of phosphate, and low nitrate concentrations may have contributed to the formation of these blooms. MCs were detected in well waters at concentrations (0.3–1.8 g L^{-1}), which is higher than the WHO guideline level (1 gL^{-1}) in some wells (Mohamed and Al Shehri 2009).

References

Abdallah MF, Van Hassel WH, Andjelkovic M, et al. Cyanotoxins and food contamination in developing countries: review of their types, toxicity, analysis, occurrence and mitigation strategies. Toxins. 2021;13:786.

Adekoya I, Njobeh P, Obadina A, et al. Awareness and prevalence of mycotoxin contamination in selected Nigerian fermented foods. Toxins. 2017;9:363.

Ahmad MM, Qamar F, Saifi M, et al. Natural inhibitors: A sustainable way to combat aflatoxins. Front Microbiol. 2022;13:993834.

Ahmed RB, Sharkawy AA, Elsharkwy EE. Seasonal monitoring of Aflatoxin M1 in row milk samples at Sohag governorate. Assiut Vet Med J. 2023;69:88–97.

Akcaalan R, Köker L, Oğuz A, et al. First report of cylindrospermopsin production by two cyanobacteria (Dolichospermum mendotae and Chrysosporum ovalisporum) in Lake Iznik, Turkey. Toxins. 2014;6:3173–86.

Alberts CJ, Clifford GM, Georges D, et al. Worldwide prevalence of hepatitis B virus and hepatitis C virus among patients with cirrhosis at country, region, and global levels: a systematic review, vol. 7. Lancet Gastroenterol Hepatol; 2022. p. 724.

Algabr HM, Alwaseai A, Alzumir M, et al. Occurrences and frequency of fungi and detection of mycotoxins on poultry rations in Yemen. Bull Natl Res Cent. 2018;42:1–12.

Alshannaq A, Yu J-H. Occurrence, toxicity, and analysis of major mycotoxins in food. Int J Environ Res Public Health. 2017;14:632.

Álvarez-Días F, Torres-Parga B, Valdivia-Flores AG, et al. Aspergillus flavus and Total aflatoxins occurrence in dairy feed and aflatoxin M1 in bovine Milk in Aguascalientes, Mexico. Toxins. 2022;14:292.

Amorim CA, do Nascimento Moura A. Ecological impacts of freshwater algal blooms on water quality, plankton biodiversity, structure, and ecosystem functioning. Sci Total Environ. 2021;758:143605.

Amrani A, Nasri H, Azzouz A, et al. Variation in cyanobacterial hepatotoxin (microcystin) content of water samples and two species of fishes collected from a shallow lake in Algeria. Arch Environ Contam Toxicol. 2014;66:379–89.

ATSDR. Toxicological profile for toxicological profile for polycyclic aromatic hydrocarbons. 1995.

Ayo EM, Matemu A, Laswai G, et al. Socioeconomic characteristics influencing level of awareness of aflatoxin contamination of feeds among livestock farmers in Meru District of Tanzania. Scientifica. 2018;2018:1.

Azziz-Baumgartner E, Lindblade K, Gieseker K, et al. Case–control study of an acute aflatoxicosis outbreak, Kenya, 2004. Environ Health Perspect. 2005;113:1779–83.

Bani Ismail Z, Al-Nabulsi F, Abu-Basha E, et al. Occurrence of on-farm risk factors and health effects of mycotoxins in dairy farms in Jordan. Trop Anim Health Prod. 2020;52:2371–7.

Barsouk A, Thandra KC, Saginala K, et al. Chemical risk factors of primary liver cancer: an update. Hepatic Med Eviden Res. 2021;12:179–88.

Bates M, Smith A, Hopenhayn-Rich C. Arsenic toxicity. Am J Epidemiol. 1994;135:462.

Bouaïcha N, Corbel S. Cyanobacterial toxins emerging contaminants in soils: a review of sources, fate and impacts on ecosystems, plants and animal and human health. InTech Rijeka. 2016;21:105–26.

Bouaïcha N, Miles CO, Beach DG, et al. Structural diversity, characterization and toxicology of microcystins. Toxins. 2019;11:714.

Boyd ML, Cotty PJ. Aspergillus flavus and aflatoxin contamination of leguminous trees of the Sonoran Desert in Arizona. Phytopathology. 2001;91:913–9.

Brahmi D, Bouaziz C, Ayed Y, et al. Chemopreventive effect of cactus Opuntia ficus indica on oxidative stress and genotoxicity of aflatoxin B1. Nutrit Metab. 2011;8:1–16.

Bressac B, Kew M, Wands J, et al. Selective G to T mutations of p53 gene in hepatocellular carcinoma from southern Africa. Nature. 1991;350:429–31.

Carmichael WW, Boyer GL. Health impacts from cyanobacteria harmful algae blooms: implications for the north American Great Lakes. Harmful Algae. 2016;54:194–212.

Caulfeld CD, Cassidy JP, Kelly JP. Effects of gamma irradiation and pasteurization on the nutritive composition of commercially available animal diets. J Am Assoc Lab Anim Sci. 2008;47:61–6.

Cavin C, Marin-Kuan M, Langouët S, et al. Induction of Nrf2-mediated cellular defenses and alteration of phase I activities as mechanisms of chemoprotective effects of coffee in the liver. Food Chem Toxicol. 2008;46:1239–48.

Chain EPCF, Schrenk D, Bignami M, et al. Risk assessment of aflatoxins in food. EFSA J. 2020;18:e06040.

Chang J, Chen Z-l, Wang Z, et al. Oxidation of microcystin-LR in water by ozone combined with UV radiation: the removal and degradation pathway. Chem Eng J. 2015;276:97–105.

Chen J, Xie P, Zhang D, et al. In situ studies on the bioaccumulation of microcystins in the phytoplanktivorous silver carp (Hypophthalmichthys molitrix) stocked in Lake Taihu with dense toxic Microcystis blooms. Aquaculture. 2006;261:1026–38.

Chen J, Xie P, Zhang D, et al. In situ studies on the distribution patterns and dynamics of microcystins in a biomanipulation fish–bighead carp (Aristichthys nobilis). Environ Pollut. 2007;147:150–7.

Chen R, Seaton A. A meta-analysis of mortality among workers exposed to organic solvents. Occup Med. 1996;46:337–44.

Chen Y, Qin B, Teubner K, et al. Long-term dynamics of phytoplankton assemblages: Microcystis-domination in Lake Taihu, a large shallow lake in China. J Plankton Res. 2003;25:445–53.
Cicalese L, Curcuru G, Montalbano M, et al. Hazardous air pollutants and primary liver cancer in Texas. PLoS One. 2017a;12:e0185610.
Cicalese L, Raun L, Shirafkan A, et al. An ecological study of the association between air pollution and hepatocellular carcinoma incidence in Texas. Liver Cancer. 2017b;6:287–96.
Clemens S, Aarts MG, Thomine S, et al. Plant science: the key to preventing slow cadmium poisoning. Trends Plant Sci. 2013;18:92–9.
Coles JF, Jones RC. Effect of temperature on photosynthesis-light response and growth of four phytoplankton species isolated from a tidal freshwater river. J Phycol. 2000;36:7–16.
Copetti D, Finsterle K, Marziali L, et al. Eutrophication management in surface waters using lanthanum modified bentonite: a review. Water Res. 2016;97:162–74.
Cordeiro-Araújo MK, Chia MA, de Toledo Arruda-Neto JD, et al. Microcystin-LR bioaccumulation and depuration kinetics in lettuce and arugula: human health risk assessment. Sci Total Environ. 2016;566:1379–86.
Cotty P. Effect of harvest date on aflatoxin contamination of cottonseed. Plant Dis. 1991;75:312–4.
Cotty PJ, Cardwell KF. Divergence of west African and north American communities of aspergillus section flavi. Appl Environ Microbiol. 1999;65:2264–6.
Crush J, Briggs L, Sprosen J, et al. Effect of irrigation with lake water containing microcystins on microcystin content and growth of ryegrass, clover, rape, and lettuce. Environ Toxicol Int J. 2008;23:246–52.
D'Anglada LV, Donohue JM, Strong J, et al. Health effects support document for the cyanobacterial toxin microcystins. US Environmental Protection Agency, Office of Water; 2015.
Daou R, Joubrane K, Maroun RG, et al. Mycotoxins: factors influencing production and control strategies. AIMS Agri Food. 2021;6:416–47.
De Figueiredo DR, Azeiteiro UM, Esteves SM, et al. Microcystin-producing blooms—a serious global public health issue. Ecotoxicol Environ Saf. 2004;59:151–63.
Dehghani MH. Removal of cyanobacterial and algal cells from water by ultrasonic waves—A review. J Mol Liq. 2016;222:1109–14.
Diao E, Hou H, Dong H. Ozonolysis mechanism and influencing factors of aflatoxin B1: A review. Trends Food Sci Technol. 2013;33:21–6.
Dickens J, Whitaker T. Efficacy of electronic color sorting and hand picking to remove aflatoxin contaminated kernels from commercial lots of shelled peanuts. Peanut Science. 1975;2:45–50.
Díez-Quijada L, Prieto AI, Guzmán-Guillén R, et al. Occurrence and toxicity of microcystin congeners other than MC-LR and MC-RR: A review. Food Chem Toxicol. 2019a;125:106–32.
Díez-Quijada L, Puerto M, Gutiérrez-Praena D, et al. Microcystin-RR: occurrence, content in water and food and toxicological studies. A review, Environmental research. 2019b;168:467–89.
Ding W-X, Nam Ong C. Role of oxidative stress and mitochondrial changes in cyanobacteria-induced apoptosis and hepatotoxicity. FEMS Microbiol Lett. 2003;220:1–7.
Dohlman E. Mycotoxin hazards and regulations. Int Trade Food Safe. 2003;97
Du X, Liu H, Yuan L, et al. The diversity of cyanobacterial toxins on structural characterization, distribution and identification: A systematic review. Toxins. 2019;11:530.
Echenique R, Rodríguez J, Caneo M, et al. Microcystins in the drinking water supply in the cities of Ensenada and La Plata (Argentina). In: Congresso Brasileiro de Ficología & Simposio Latino-Americano de Algas Nocivas; 2006.
El Khalloufi F, Oufdou K, Lahrouni M, et al. Physiological and antioxidant responses of Medicago sativa-rhizobia symbiosis to cyanobacterial toxins (microcystins) exposure. Toxicon. 2013;76:167–77.
Ezzat S, Abdel-Hamid M, Eissa SA-L, et al. Associations of pesticides, HCV, HBV, and hepatocellular carcinoma in Egypt. Int J Hyg Environ Health. 2005;208:329–39.
Falconer I, Bartram J, Chorus I, et al. Safe levels and safe practices. Toxic cyanobacteria in water. 1999:155–78.
Fan X, Huang R, Chen H. Application of ultraviolet C technology for surface decontamination of fresh produce. Trends Food Sci Technol. 2017;70:9–19.

Fattovich G, Bortolotti F, Donato F. Natural history of chronic hepatitis B: special emphasis on disease progression and prognostic factors. J Hepatol. 2008;48:335–52.
FDA. GRAS status of ozone. Fed Regist. 1982;47(215):50209–10.
FDA. Code of federal regulations (Title 21, Vol. 3), 21CFR179.41. Silver Spring, MD: United States Government Printing; 1996.
FDA. FDA compliance policy guides: CPG Sec. 527.400, whole milk, low fat milk, skim milk aflatoxin M1. Silver Spring, MD: Food and Drug Administration; 2005.
Fedeli U, Mastrangelo G. Vinyl chloride industry in the courtroom and corporate influences on the scientific literature. Am J Ind Med. 2011;54:470–3.
Ferrín G, Guerrero M, Amado V, et al. Activation of mTOR signaling pathway in hepatocellular carcinoma. Int J Mol Sci. 2020;21:1266.
Frias HV, Mendes MA, Cardozo KHM, et al. Use of electrospray tandem mass spectrometry for identification of microcystins during a cyanobacterial bloom event. Biochem Biophys Res Commun. 2006;344:741–6.
Gayán E, Condón S, Álvarez I. Biological aspects in food preservation by ultraviolet light: A review. Food Bioprocess Technol. 2014;7:1–20.
Georges des Aulnois M, Roux P, Caruana A, et al. Physiological and metabolic responses of freshwater and brackish-water strains of Microcystis aeruginosa acclimated to a salinity gradient: insight into salt tolerance. Appl Environ Microbiol. 2019;85:e01614–9.
Giannuzzi L, Sedan D, Echenique R, et al. An acute case of intoxication with cyanobacteria and cyanotoxins in recreational water in Salto Grande dam. Argentina, Marine Drugs. 2011;9:2164–75.
Gong Y, Egal S, Hounsa A, et al. Determinants of aflatoxin exposure in young children from Benin and Togo, West Africa: the critical role of weaning. Int J Epidemiol. 2003;32:556–62.
Guchi E. Stakeholders' perception about aflatoxin contamination in groundnut (arachis hypogaea L.) along the value chain actors in eastern Ethiopia. Int J Food Contam. 2015;2:1–7.
Guo Y, Zhao L, Ma Q, et al. Novel strategies for degradation of aflatoxins in food and feed: A review. Food Res Int. 2021;140:109878.
Gurbuz F, Uzunmehmetoğlu OY, Diler Ö, et al. Occurrence of microcystins in water, bloom, sediment and fish from a public water supply. Sci Total Environ. 2016;562:860–8.
Harvey RW, Metge DW, LeBlanc DR, et al. Importance of the colmation layer in the transport and removal of cyanobacteria, viruses, and dissolved organic carbon during natural lake-bank filtration. J Environ Qual. 2015;44:1413–23.
He X, de la Cruz AA, Hiskia A, et al. Destruction of microcystins (cyanotoxins) by UV-254 nm-based direct photolysis and advanced oxidation processes (AOPs): influence of variable amino acids on the degradation kinetics and reaction mechanisms. Water Res. 2015;74:227–38.
He X, Liu Y-L, Conklin A, et al. Toxic cyanobacteria and drinking water: impacts, detection, and treatment. Harmful Algae. 2016;54:174–93.
Hell K, Cardwell KF, Setamou M, et al. The influence of storage practices on aflatoxin contamination in maize in four agroecological zones of Benin, West Africa. J Stored Prod Res. 2000;36:365–82.
Hernandez BY, Zhu X, Nagata M, et al. Cyanotoxin exposure and hepatocellular carcinoma. Toxicology. 2023;487:153470.
Huang Q, Li J, Zheng J, et al. The carcinogenic role of the notch signaling pathway in the development of hepatocellular carcinoma. J Cancer. 2019;10:1570.
Humpage A, Falconer I. Oral toxicity of the cyanobacterial toxin cylindrospermopsin in male Swiss albino mice: determination of no observed adverse effect level for deriving a drinking water guideline value. Environmental Toxicology: An International Journal. 2003;18:94–103.
Humpage AR, Fontaine F, Froscio S, et al. Cylindrospermopsin genotoxicity and cytotoxicity: role of cytochrome P-450 and oxidative stress. J Toxic Environ Health A. 2005;68:739–53.
Hussein A, Abdalla M, Hussein J, et al. Antioxidants in shoe-makers exposed to organic solvents. J Appl Sci Res. 2008;4:1107–17.
IARC. Ingested nitrate and nitrite, and cyanobacterial peptide toxins. In: IARC monographs on the evaluation of carcinogenic risks to humans; 2010a. p. 94.

IARC. Some non-heterocyclic polycyclic aromatic hydrocarbons and some related exposures. IARC Monogr Eval Carcinog Risks Hum. 2010b;92:1–853.
IARC. IARC monographs on the evaluation of carcinogenic risks to humans: arsenic, metals, fibres, and dusts. World Health Organization, International Agency for Research on Cancer Lyon. 2012a;100:11–465.
IARC. Chemical agents and related occupations. IARC Monogr Eval Carcinog Risks Hum. 2012b;100:9–562.
Im H, Oh E, Mun J, et al. Evaluation of toxicological monitoring markers using proteomic analysis in rats exposed to formaldehyde. J Proteome Res. 2006;5:1354–66.
Ito E, Kondo F, Harada K-I. First report on the distribution of orally administered microcystin-LR in mouse tissue using an immunostaining method. Toxicon. 2000;38:37–48.
Jackson LW, Pryor BM. Degradation of aflatoxin B 1 from naturally contaminated maize using the edible fungus Pleurotus ostreatus. AMB Express. 2017;7:1–7.
Jalilzadeh-Amin G, Dalir-Naghadeh B, Ahmadnejad-Asl-Gavgani M, et al. Prevalence and concentration of mycotoxins in animal feed in the Middle East and North Africa (MENA): A systematic review and meta-analysis. Toxins. 2023;15:214.
Ji X, Li Y, He J, et al. Depletion of mitochondrial enzyme system in liver, lung, brain, stomach and kidney induced by benzo (a) pyrene. Environ Toxicol Pharmacol. 2016;43:83–93.
Jin J, Kouznetsova VL, Kesari S, et al. Synergism in actions of HBV with aflatoxin in cancer development. Toxicology. 2023;153652
Kanoshina I, Lips U, Leppänen J-M. The influence of weather conditions (temperature and wind) on cyanobacterial bloom development in the Gulf of Finland (Baltic Sea). Harmful Algae. 2003;2:29–41.
Kapka-Skrzypczak L, Cyranka M, Skrzypczak M, et al. Biomonitoring and biomarkers of organophosphate pesticides exposure-state of the art. Ann Agric Environ Med. 2011;18:304.
Kensler TW, Qian G-S, Chen J-G, et al. Translational strategies for cancer prevention in liver. Nat Rev Cancer. 2003;3:321–9.
Kew MC. Aflatoxins as a cause of hepatocellular carcinoma. Journal of Gastrointestinal & Liver Diseases. 2013;22:305.
Khan NG, Correia J, Adiga D, et al. A comprehensive review on the carcinogenic potential of bisphenol A: clues and evidence. Environ Sci Pollut Res. 2021;28:19643–63.
Kirk GD, Bah E, Montesano R. Molecular epidemiology of human liver cancer: insights into etiology, pathogenesis and prevention from The Gambia. West Africa, Carcinogenesis. 2006;27:2070–82.
Kogelschatz U. Atmospheric-pressure plasma technology. Plasma Physics and Controlled Fusion. 2004;46:B63.
Koker L, Akcaalan R, Oguz A, et al. Distribution of toxic cyanobacteria and cyanotoxins in Turkish waterbodies. J Environ Prot Ecol. 2017;18:425–32.
Kotut K, Ballot A, Krienitz L. Toxic cyanobacteria and their toxins in standing waters of Kenya: implications for water resource use. J Water Health. 2006;4:233–45.
Kranz J, Hessel S, Aretz J, et al. The role of the efflux carriers Abcg2 and Abcc2 for the hepatobiliary elimination of benzo [a] pyrene and its metabolites in mice. Chem Biol Interact. 2014;224:36–41.
Kumar P, Hegde K, Brar SK, et al. Co-culturing of native bacteria from drinking water treatment plant with known degraders to accelerate microcystin-LR removal using biofilter. Chem Eng J. 2020a;383:123090.
Kumar P, Pérez JAE, Cledon M, et al. Removal of microcystin-LR and other water pollutants using sand coated with bio-optimized carbon submicron particles: graphene oxide and reduced graphene oxide. Chem Eng J. 2020b;397:125398.
Lawton LA, Robertson PK. Physico-chemical treatment methods for the removal of microcystins (cyanobacterial hepatotoxins) from potable waters. Chem Soc Rev. 1999;28:217–24.
Lee HS, Nguyen-Viet H, Lindahl J, et al. A survey of aflatoxin B1 in maize and awareness of aflatoxins in Vietnam. World Mycotoxin J. 2017;10:195–202.

Lee J, Her J-Y, Lee K-G. Reduction of aflatoxins (B1, B2, G1, and G2) in soybean-based model systems. Food Chem. 2015;189:45–51.
Lee J, Walker HW. Adsorption of microcystin-Lr onto iron oxide nanoparticles. Colloids Surf A Physicochem Eng Asp. 2011;373:94–100.
Lewis L, Onsongo M, Njapau H, et al. Aflatoxin contamination of commercial maize products during an outbreak of acute aflatoxicosis in eastern and Central Kenya. Environ Health Perspect. 2005;113:1763–7.
Li J, Li R, Li J. Current research scenario for microcystins biodegradation–a review on fundamental knowledge, application prospects and challenges. Sci Total Environ. 2017;595:615–32.
Li K, Geng Y, Lin B, et al. Molecular mechanisms underlying mitochondrial damage, endoplasmic reticulum stress, and oxidative stress induced by environmental pollutants. Toxicology Research. 2023;12:1014–23.
Li X, Chen S, Zeng J, et al. Impact of chlorination on cell inactivation, toxin release and degradation of cyanobacteria of development and maintenance stage. Chem Eng J. 2020;397:125378.
Lian L, Cao X, Wu Y, et al. A green synthesis of magnetic bentonite material and its application for removal of microcystin-LR in water. Appl Surf Sci. 2014;289:245–51.
Lim MH, Tay HSM, Devotta DA, et al. Risk Management of Cyanotoxins in Singapore. Journal of Water Resource and Protection. 2020;12:512–25.
Lindahl JF, Kagera I, Grace D. Aflatoxin M1 levels in different marketed milk products in Nairobi. Kenya, Mycotoxin Research. 2018;34:289–95.
Liu J, Sun Y. The role of PP2A-associated proteins and signal pathways in microcystin-LR toxicity. Toxicol Lett. 2015;236:1–7.
Liu R, Jin Q, Tao G, et al. Photodegradation kinetics and byproducts identification of the aflatoxin B1 in aqueous medium by ultra-performance liquid chromatography–quadrupole time-of-flight mass spectrometry. J Mass Spectrom. 2010;45:553–9.
Liu R, Wang R, Lu J, et al. Degradation of AFB1 in aqueous medium by electron beam irradiation: kinetics, pathway and toxicology. Food Control. 2016;66:151–7.
Liu Y, Wu F. Global burden of aflatoxin-induced hepatocellular carcinoma: a risk assessment. Environ Health Perspect. 2010;118:818–24.
Llana-Ruiz-Cabello M, Jos A, Cameán A, et al. Analysis of the use of Cylindrospermopsin and/or microcystin-contaminated water in the growth, mineral content, and contamination of Spinacia oleracea and Lactuca sativa. Toxins. 2019;11:624.
Lu K, Boysen G, Gao L, et al. Formaldehyde-induced histone modifications in vitro. Chem Res Toxicol. 2008;21:1586–93.
Luevano J, Damodaran C. A review of molecular events of cadmium-induced carcinogenesis. J Environ Pathol Toxicol Oncol. 2014;33:183.
Ma M, Liu R, Liu H, et al. Chlorination of Microcystis aeruginosa suspension: cell lysis, toxin release and degradation. J Hazard Mater. 2012;217:279–85.
Machado J, Campos A, Vasconcelos V, et al. Effects of microcystin-LR and cylindrospermopsin on plant-soil systems: A review of their relevance for agricultural plant quality and public health. Environ Res. 2017;153:191–204.
Magalhaes V, Marinho M, Domingos P, et al. Microcystins (cyanobacteria hepatotoxins) bioaccumulation in fish and crustaceans from Sepetiba Bay (Brasil, RJ). Toxicon. 2003;42:289–95.
Magzoub R, Yassin A, Abdel-Rahim A, et al. Photocatalytic detoxification of aflatoxins in Sudanese peanut oil using immobilized titanium dioxide. Food Control. 2019;95:206–14.
Massey IY, Yang F, Ding Z, et al. Exposure routes and health effects of microcystins on animals and humans: A mini-review. Toxicon. 2018;151:156–62.
Matthijs HC, Visser PM, Reeze B, et al. Selective suppression of harmful cyanobacteria in an entire lake with hydrogen peroxide. Water Res. 2012;46:1460–72.
Mchau GJ, Machunda R, Kimanya M, et al. First report of the co-occurrence of cylindrospermopsin, nodularin and microcystins in the freshwaters of Lake Victoria. Tanzania, Exposure and Health. 2021;13:185–94.

Medalcho TH, Abegaz K, Dessalegn E, et al. Aflatoxin B1 detoxification potentials of garlic, ginger, cardamom, black cumin, and sautéing in ground spice mix red pepper products. Toxins. 2023;15:307.
Medina Á, Rodríguez A, Magan N. Climate change and mycotoxigenic fungi: impacts on mycotoxin production. Curr Opin Food Sci. 2015;5:99–104.
Melaram R, Newton AR, Chafin J. Microcystin contamination and toxicity: implications for agriculture and public health. Toxins. 2022;14:350.
Menon A, Stojceska V, Tassou SA. A systematic review on the recent advances of the energy efficiency improvements in non-conventional food drying technologies. Trends Food Sci Technol. 2020;100:67–76.
Miyata M, Takano H, Guo LQ, et al. Grapefruit juice intake does not enhance but rather protects against aflatoxin B 1-induced liver DNA damage through a reduction in hepatic CYP3A activity. Carcinogenesis. 2004;25:203–9.
Modley L-AS, Rampedi IT, Avenant-Oldewage A, et al. Microcystin concentrations and liver histopathology in Clarias gariepinus and Oreochromis mossambicus from three impacted rivers flowing into a hyper-eutrophic freshwater system: A pilot study. Environ Toxicol Pharmacol. 2019;71:103222.
Mohamed Z, Carmichael W, An J, et al. Activated carbon removal efficiency of microcystins in an aqueous cell extract of Microcystis aeruginosa and Oscillatoria tenuis strains isolated from Egyptian freshwaters. Environmental Toxicology: An International Journal. 1999;14:197–201.
Mohamed ZA, Al Shehri AM. Microcystins in groundwater wells and their accumulation in vegetable plants irrigated with contaminated waters in Saudi Arabia. J Hazard Mater. 2009;172:310–5.
Mohamed ZA, Alamri S, Hashem M. The link between microcystin levels in groundwater and surface Nile water, and assessing their potential risk to human health. J Contam Hydrol. 2022;244:103921.
Mohamed ZA, Deyab MA, Abou-Dobara MI, et al. Occurrence of cyanobacteria and microcystin toxins in raw and treated waters of the Nile River, Egypt: implication for water treatment and human health. Environ Sci Pollut Res. 2015;22:11716–27.
Mohamed ZA, El-Sharouny HM, Ali WS. Microcystin production in benthic mats of cyanobacteria in the Nile River and irrigation canals. Egypt, Toxicon. 2006;47:584–90.
Mokhles M, Abd El Wahhab M, Tawfik M, et al. Detection of aflatoxin among hepatocellular carcinoma patients in Egypt. Pakistan Journal of Biological Sciences: PJBS. 2007;10:1422–9.
Mutoti MI, Edokpayi J, Mutileni N, et al. Cyanotoxins in groundwater; occurrence, potential sources, health impacts and knowledge gap for public health. Toxicon. 2023;107077
Nakavuma JL, Kirabo A, Bogere P, et al. Awareness of mycotoxins and occurrence of aflatoxins in poultry feeds and feed ingredients in selected regions of Uganda. Int J Food Contam. 2020;7:1–10.
Neilan BA, Pearson LA, Muenchhoff J, et al. Environmental conditions that influence toxin biosynthesis in cyanobacteria. Environ Microbiol. 2013;15:1239–53.
Nielsen MC, Jiang SC. Can cyanotoxins penetrate human skin during water recreation to cause negative health effects? Harmful Algae. 2020;98:101872.
Nisa A, Zahra N, Hina S. Detection of aflatoxins in rice samples, Bangladesh. J Sci Ind Res. 2014;49:189–94.
Niture S, Gadi S, Lin M, et al. Cadmium modulates steatosis, fibrosis, and oncogenic signaling in liver cancer cells by activating notch and AKT/mTOR pathways. Environ Toxicol. 2023;38:783–97.
Niture S, Gyamfi MA, Lin M, et al. TNFAIP8 regulates autophagy, cell steatosis, and promotes hepatocellular carcinoma cell proliferation. Cell Death Dis. 2020;11:178.
Nutrition E. 2022. https://ew-nutrition.com/mycotoxin-report-2021/
Nyakairu GWA, Nagawa CB, Mbabazi J. Assessment of cyanobacteria toxins in freshwater fish: a case study of Murchison Bay (Lake Victoria) and Lake Mburo, Uganda. Toxicon. 2010;55:939–46.
Ohad I, Raanan H, Keren N, et al. Light-induced changes within photosystem II protects Microcoleus sp. in biological desert sand crusts against excess light. PLoS One. 2010;5:e11000.

Organization WH. High-dose irradiation: wholesomeness of food irradiatied with doses above 10 kGy, vol. 890. World Health Organization; 1999.
Oudra B, Loudiki M, Sbiyyaa B, et al. Isolation, characterization and quantification of microcystins (heptapeptides hepatotoxins) in Microcystis aeruginosa dominated bloom of Lalla Takerkoust lake–reservoir (Morocco). Toxicon. 2001;39:1375–81.
Padedda BM, Sechi N, Lai GG, et al. Consequences of eutrophication in the management of water resources in Mediterranean reservoirs: A case study of Lake Cedrino (Sardinia, Italy). Global Ecology and Conservation. 2017;12:21–35.
Paerl HW, Paul VJ. Climate change: links to global expansion of harmful cyanobacteria. Water Res. 2012;46:1349–63.
Park J-A, Jung S-M, Choi J-W, et al. Mesoporous carbon for efficient removal of microcystin-LR in drinking water sources, Nak-Dong River, South Korea: application to a field-scale drinking water treatment plant. Chemosphere. 2018;193:883–91.
Parkin DM. The global health burden of infection-associated cancers in the year 2002. Int J Cancer. 2006;118:3030–44.
Peeters F, Straile D, Lorke A, et al. Earlier onset of the spring phytoplankton bloom in lakes of the temperate zone in a warmer climate. Glob Chang Biol. 2007;13:1898–909.
Peterson S, Lampe JW, Bammler TK, et al. Apiaceous vegetable constituents inhibit human cytochrome P-450 1A2 (hCYP1A2) activity and hCYP1A2-mediated mutagenicity of aflatoxin B1. Food Chem Toxicol. 2006;44:1474–84.
Pham TL, Shimizu K, Dao TS, et al. First report on free and covalently bound microcystins in fish and bivalves from Vietnam: assessment of risks to humans. Environ Toxicol Chem. 2017;36:2953–7.
Poste AE, Hecky RE, Guildford SJ. Evaluating microcystin exposure risk through fish consumption. Environ Sci Technol. 2011;45:5806–11.
Prandini A, Tansini G, Sigolo S, et al. On the occurrence of aflatoxin M1 in milk and dairy products. Food Chem Toxicol. 2009;47:984–91.
Probst C, Njapau H, Cotty PJ. Outbreak of an acute aflatoxicosis in Kenya in 2004: identification of the causal agent. Appl Environ Microbiol. 2007;73:2762–4.
Puga-Torres B, Salazar D, Cachiguango M, et al. Determination of aflatoxin M1 in raw milk from different provinces of Ecuador. Toxins. 2020;12:498.
Rahmani J, Alipour S, Miri A, et al. The prevalence of aflatoxin M1 in milk of Middle East region: A systematic review, meta-analysis and probabilistic health risk assessment. Food Chem Toxicol. 2018;118:653–66.
Rapisarda V, Loreto C, Malaguarnera M, et al. Hepatocellular carcinoma and the risk of occupational exposure. World J Hepatol. 2016;8:573.
Rezaitabar S, Sari AE, Bahramifar N, et al. Transfer, tissue distribution and bioaccumulation of microcystin LR in the phytoplanktivorous and carnivorous fish in Anzali wetland, with potential health risks to humans. Sci Total Environ. 2017;575:1130–8.
Roegner AF, Brena B, González-Sapienza G, et al. Microcystins in potable surface waters: toxic effects and removal strategies. J Appl Toxicol. 2014;34:441–57.
Romero-Oliva CS, Contardo-Jara V, Block T, et al. Accumulation of microcystin congeners in different aquatic plants and crops–A case study from Lake Amatitlán. Guatemala, Ecotoxicology and environmental safety. 2014;102:121–8.
Rose AK, Fabbro L, Kinnear S. Cyanobacteria breakthrough: effects of Limnothrix redekei contamination in an artificial bank filtration on a regional water supply. Harmful Algae. 2018;76:1–10.
Ruangrit K, Peerapornpisal Y, Pekkoh J, et al. Microcystin accumulation in Nile tilapia, Oreochromis niloticus and giant freshwater prawns, Macrobrachium rosenbergii in green water system cultivation. Int J Geosci. 2013;4:60–3.
Saad-Hussein A, Beshir S, Taha MM, et al. Early prediction of liver carcinogenicity due to occupational exposure to pesticides. Mutation Research/Genetic Toxicology and Environmental Mutagenesis. 2019;838:46–53.

Saad-Hussein A, Noshy M, Taha M, et al. GSTP1 and XRCC1 polymorphisms and DNA damage in agricultural workers exposed to pesticides. Mutation Research/Genetic Toxicology and Environmental Mutagenesis. 2017;819:20–5.
Saad-Hussein A, Ramadan HK-A. Impacts of climate change on environmental toxins and pollutants causing liver health problems. In: Saad-Hussein A, Elwakil R, Khomsi K, editors. Impact of climate change on health in Africa: A focus on liver and gastrointestinal tract. Cham: Springer; 2023. p. 53–78.
Saad-Hussein A, Shahy EM, Ibrahim KS, et al. Influence of GSTM1, T1 genes polymorphisms on oxidative stress and liver enzymes in rural and urban pesticides-exposed workers. Arch Environ Occup Health. 2022;77:800–8.
Saad AA-AM, El-Desokky SA, Sharada HM, Fouad MM. Hepatic health hazards of occupational exposure to products of polyurethane thermal degradations. Central European Journal of Occupational and Environmental Medicine (CEJOEM). 2004;10:319–32.
Saad A, Beshir S, Baathallah S. Prediction of respiratory hazards, cytotoxicity, and carcinogenicity of occupational exposure to formaldehyde in pathology laboratories. JASMR. 2006;1
Saad A, Hassanien MA. Assessment of arsenic level in the hair of the nonoccupational Egyptian population: pilot study. Environ Int. 2001;27:471–8.
Sagnelli E, Macera M, Russo A, et al. Epidemiological and etiological variations in hepatocellular carcinoma. Infection. 2020;48:7–17.
Satarug S. Long-term exposure to cadmium in food and cigarette smoke, liver effects and hepatocellular carcinoma. Curr Drug Metab. 2012;13:257–71.
Semyalo R, Rohrlack T, Naggawa C, et al. Microcystin concentrations in Nile tilapia (Oreochromis niloticus) caught from Murchison Bay. Lake Victoria and Lake Mburo: Uganda, Hydrobiologia. 2010;638:235–44.
Shearer J, Sweets L, Baker N, et al. A study of aspergillus flavus/parasiticus in Iowa crop fields: 1988-1990. Plant Dis. 1992;76:19–22.
Sherman M. Vinyl chloride and the liver. J Hepatol. 2009;51:1074–81.
Shi J, Zhu L, Liu S, et al. A meta-analysis of case–control studies on the combined effect of hepatitis B and C virus infections in causing hepatocellular carcinoma in China. Br J Cancer. 2005;92:607–12.
Shuib NS, Makahleh A, Salhimi SM, et al. Natural occurrence of aflatoxin M1 in fresh cow milk and human milk in Penang. Malaysia, Food Control. 2017;73:966–70.
Silva CF, Batista LR, Schwan RF. Incidence and distribution of filamentous fungi during fermentation, drying and storage of coffee (Coffea arabica L.) beans. Braz J Microbiol. 2008;39:521–6.
Simiyu BM, Oduor SO, Rohrlack T, et al. Microcystin content in phytoplankton and in small fish from eutrophic Nyanza gulf, Lake Victoria, Kenya. Toxins. 2018;10:275.
Singh S, Asthana RK. Assessment of microcystin concentration in carp and catfish: a case study from Lakshmikund Pond, Varanasi, India. Bull Environ Contam Toxicol. 2014;92:687–92.
Soni A, Smith J, Thompson A, et al. Microwave-induced thermal sterilization-A review on history, technical progress, advantages and challenges as compared to the conventional methods. Trends Food Sci Technol. 2020;97:433–42.
Steenland K, Palu S. Cohort mortality study of 57,000 painters and other union members: a 15 year update. Occup Environ Med. 1999;56:315.
Stepman F. Scaling-up the impact of aflatoxin research in Africa. The role of social sciences. Toxins. 2018;10:136.
Su PF, Lee TC, Lin PJ, et al. Differential DNA methylation associated with hepatitis B virus infection in hepatocellular carcinoma. Int J Cancer. 2007;121:1257–64.
Su Y, Zhao B, Guo F, et al. Interaction of benzo [a] pyrene with other risk factors in hepatocellular carcinoma: a case-control study in Xiamen. China, Annals of Epidemiology. 2014;24:98–103.
Sun S, Zhao R, Xie Y, et al. Photocatalytic degradation of aflatoxin B1 by activated carbon supported TiO2 catalyst. Food Control. 2019;100:183–8.
Sun X, Sun C, Zhang X, et al. Aflatoxin B1 decontamination by UV-mutated live and immobilized aspergillus Niger. Food Control. 2016;61:235–42.

Tamele IJ, Vasconcelos V. Microcystin incidence in the drinking water of Mozambique: challenges for public health protection. Toxins. 2020;12:368.
Thongkorn S, Kanlayaprasit S, Jindatip D, et al. Sex differences in the effects of prenatal bisphenol A exposure on genes associated with autism spectrum disorder in the hippocampus. Sci Rep. 2019;9:3038.
Tian M, Zhao B, Zhang J, et al. Association of environmental benzo [a] pyrene exposure and DNA methylation alterations in hepatocellular carcinoma: a Chinese case–control study. Sci Total Environ. 2016;541:1243–52.
Trung B, Dao T-S, Faassen E, et al. Cyanobacterial blooms and microcystins in Southern Vietnam. Toxins. 2018;10:471.
Tsai W-T. Human health risk on environmental exposure to Bisphenol-A: a review. J Environ Sci Health C. 2006;24:225–55.
Turner P, Mendy M, Whittle H, et al. Hepatitis B infection and aflatoxin biomarker levels in Gambian children. Trop Med Int Health. 2000;5:837–41.
Uccello M, Malaguarnera G, Corriere T, et al. Risk of hepatocellular carcinoma in workers exposed to chemicals. Hepat Mon. 2012;12:e5943.
USEPA. Drinking water health advisory for the cyanobacterial microcystin toxins. Eviron Protect Agency. 2015;75:49. https://doi.org/10.1590/S1980-57642009DN30100010.
Vacchi-Suzzi C, Kruse D, Harrington J, et al. Is urinary cadmium a biomarker of long-term exposure in humans? A review. Curr Environ Heal Rep. 2016;3:450–8.
van Vliet MT, Franssen WH, Yearsley JR, et al. Global river discharge and water temperature under climate change. Glob Environ Chang. 2013;23:450–64.
VoPham T, Bertrand KA, Hart JE, et al. Pesticide exposure and liver cancer: a review. Cancer Causes Control. 2017;28:177–90.
Wagacha J, Muthomi J. Mycotoxin problem in Africa: current status, implications to food safety and health and possible management strategies. Int J Food Microbiol. 2008;124:1–12.
Walsby AE, Schanz F, Schmid M. The Burgundy-blood phenomenon: a model of buoyancy change explains autumnal waterblooms by Planktothrix rubescens in Lake Zürich. New Phytol. 2006;169:109–22.
Wang B, Mahoney NE, Pan Z, et al. Effectiveness of pulsed light treatment for degradation and detoxification of aflatoxin B1 and B2 in rough rice and rice bran. Food Control. 2016;59:461–7.
Wang W, Wang P, Wang S, et al. Benchmark dose assessment for coke oven emissions-induced telomere length effects in occupationally exposed workers in China. Ecotoxicol Environ Saf. 2019;182:109453.
WHO. Arsenic. In: Toxicological evaluation of certain food additives and contaminants, WHO food additives series 18. Geneva: WHO's Office of Public Information; 1983. p. 176–202.
WHO. Water safety plan manual. World Health Organization; 2009.
Wild C, Turner P. The toxicology of aflatoxins as a basis for public health decisions. Mutagenesis. 2002;17:471–81.
Wild CP. Aflatoxin exposure in developing countries: the critical interface of agriculture and health. Food Nutr Bull. 2007;28:S372–80.
Wild CP, Fortuin M, Donato F, et al. Aflatoxin, liver enzymes, and hepatitis B virus infection in Gambian children, cancer epidemiology, biomarkers & prevention: a publication of the American Association for Cancer Research, cosponsored by the American Society of Preventive. Oncology. 1993;2:555–61.
Williams JH, Phillips TD, Jolly PE, et al. Human aflatoxicosis in developing countries: a review of toxicology, exposure, potential health consequences, and interventions. Am J Clin Nutr. 2004;80:1106–22.
Withers PJ, Neal C, Jarvie HP, et al. Agriculture and eutrophication: where do we go from here? Sustain For. 2014;6:5853–75.
Wu H, Wei G, Tan X, et al. Species-dependent variation in sensitivity of Microcystis species to copper sulfate: implication in algal toxicity of copper and controls of blooms. Sci Rep. 2017;7:40393.

Xiang L, Li Y-W, Wang Z-R, et al. Bioaccumulation and phytotoxicity and human health risk from microcystin-LR under various treatments: a pot study. Toxins. 2020;12:523.
Xie G, Hu X, Du Y, et al. Light-driven breakdown of microcystin-LR in water: a critical review. Chem Eng J. 2021;417:129244.
Yang Y, Yu G, Chen Y, et al. Four decades of progress in cylindrospermopsin research: the ins and outs of a potent cyanotoxin. J Hazard Mater. 2021;406:124653.
Yu SZ. Primary prevention of hepatocellular carcinoma. J Gastroenterol Hepatol. 1995;10:674–82.
Zamora-Barrios CA, Nandini S, Sarma S. Bioaccumulation of microcystins in seston, zooplankton and fish: A case study in Lake Zumpango, Mexico. Environ Pollut. 2019;249:267–76.
Zamyadi A, Greenstein KE, Glover CM, et al. Impact of hydrogen peroxide and copper sulfate on the delayed release of microcystin. Water. 2020;12:1105.
Zewde TW, Johansen JA, Kifle D, et al. Concentrations of microcystins in the muscle and liver tissues of fish species from Koka reservoir, Ethiopia: A potential threat to public health. Toxicon. 2018;153:85–95.
Zhang Y, Whalen JK, Sauvé S. Phytotoxicity and bioconcentration of microcystins in agricultural plants: meta-analysis and risk assessment. Environ Pollut. 2021;272:115966.
Zhao X, Liu Y, Guo Y-M, et al. Meta-analysis reveals cyanotoxins risk across African inland waters. J Hazard Mater. 2023;451:131160.

Imaging of HCC

5

Rasha S. Hussein

Abstract

Hepatocellular carcinoma (HCC) is a malignant primary hepatic tumor. It develops in cirrhotic liver. HCC generally presents late in the disease process and as a result the associated mortality is relatively high, with sources estimating it to be the third or fourth most common cause of death due to cancer worldwide. Imaging is the cornerstone for diagnosis of HCC. Screening is usually performed by using ultrasound examination. Ultrasonography surveillance for early detection of HCC improves survival in a cost-effective way and is endorsed by major practice guidelines. If imaging criteria is suggestive for HCC diagnosis, biopsy could be avoided. Multiple imaging modalities are available for assessing HCC at different stages either screening, diagnosis, staging and post-treatment evaluation. Diagnosis and staging are usually performed by cross-sectional imaging either CT or MRI. Sometimes PET-CT imaging could be used in initial staging especially prior to liver transplantation. Multiple imaging methods are also utilized for the evaluation of treatment response either after local regional treatment or systemic therapy.

Keywords

CT · MRI · HCC · LI-RADS · PET-CT · DWI · Loco-reginal treatment of HCC

R. S. Hussein (✉)
Department of Radiology, Interventional Radiology and Molecular Imaging, Faculty of Medicine, Ain Shams University, Cairo, Egypt
e-mail: rashasalah@med.asu.edu.eg

R. Elwakil et al. (eds.), *Approach to Hepatocellular Carcinoma (HCC) Management in Low/Middle-Income Countries*,
https://doi.org/10.1007/978-981-96-3894-9_5

Abbreviations

ACR	American College of Radiology
ADC	Apparent diffusion coefficient
AFP	Alpha-fetoprotein
APHE	Arterial phase hyperenhancement
CT	Computed tomography
DWI	Diffusion-weighted images
HCC	Hepatocellular carcinoma
IVC	Inferior vena cava
LI-RADS	Liver imaging reporting and data system
LMICs	Low/middle income countries
MPV	Main portal vein
MRI	Magnetic resonance imaging
PET	Positron emission tomography
RECIST	Response Evaluation Criteria in Solid Tumors
RFA	Radiofrequency ablation
SMA	Superior mesenteric artery
TACE	Trans-arterial chemoembolization
TARE	Trans-arterial radio embolization
US	Ultrasound

5.1 Introduction

Hepatocellular carcinoma (HCC) is the commonest primary liver tumor, comprising 75–85% of cases. HCC ranks sixth in global incidence after breast, lung, colorectal, prostate, and gastric cancer. In terms of mortality, it ranks third for both genders, and rates of incidence and mortality are 2–3 times higher in men than in women (Global Cancer Observatory 2024).

HCC generally presents late in the disease process and as a result the associated mortality is relatively high, with sources estimating it to be the third or fourth most common cause of death due to cancer worldwide (Altekruse et al. 2009; Akinyemiju et al. 2017). Five-year survival is <16%; however, when identified at an earlier stage, the 5-year survival rates have been as high as 93% (Siegel et al. 2013; Takayama et al. 2008).

Imaging plays a key role in surveillance, diagnosis, and staging as well as post-treatment follow-up. It was proved that ultrasound surveillance improves survival in a cost-effective way and is endorsed by major practice guidelines (Marrero et al. 2018; Galle et al. 2018; Omata et al. 2017). On the other hand, dynamic contrast-enhanced computed tomography (CT) takes advantage of the hemodynamic changes that occur in the cirrhotic nodule as it progresses to early HCC during the multistep process of hepatocarcinogenesis (Chartampilas et al. 2022).

This chapter highlights different imaging methods used for the diagnosis of HCC. All the figures in this chapter are Courtesy of the author except Fig. 5.8.

5.2 Screening

Patients with liver cirrhosis are at great risk to develop hepatocellular carcinoma (HCC) (Choi et al. 2014a, b). Early detection of HCC is crucial for prognosis and survival because in the early stages of HCC it is potentially curable. Commonly, HCC does not have specific symptoms. Surveillance strategy is important to detect HCC in its early stages and it is recommended by many societies (Bruix and Sherman 2011; Llovet and Bruix 2012). All guidelines recommend ultrasound (US) for surveillance. CT and MRI are not routinely used in surveillance except for limited situations, e.g., obesity (Omata et al. 2010). The American Association for the Study of Liver Diseases recommends US screening every 6 months (Bruix and Sherman 2011; Llovet et al. 2012; Esfeh et al. 2020). Advantages of US include noninvasive technique, accepted by the patients, and relatively low-cost (Cassinottoa et al. 2017).

In 2018, our department started surveillance for our patients with liver cirrhosis in Ain Shams University Hospitals, Cairo, Egypt by using LI-RADS v2017 screening protocol (LI-RADS US Algorithm Portrait 2017). The recommended views by the ACR guidelines are as follows for longitudinal images; left lobe: left of midline, at midline; include proximal abdominal aorta, celiac artery, and SMA, with IVC; include caudate lobe, MPV, and pancreatic head, with left portal vein and for right lobe: with gallbladder, with right kidney, including right hemidiaphragm and adjacent pleural space, far lateral, main portal vein; include grayscale and color Doppler, common bile duct at porta hepatis; include diameter measurement. As regards the transverse images, dome with hepatic veins, include entire right and left lobe with medial and lateral liver edges (on separate images as needed), left lobe: with left portal vein; falciform ligament to evaluate for the presence of patent paraumbilical vein, Main portal vein bifurcation; right lobe: with right portal vein, with main portal vein, with gallbladder, with right kidney and near liver tip (LI-RADS US Algorithm Portrait 2017).

In the Radiodiagnosis Department, Ain Shams University Hospitals, we apply "US visualization score"; A: No or minimal limitations; B: Moderate limitations; and C: severe limitations. This was mainly based on liver heterogenicity, beam attenuation and visualization of the entire hepatic parenchyma (LI-RADS US Algorithm Portrait 2017). We do "US category"; US-1; negative (No observation OR only definitely benign observation(s), repeat surveillance after 6 months), US-2; subthreshold (Observation(s) < 10 mm in diameter, not definitely benign, need short-term US follow-up in 3–6 months; and US-3; positive (observation(s) ≥ 10 mm in diameter, not definitely benign OR new thrombus in vein, needs further imaging assessment either CT or MRI) (LI-RADS US Algorithm Portrait 2017).

As reported by Son et al.; LI-RADS US scoring system, US-3 category demonstrated a high specificity yet with a low sensitivity for diagnosis of HCC. The US limitations includes increased body weight, Child-Pugh score B, and moderate to severe fatty liver (Son et al. 2019).

5.3 HCC Diagnosis and Staging

Diagnostic imaging tools are used to characterize positive surveillance tests or to characterize incidentally detected observations (Park and Kim 2020). In Egypt, the most frequently used diagnostic imaging is either contrast-enhancing CT or MRI. CT and MRI replaced tissue biopsy in most of the cases with liver cirrhosis and developing hepatic focal lesions (Hennedige and Venkatesh 2012).

5.3.1 Triphasic CT

For a long time, CT was the preferred imaging modality for the evaluation of patients with liver cirrhosis with hepatic focal lesions. The advantage of CT is that it is widely available, easy to perform and of the lower cost compared to MRI (Crocetti et al. 2011; Ayuso et al. 2012; Cunha et al. 2022). In Egypt, CT is the widely used imaging modality for evaluating hepatic focal lesions in cirrhotic patients. Classic HCC in CT shows early arterial enhancement followed by washout in portal/delayed phase with delayed pseudocapsular enhancement (Fig. 5.1) (Shah et al. 2007).

Unfortunately, there is atypical appearance of HCC in imaging as well. Atypical features in CT, e.g., fat content makes diagnosis of HCC more challenging (Fig. 5.2).

So, the diagnostic algorithm was made by American College of Radiology (ACR) to facilitate interpretation of atypical appearance of HCC, and it was called Liver Imaging Reporting and Data System (LI-RADS) (American College of Radiology. CT/MRI LI-RADS v2018 core). It started in 2011 and continuously updated till 2018. In our practice, we used LI-RADS for the evaluation of hepatic focal lesion in cirrhotic patient. It is a simple and a comprehensive method to communicate with our hepatologists. It minimized interobserver variability and improves communication (Cunha et al. 2022).

Triphasic CT is performed in three phases: late arterial phase, to visualize the peak of tumor enhancement; portal venous phase (60–70 sec post-injection) corresponding to the peak of parenchymal enhancement and peak to evaluate portal vein; and the delayed venous phase (180 s post-injection) for detection of washout and pseudocapsule enhancement (Choi et al. 2014a, b). The HCC diagnosis main features in LI-RADS are arterial phase hyperenhancement (APHE), lesion size, washout, capsule enhancement, and threshold growth. The LI-RADS classified detected observations from definitely benign (LR-1) to definitely HCC (LR-5). Other categories include tumor-in-vein (LR-TIV) and observation that is probably or definitely malignant but not HCC specific (LR-M).

CT sensitivity for lesions 2 cm or more is high (90%) and this sensitivity decreases with decrease of size; lesions measures 1–2 cm, CT sensitivity is 40–44% and lesions <1 cm have sensitivity of 10–33% (Choi et al. 2014a, b).

HCC could be solitary. But HCC are multifocal in about one-third of the patients (Okusaka et al. 2002). Multifocal HCC may be due to synchronous development of multiple, independent hepatic focal lesions or intrahepatic metastases from the

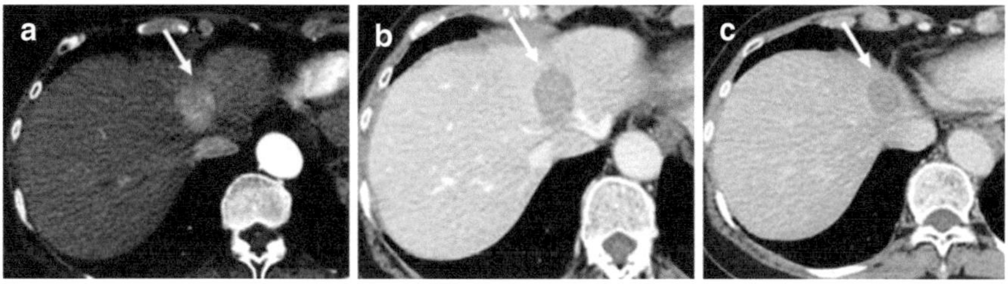

Fig. 5.1 Classic HCC. Triphasic CT in the arterial (**a**), portal venous (**b**), and delayed images (**c**). Hyper-enhancing left lobe focal lesion followed by washout is noted; classic appearance of HCC

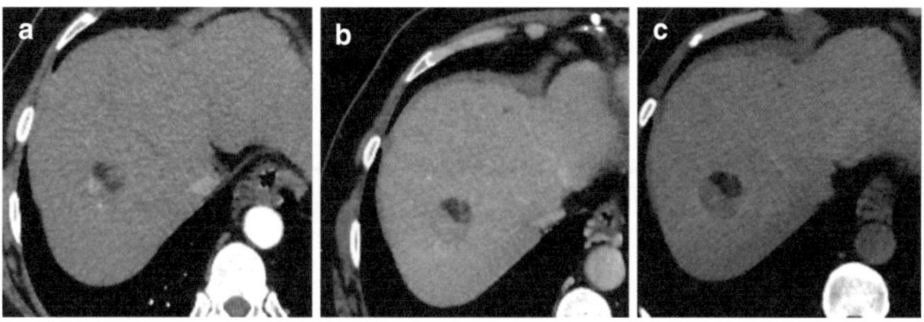

Fig. 5.2 Fat-containing HCC. Triphasic CT in the arterial (**a**), portal venous (**b**), and delayed images (**c**). Heterogeneously enhancing focal lesion is noted followed by washout. Noted the fat content of the focal lesion

primary tumor (Trevisani et al. 2008). Moreover, HCC can infiltrate venous drainage around the primary tumor to perform an infiltrative appearance. In the early stage of this infiltration, they appear as small satellites adjacent to the primary focal lesion (Jha et al. 2018).

HCC could infiltrate adjacent to vascular structures, e.g., portal vein, hepatic veins, and even IVC (Fig. 5.3). Hepatic arteries are not infiltrated (Kneuertz et al. 2012). This is one of the characteristic features for HCC diagnosis. The presence of the expansile, enhancing vascular thrombus within the portal vein or its branches is more diagnostic for HCC rather than other malignancy, e.g., cholangiocarcinoma or metastatic lesion, where in the latter tumoral thrombosis showed no expansion of the infiltrated vein. This vascular invasion is having a poor prognosis (Arif-Tiwari et al. 2014; Jha et al. 2018). Also, HCC can infiltrate adjacent biliary tree although not common (Wu et al. 2021).

5.3.2 Magnetic Resonance Imaging (MRI)

MRI could be recommended to evaluate the possibility of having small HCC in high-risk patients or if the CT is not conclusive. MRI has a higher sensitivity compared CT (84–90% compared to 47% with MRI and CT, respectively) (Ayuso et al.

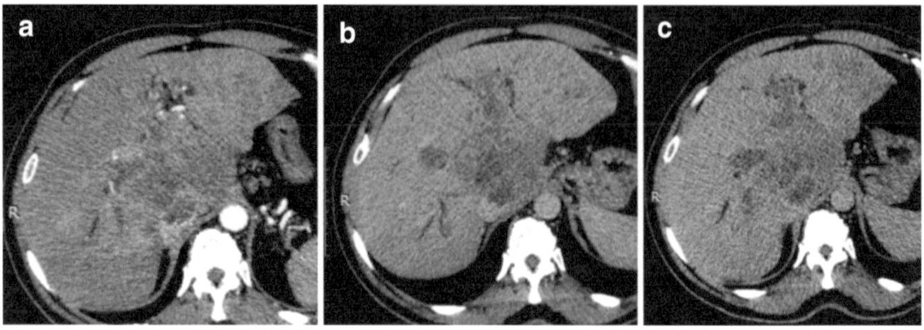

Fig. 5.3 Infiltrative HCC with associated LR-TIV. Triphasic CT in the arterial (**a**), portal venous (**b**), and delayed images (**c**). Diffuse infiltrative hepatic focal lesion is seen involving both hepatic lobes showing early heterogeneous enhancement followed by washout. Infiltration of the portal vein branches and the IVC are also noted by tumoral thrombus which is showing early enhancement followed by washout. Note the intra hepatic biliary dilatation as well as secondary to mass-effect/infiltration of the central biliary

2012; Liu et al. 2018; Kovac et al. 2020). But MRI is more expensive and not widely available, so it is resolved as a problem-solving tool.

Due to our relative limited resources in Egypt, MRI in initial staging is performed only in equivocal cases with discordant CT results with the clinical data. Also, it is performed for patients eligible for surgical intervention either resection or liver transplant to evaluate the true extent of the disease.

We perform the MRI on either 1.5 T or 3 T machine according to the availability. Our MR imaging protocol includes T2-weighted images, T1-weighted images (in phase–out of phase), heavy T2-weighted images, diffusion-weighted image (DWI), and ADC. Triphasic T1-weighted 3D GRE sequences using extracellular contrast agents (Fig. 5.4). We also add the subtracted images to discriminate between true enhancing lesions and/or hemorrhagic or intrinsically high signal nodules in pre-contrast T1-weighted images.

We do apply the LI-RADS scoring to evaluate any observation within the hepatic parenchyma. MRI is more helpful in evaluating the tumor heterogenicity regarding hemorrhagic content, fat content or cystic changes. We use the ancillary features, e.g., T2 signal, DWI signal, fat content (Fig. 5.5), nodule-in-nodule appearance (Fig. 5.6) to assess hepatic focal lesions.

Nodule-in-nodule appearance refers to malignant transformation of one of the regenerative nodules. However, the malignant part shows hyperintensity on the T2-weighted images, low signal on the T1-weighted image, restricted diffusion and the corresponding hyperenhancement on the dynamic study compared to the surrounding the appearance of the regenerative nodules being of low signal on the T2 weighted image, high signal on the T1-weighted images, no restricted diffusion and no appreciable enhancement (Fig. 5.6).

It is important to evaluate thrombosis of the portal vein and to discriminate between non-tumoral (bland) thrombus and tumoral thrombus. Discrimination

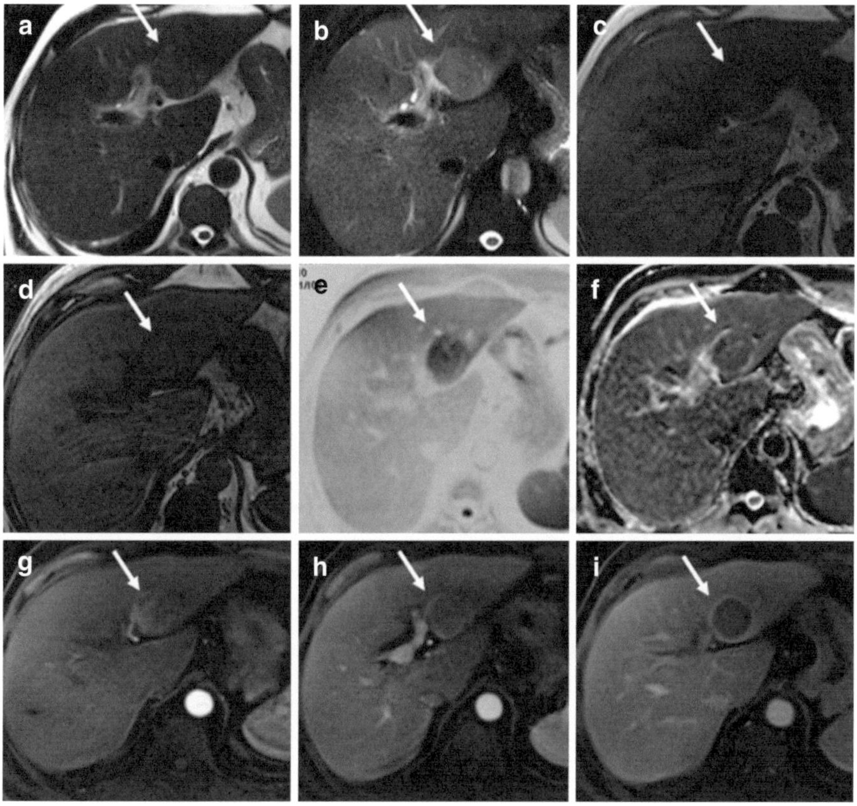

Fig. 5.4 Classic HCC in MRI. T2WI (**a**), T2 fat sat (**b**), T1 WI in-phase (**c**), T1 WI out-of-phase (**d**), inverse of DWI (**e**), ADC (**f**), dynamic study in the arterial (**g**), portal venous (**h**), and delayed images (**i**). Segment III focal lesion with intermediated signal on T2 and T2 fat sat, no dropped signal on out-of-phase. It shows restricted DWI. On dynamic study, it shows early enhancement followed by washout with delayed capsular enhancement

between both types of thrombi based on the T1 and T2 signal is difficult but the addition of the contrast-enhanced images allows better discrimination between both entities (Saddik et al. 1999) (Fig. 5.7).

In spite of that hepatobiliary contrast agents improves the detection of precancerous lesions and early stage of HCCs, we do not have these contrast materials (Zhou et al. 2017; Kogita et al. 2010).

DWI is a very helpful tool in the evaluation and detection of hepatic focal lesions as well as at its extension into the adjacent vascular structures. Diffusion gives an idea about the tissue cellularity and necrosis based on apparent diffusion coefficient (ADC) values. So, it can predict the degree of differentiation of the tumor. In spite of its high sensitivity, yet it shows low specificity to differentiate between benign and malignant tumoral thrombus. It does not add extra cost to MR technique (Granata et al. 2016; Li et al. 2016; Horvat et al. 2018).

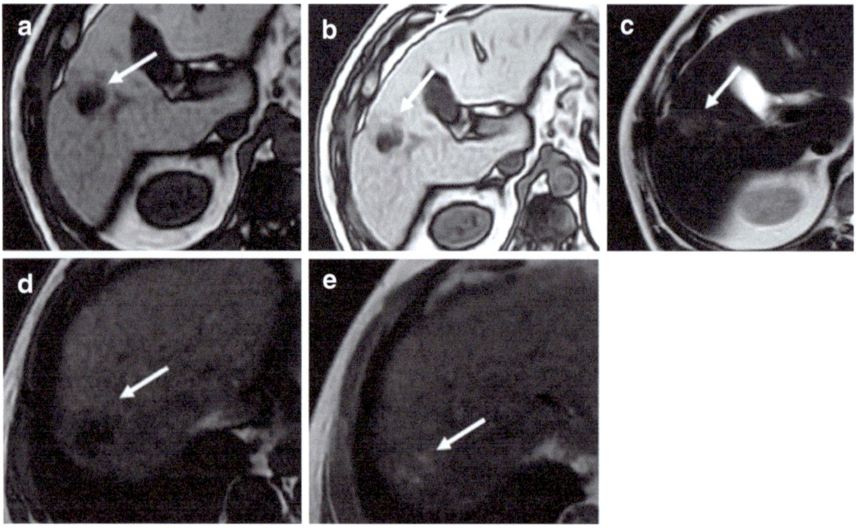

Fig. 5.5 Two patients with fat-containing HCC. First patient (upper raw): Dropped signal is noted on the out-of-phase imaging (**a**) compared to in phase image (**b**). The focal lesion is showing intermediate to high signal on T2-weighted images (**c**). Second patient (lower raw): Dropped signal is noted on the out-of-phase imaging (**d**) compared to in phase image (**e**)

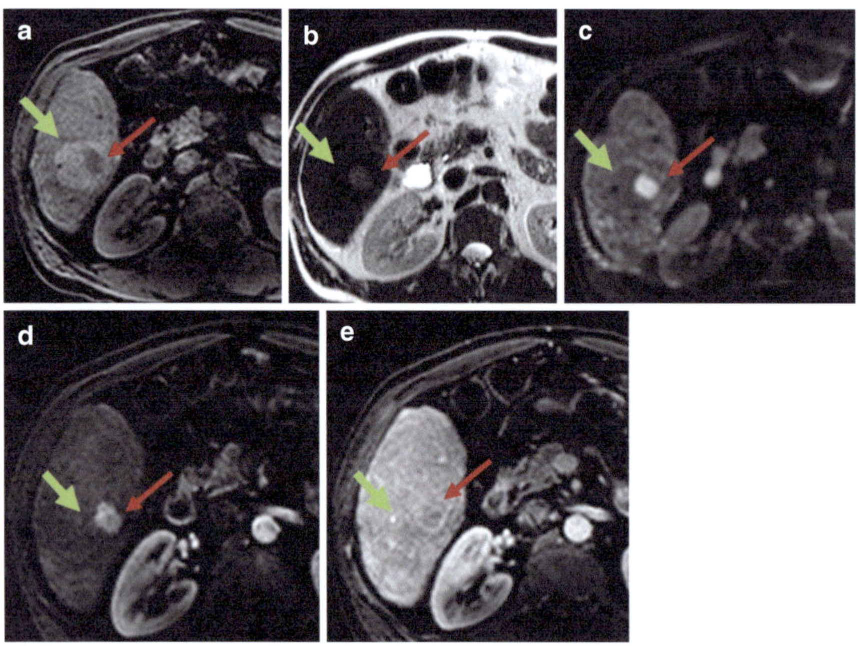

Fig. 5.6 Nodule-in-nodule: T1 fat sat (**a**), T2WI (**b**), DWI (**c**), arterial phase enhancement (**d**), and delayed image (**e**). There is a malignant transformation (red arrows) noted within regenerative nodules (green arrows) where there is malignant transformation show low signal on the T1-WI, high signal on the T2-WI, restricted diffusion with early enhancement and the followed by washout (red arrows). While the rest of the regenerative nodules show high signal on T1-WI, low signal on T2-WI, no restricted diffusion and isointense enhancement on the dynamic study (green arrows)

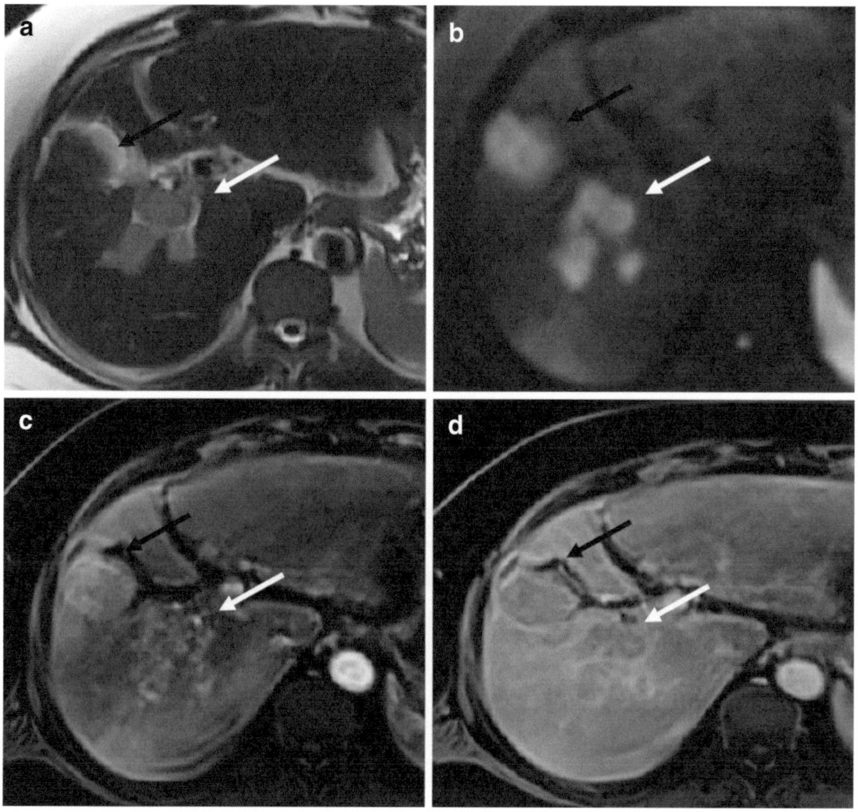

Fig. 5.7 LR-TIV. Tumoral thrombosis was seen at right portal vein and its branches (white arrows) showing intermediate signal on the T2-weighted image (**a**), restricted diffusion (**b**), with early enhancement (**c**) followed by washout (**d**). HCC with similar imaging pattern of the tumoral thrombus at right portal vein and its branch (black arrows)

DWI is a very helpful and sensitive tool in evaluating peritoneal deposits associated with the HCC (Gluskin et al. 2016; Ablefoni et al. 2022).

5.3.3 Positron Emission Tomography (PET) Imaging

PET-CT has a limited role in evaluating small, low-grade, well differentiated HCCs which appear to be negative on the PET image as it is masked by increased background liver activity (Hayakawa et al. 2014; Shaban 2018) (Fig. 5.8). It is more valuable in evaluating undifferentiated HCC, and this appears to be significantly avid on PET imaging. PET imaging can be used in initial staging of HCC. Some authors find that adding quantitative data to PET visual assessment can help in evaluation of low-grade metabolically active lesion. They assess the SUV ratio (tumor SUV_{max}/liver SUV_{mean}) and it was helpful in evaluating low grade tumors after treatment (Abdelhalim et al. 2020, Adbelrahman et al. 2021).

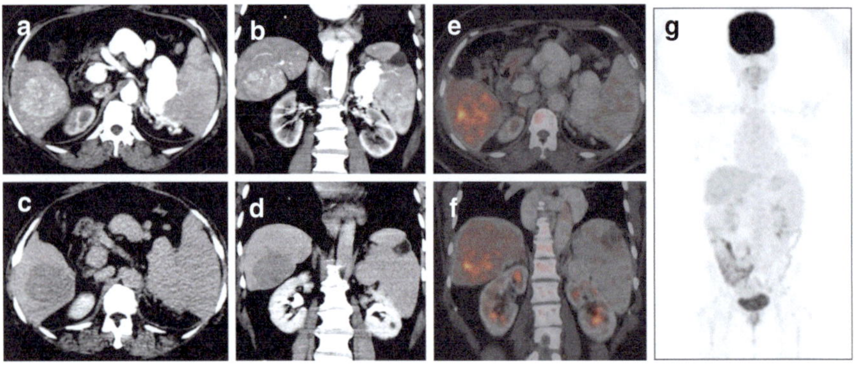

Fig. 5.8 PET/CT showing right hepatic focal lesion at segment VI. Arterial phases in axial (**a**) and coronal (**b**) show early enhancement. Delayed images in axial (**c**) and coronal (**d**) show washout. Fused PET-CT axial (**e**) and coronal (**f**) showed no significant FDG uptake which was confirmed in 3D-PET image (**g**).(Courtesy of Dr. Yehia Omar, MD, Radiology Consultant, Misr Radiology Center, Cairo, Egypt)

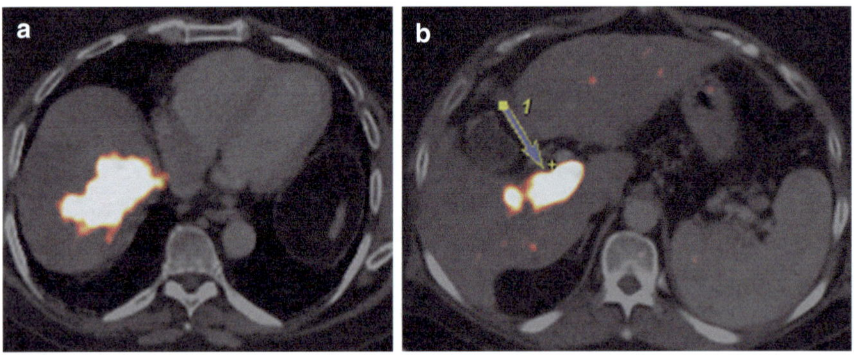

Fig. 5.9 Fused PET/CT showing infiltrative hepatic focal lesion at right lobe (**a**) associated with the tumoral thrombosis of the right portal vein (**b**) (arrow)

PET-CT is not used to evaluate the actual extent of the HCC in the hepatic parenchyma, but it is valuable in the evaluation of extrahepatic disease. PET imaging is used in evaluating patients who are prepared for liver transplantation to exclude extrahepatic disease, e.g., pulmonary, osseous, nodal, peritoneal deposits, soft tissue metastases, and bone metastases (Xia et al. 2014; Divisi et al. 2017). Also, PET imaging is very helpful in discriminating benign from malignant tumoral thrombus of the portal vein and its branches (Fig. 5.9).

5.4 Treatment Response Assessment

Multiple locoregional treatment options are available in our country and accepted by the patients including thermal ablation (radiofrequency ablation and microwave ablation), trans-arterial chemoembolization (TACE) and radio embolization (TARE). The policy in our hospital, Ain Shams University Hospital, is to perform the evaluation after one month of locoregional treatment whether it is thermal ablation or TACE. Longer time is needed after radio embolization to allow subsidence of the extensive inflammatory process induced and it is usually between 2 and 3 months after the procedure.

Proper evaluation after treatment is mandatory to plan further management strategy. Multiple evaluation systems are implemented to evaluate treatment response for solid tumors, e.g., World Health Organization criteria and Response Evaluation Criteria in Solid Tumors (RECIST) classification (Yaghmai et al. 2011). Both systems based on the change in size of the tumor after treatment. This is not proper for evaluating treatment response in HCC because of the change in size is not an indicator for proper treatment response after local regional treatment. Sometimes after local regional treatment the tumor becomes larger in size due to the post-treatment induced surrounding inflammation. Dedicated system for assessing post-treatment changes for HCC was used such as mRECIST. The system is depending mainly on the deep evaluation of the residual enhancing component rather than evaluating the size change of the tumor (Bruix et al. 2001; Lencioni and Llovet 2010). Evaluation of HCC treatment response after local regional treatment is relatively challenging in some cases. So, we also use the LI-RADS v2018 for the evaluation of treatment response either in the CT or MRI images to minimize inter-observer variability. MRI is also used in equivocal appearance in CT (Hussein et al. 2019).

LI-RADS treatment response algorithm includes LR-TR nonevaluable (inadequate image quality), LR-TR nonviable (no residual enhancing tumor), LR-TR viable (residual enhancing tumor), and LR-TR equivocal (when it is difficult to discriminate between the post-treatment inflammatory changes and the true residual viable tumor and in such cases we either refer to another imaging modality for discrimination between both entities or wait for the next follow-up). The evaluation is based on assessing the residual enhancing viable tumor. The residual tumor is usually seen at the periphery of the lesion and measuring the largest size of the viable nodules (Hussein et al. 2019).

Due to change in tumor vascular kinetics after treatment, the appreciable washout can be difficultly evaluated on the dynamic study. So proper evaluation of residual viable tumor could be evaluated by the presence of early arterial enhancement (Polikoff et al. 2022).

Most commonly, we use triphasic CT study to evaluate treatment response especially after thermal ablation. After TACE, we can use triphasic CT if the used substance in the procedure did not contain lipidol, e.g., drug-eluting beads. However, if lipidol was used, beaming artifacts of lipiodol hinder the proper evaluation of residual viable tumor (Fig. 5.10); then MRI is preferably performed (Fig. 5.11). In MRI, DWI can be helpful in discriminating viable from nonviable tumor.

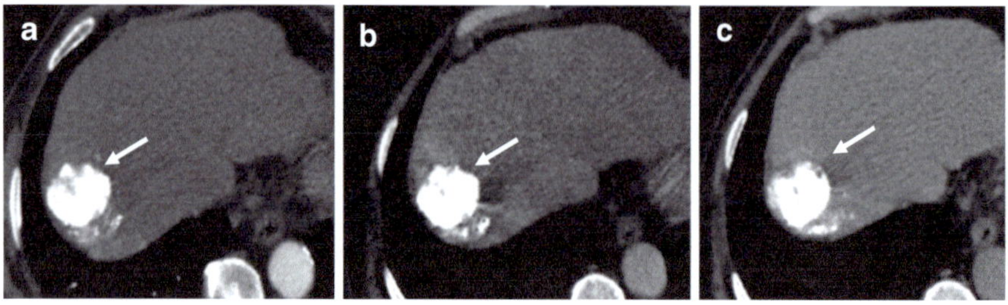

Fig. 5.10 Triphasic CT after TACE with Lipidol. Arterial phase (**a**), Venous (**b**), and delayed images (**c**) are showing dense lipidol concentration with surrounding beaming artifact hindering proper evaluation of any appreciable enhancing component

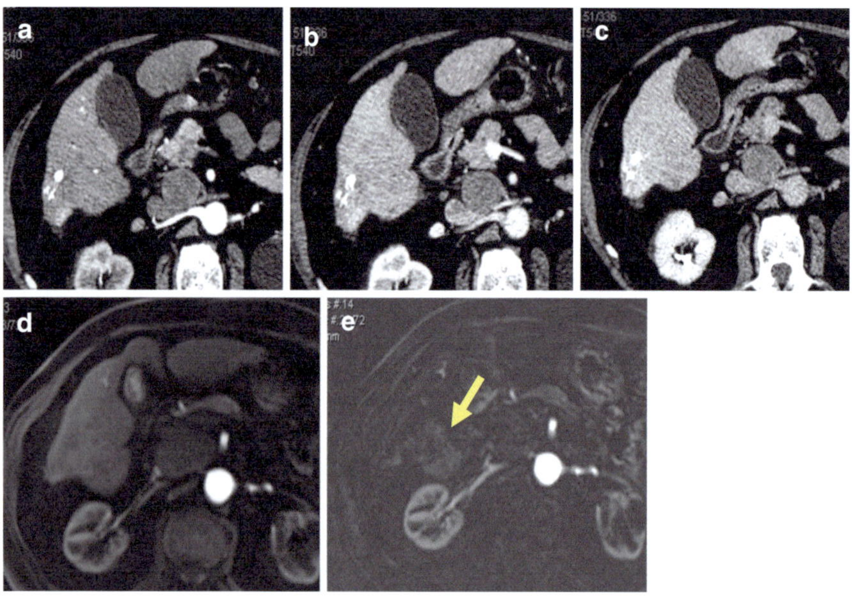

Fig. 5.11 Triphasic CT after TACE with lipidol. Arterial phase (**a**), Venous (**b**), and delayed images (**c**) are showing heterogeneous lipidol concentration with no definite enhancing component. Due to still high alpha-fetoprotein after TACE, MRI was done. Arterial phase (**a**) and subtraction (**e**) show enhancement at the exophytic component, denoting residual viable tumor that was not visualized on the triphasic CT

5.4.1 Post-Thermal Ablation Assessment

After thermal ablation, the coagulative necrosis remnant appears to be slightly hyperdense on the CT with no appreciable enhancement noted. Sometimes fainter wedge enhancement seen around the treated lesion attributed to a surrounding inflammation. On MRI, well-treated lesion appears to be hypointense on T1-weighted images due to coagulative necrosis with low signal on the T2-weighted images. After contrast injection no appreciable enhancement noted within the lesion and this is best seen on the subtracted images. In the immediate post-treatment evaluation, the treated lesion may appear to be larger than the initial primary tumor, then it becomes smaller in size over time (Mendiratta-Lala et al. 2020). Immediately after ablation, there is smooth thin peripheral wall enhancement noted. This peripheral enhancement is seen in the arterial phase and becomes isointense to the hepatic parenchyma on delayed images (Goldberg et al. 2000; Young et al. 2018). Also, wedged enhancement is seen around the treated lesion due to surrounding inflammation/small AV fistula.

In viable tumors, there are viable components that are seen mainly at the periphery of the treated lesion and not at the central part. The viable tumor may show early enhancement only or washout only. Thickened and irregular peripheral enhancement of the wall of the treated lesion is an another sign for viable tumor. Correlation with hyperintense signal on the T2-weighted images, impeded DWI and enlargement of the lesion could be helpful in the discriminating post-treatment changes from viable tumor. Sometimes follow-up every 3 months as indicated to discriminate between both entities (Crocetti et al. 2011; Mahmoud et al. 2016; Mahmoud et al. 2021).

Post-TACE Assessment

Chemoembolization induced necrosis of the tumor occurs either by induction of ischemic changes or by cytotoxic effect of the chemotherapeutic agents (Polikoff et al. 2022). Post-treatment hemorrhage, liquefactive necrosis, and edema may cause increase in the size of the tumor. Evaluation of treatment response is mainly based upon the absence of nodular enhancing components at the periphery of the lesion. Signal intensity of the lesion on the T1 and T2 MRI is valuable according to the content of the central part of the lesion. Subtracted images is very helpful in evaluating true treatment response especially if there is hemorrhagic content within the lesion with high signal on the precontrast T1-weighted images to discriminate between the enhancing components and the intrinsic high signal on T1-weighted (Chiu et al. 2016). Inflammatory changes appear as an area of the wedged enhancement around the treated focal lesion which may persist up to 1 year post-treatment.

5.4.2 Post-TARE Assessment

Post-radio embolization is more challenging in the evaluation of treatment response because of the extensive inflammatory process induced by the radioactive material. The evaluation after radio embolization should be postponed up to 3 months as post-treatment (Singh and Anil 2014). Variable degree of enhancement is encountered after TARE. Viable tumor is diagnosed by the presence of intralesional enhancement, peripheral nodular enhancement. If enhancement is present, follow-up should be considered to evaluate the size of the enhancing component to discriminate between the post-treatment enhancing part and the residual viable tumor. Also the presence of washout, restricted diffusion and high signal on T2 can suggest residual viable tumor rather than post-treatment changes.

Also, complications as post-treatment changes, e.g., biliary injury, infection or AV fistula should be evaluated (Hussein et al. 2019). The rare complication of HCC rupture after TACE should be taken into consideration.

5.4.3 Role of PET-CT in Post-Treatment Assessment

In Egypt which is one of the low/middle-income countries (LMICs), PET-CT is used as post-treatment tool in patients who were subjected to locoregional treatment, as bridge therapy, and are waiting for liver transplantation with rising serum AFP levels (Refaat et al. 2018).

5.4.4 Evaluation after Systemic Therapy Is Challenging

With the New era of using systemic/immune therapy for treatment of unresectable HCC, the evaluation of treatment response is crucial for continuation of the treatment. Evaluation is difficult as the reduction in size is relatively slow. Specific system is used for evaluation of the treatment response after immunotherapy named the revised Choi (rChoi). The evaluation is based on assessing the size of the tumor as well as its attenuation in CT. It defines partial response (PR) as both a 10% decrease in the tumor size and a 15% decrease in the tumor density of the target lesions (Xu et al. 2022).

5.5 Conclusion

HCC is a challenging healthcare problem in the low-income countries. Imaging is corner stone in the surveillance of the patients with liver cirrhosis for early detection of HCC. Ultrasound is the best imaging modality used in surveillance due to its low cost and availability. In spite of its availability, yet it lacks the sensitivity. Effect suspected the hepatic focal lesion in ultrasound; further cross-sectional imaging is advised for proper characterization. Initial characterization methodology is seen by triphasic CT due to its lower course compared to MRI and also due to its more availability. Characterization of the detected hepatic focal lesion is made by using LIRADS v2018. It categorized lesions from benign lesions show definite HCC. It also discriminate HCC from other malignant hepatic focal lesions and it is used to evaluate the tumoral thrombosis. If CT is the inconclusive in a high-risk patient, then MRI could be used for proper characterization of the hepatic focal lesion. Also,

LIRADS v2018 is used. PET-CT has limited role for evaluation of primary hepatic tumor or its extent within the hepatic parenchyma. The role of PET-CT is in staging for extrahepatic disease.

Multiple locoregional treatments are available and accepted by patients. According to tumor size and location, the best modality is selected for proper treatment. Evaluation of the treatment response after local regional treatment is mandatory. It could be performed either by CT or MRI. In post-TACE procedure, MRI is preferred. Sometimes PET CT could be used if local regional treatment was performed as bridge therapy prior to liver transplantation.

References

Abdelhalim H, Houseni M, Elsakhaw M, et al. Role of 18F-FDG PET-CT in initial staging of hepatocellular carcinoma and its impact on changing clinical decision. Egypt Liver Journal. 2020;10:3.

Abdelrahman AS, Abdel-Rahman AS, Taha NM. The role of functional imaging; DWI, ADC and 18F-FDG PET/CT in the evaluation of HCC treatment response after transarterial chemoembolization. Egypt J Radiol Nucl Med. 2021;52:217.

Ablefoni M, Leonhardi J, Ehrengut C, et al. Magnetic resonance imaging of peritoneal Carcinomatosis: evaluation of high b-value computed diffusion-weighted imaging. Imaging Curr Oncol. 2022;29:4593–603.

Akinyemiju T, Abera S, Ahmed M, et al. The burden of primary liver cancer and underlying etiologies from 1990 to 2015 at the global, regional, and national level: results from the global burden of disease study 2015. JAMA Oncol. 2017;3:1683–91.

Altekruse SF, McGlynn KA, Reichman ME. Hepatocellular carcinoma incidence, mortality, and survival trends in the United States from 1975 to 2005. J Clin Oncol. 2009;27:1485–91.

American College of Radiology. CT/MRI LI-RADS v2018 core. https://www.acr.org/-/media/ACR/Files/RADS/LI-RADS/LI-RADS-2018-Core.pdf

Arif-Tiwari H, Kalb B, Chundru S, et al. MRI of hepatocellular carcinoma: an update of current practices. Diagn Interv Radiol. 2014;2014(20):209–21.

Ayuso C, Rimola J, Garcia-Criado A. Imaging of HCC. Abdom Imaging. 2012;37:215–30.

Bruix J, Sherman M. American Association for the Study of Liver Diseases. Management of hepatocellular carcinoma: an update. Hepatology. 2011;53(3):1020–1022. 13.

Bruix J, Sherman M, Llovet JM, et al. Clinical Management of Hepatocellular Carcinoma. Conclusions of the Barcelona-2000 EASL conference. J Hepatol. 2001;35(3):421–30.

Cassinottoa C, Aubéb C, Dohanc A. Diagnosis of hepatocellular carcinoma: an update on international guidelines. Diagn Interv Imaging. 2017;9:379–91.

Chartampilas E, Rafailidis V, Georgopoulou V, et al. Current imaging diagnosis of hepatocellular carcinoma. Cancers (Basel). 2022;14(16):3997.

Chiu RYW, Yap WW, Patel R, et al. Hepatocellular carcinoma post Embolotherapy: imaging appearances and pitfalls on com-puted tomography and magnetic resonance imaging. Can Assoc Radiol J. 2016;67(2):158–72.

Choi JY, Lee JM, Sirlin C. CT and MR imaging diagnosis and staging of hepatocellular carcinoma: part I. Development, growth, and spread: key pathologic and imaging aspects. Radiology. 2014a;272:635–54.

Choi JY, Lee JM, Sirlin CB. CT and MR imaging diagnosis and staging of hepatocellular carcinoma: part II. Extracellular agents, hepatobiliary agents, and ancillary imaging features. Radiology. 2014b;273(1):30–50.

Crocetti L, Della Pina C, et al. Peri-intraprocedural imaging: US, CT, and MRI. Abdom Imaging. 2011;36(6):648–60.

Cunha GM, Hosseini M, Furlan A, et al. Hepatocellular carcinoma staging: differences between radiologic and pathologic systems and relevance to patient selection and outcomes in liver transplantation. AJR. 2022;218:77–87.

Divisi D, Barone M, Bertolaccini L, et al. Standardized uptake value and radiological density attenuation as predictive and prognostic factors in patients with solitary pulmonary nodules: our experience on 1,592 patients. J Thorac Dis. 2017;9(8):2551–9.

Esfeh JM, Hajifathalian K, Ansari-Gilani K. Sensitivity of ultrasound in detecting hepatocellular carcinoma in obese patients compared to explant pathology as the gold standard. Clin Mol Hepatol. 2020;26:54–9.

Galle PR, Forner A, Llovet JM, et al. EASL clinical practice guidelines: management of hepatocellular carcinoma. J Hepatol. 2018;69:182–236.

Global Cancer Observatory. Available online: http://globocan.iarc.fr/Default.aspx. Accessed on March 2024.

Gluskin J, Chegai F, Monti S, Squillaci E, Mannelliet L. Hepatocellular carcinoma and diffusion-weighted MRI: detection and evaluation of treatment response. J Cancer. 2016;7(11):1565–70.

Goldberg SN, Gazelle GS, Mueller PR. Thermal ablation therapy for focal malignancy: a unified approach to underlying principles, techniques, and diagnostic imaging guidance. AJR Am J Roentgenol. 2000;174(2):323–31.

Granata V, Fusco R, Catalano O, et al. Intravoxel incoherent motion (IVIM) in diffusion-weighted imaging (DWI) for hepatocellular carcinoma: correlation with histologic grade. Oncotarget. 2016;7:79357–64.

Hayakawa N, Nakamoto Y, Nakatani K, et al. Clinical utility and limitations of FDG PET in detecting recurrent hepatocellular carcinoma in postoperative patients. Int J Clin Oncol. 2014;19:1020–8.

Hennedige T, Venkatesh SK. Imaging of hepatocellular carcinoma: diagnosis, staging and treatment monitoring. Cancer Imaging. 2012;12(3):530–47.

Horvat N, Monti S, Oliveira BC, et al. State of the art in magnetic resonance imaging of hepatocellular carcinoma Radiol. Oncologia. 2018;52(4):353–64.

Hussein RS, Tantawy W, Abbas YA. MRI assessment of hepatocellular carcinoma after locoregional therapy. Insights Imaging. 2019;10:8.

Jha RC, Khera SS, Kalaria AD. Portal vein thrombosis: imaging the Spectrum of disease with an emphasis on MRI features. AJR. 2018;211:14–24.

Kneuertz PJ, Demirjian A, Firoozmand A, et al. Diffuse infiltrative hepatocellular carcinoma: assessment of presentation, treatment, and outcomes. Ann Surg Oncol. 2012;19(9):2897–907.

Kogita S, Imai Y, Okada M, et al. Gd-EOB-DTPA-enhanced magnetic resonance images of hepatocellular carcinoma: cor-relation with histological grading and portal blood flow. Eur Radiol. 2010;20:2405–13.

Kovac JD, Milovanovic T, Dugalic V, Dumic I. Pearls and pitfalls in magnetic resonance imaging of hepatocellular carcinoma. World J Gastroenterol. 2020;26(17):2012–29.

Lencioni R, Llovet JM. Modified RECIST (mRECIST) assessment for hepatocellular carcinoma. Semin Liver Dis. 2010;30(1):52–60.

Li X, Zhang K, Shi Y, et al. Correlations between the minimum and mean apparent diffusion coefficient values of hepatocellular carcinoma and tumor grade. J Magn Reason Imaging. 2016;44:1442–7.

LI-RADS US Algorithm Portrait 2017. https://www.acr.org/-/media/ACR/Files/RADS/LI-RADS/LI-RADS-US-Algorithm-Portrait-2017.pdf

Llovet JM, Bruix J. Hepatocellular carcinoma. Lancet. 2012;379:1245–55.

Liu W, Qin J, Guo R, et al. Accuracy of the diagnostic evaluation of hepatocellular carcinoma with LI-RADS. Acta Radiol. 2018;59(2):140–6.

Llovet JM, Ducreux M, Lencioni R, et al. European Association for the Study of the liver; European Organisation for Research and Treatment of Cancer. EASL-EORTC clinical practice guidelines: management of hepatocellular carcinoma. J Hepatol. 2012;56(4):908–43.
Mahmoud B, Elkholy SF, Nabeel M, et al. Role of MRI in the assessment of treatment response after radiofrequency and microwave ablation therapy for hepatocellular carcinoma. Egypt J Radiol Nucl Med. 2016;47(2):377–85.
Mahmoud BE, Gadalla AAEH, Elkholy SF. The role of dynamic and diffusion MR imaging in therapeutic response assessment after microwave ablation of hepatocellular carcinoma using LI-RADS v2018 treatment response algorithm. Egypt J Radiol Nucl Med. 2021;52:60.
Marrero JA, Kulik LM, Sirlin CB, et al. Diagnosis, staging, and management of hepatocellular carcinoma: 2018 practice guidance by the American Association for the Study of Liver Diseases. Hepatology. 2018;68:723–50.
Mendiratta-Lala M, Masch WR, Shamp K, et al. MRI assessment of hepatocellular carcinoma after local-regional therapy: a comprehensive review. Radiol Imaging Cancer. 2020;2:1.
Okusaka T, Okada S, Ueno H, et al. Satellite lesions in patients with small hepatocellular carcinoma with reference to clinicopathologic features. Cancer. 2002;95(9):1931–7.
Omata M, Cheng A-L, Kokudo N, et al. Asia–Pacific clinical practice guidelines on the management of hepatocellular carcinoma: a 2017 update. Hepatol Int. 2017;11:317–70.
Omata M, Lesmana LA, Tateishi R, et al. Asian Pacific Association for the Study of the Liver consensus recommendations on hepatocellular carcinoma. Hepatol Int. 2010;4(2):439–74.
Park HJ, Kim SY. Imaging modalities for hepatocellular carcinoma surveillance: expanding horizons beyond ultrasound. J Liver Cancer. 2020;20(2):99–105.
Polikoff A, Wessner CE, Rashmi Balasubramanya R, et al. Imaging appearance of residual HCC following incomplete transarterial chemoembolization on contrast-enhanced imaging. Abdom Radiol. 2022;47(1):152–60.
Refaat R, Basha MA, Hassan MS, et al. Efficacy of contrast-enhanced FDG PET/CT in patients awaiting liver transplantation with rising alpha-fetoprotein after bridge therapy of hepatocellular carcinoma. Eur Radiol. 2018;28:5356–67.
Saddik D, Frazer C, Robbins P, et al. Gadolinium-enhanced three-dimensional MR portal venography. AJR. 1999;172:413–7.
Shaban EAIN. Can fluorine-18-fluorodeoxyglucose positron emission tomography/computed tomography detect hepatocellular carcinoma and its extrahepatic metastases? The Egyptian Journal of Radiology and Nuclear Medicine. 2018;49:196–20.
Shah ZK, McKernan MG, Hahn PF, et al. Enhancing and expansile portal vein thrombosis: value in the diagnosis of hepatocellular carcinoma in patients with multiple hepatic lesions. AJR. 2007;188:1320–3.
Siegel R, Naishadham D, Jemal A. Cancer statistics, 2013. CA Cancer J Clin. 2013;63:11–30.
Singh P, Anil G. Yttrium-90 radioembolization of liver tumors: what do the images tell us? Cancer Imaging. 2014;13(4):645–57.
Son JH, Choi SH, Kim SY, et al. Validation of US liver imaging reporting and data system version 2017 in patients at high risk for hepatocellular carcinoma. Radiology. 2019;292:390–7.
Takayama T, Makuuchi M, Kojiro M, et al. Early hepatocellular carcinoma: pathology, imaging, and therapy. Ann Surg Oncol. 2008;15:972–8.
Trevisani F, Cantarini MC, Wands JR, Bernardi M. Recent advances in the natural history of hepatocellular carcinoma. Carcinogenesis. 2008;29(7):1299–305.
Wu J, Huang L, Bai Y, et al. Imaging features of hepatocellular carcinoma with bile duct tumor thrombus: a multicenter study. Front Oncol. 2021;11:723455.
Xia F, Wu L, Lau W-Y, et al. Positive lymph node metastasis has a marked impact on the long-term survival of patients with hepatocellular carcinoma with extrahepatic metastasis. PLoS One. 2014;9(4):e95889.

Xu Y, Yang Y, Li L, et al. Different radiological criteria for early tumor response evaluation in patients with Unresectable hepatocellular carcinoma treated with anti-PD-1 antibody plus bevacizumab. Front Oncol. 2022;12:848129.
Yaghmai V, Miller FH, Rezai P, et al. Response to treatment series: part 2, tumor response assessment—using new and conventional criteria. AJR. 2011;197:18–27.
Young S, Taylor AJ, Sanghvi T. Post Locoregional therapy treatment imaging in hepatocellular carcinoma patients: a literature-based review. J Clin Transl Hepatol. 2018;6(2):189–97.
Zhou W, Zhang L, Wang K, et al. Malignancy characterization of hepatocellular carcinomas based on texture analysis of contrast-enhanced MR images. J Magn Reson Imaging May. 2017;45(5):1476–84.

Surgical Management of Hepatocellular Carcinoma

6

Hany M. Dabbous and Mohamed Fathy Abdel Ghaffar

Abstract

Surgical intervention remains a primary curative option for managing hepatocellular carcinoma (HCC) in low-income countries. Liver resection is considered safer in patients without cirrhosis and in those with Child-Pugh A cirrhosis when portal hypertension is absent. However, preoperative evaluation using indocyanine green clearance is often unavailable in these settings. Instead, upper endoscopy and measurement of hepatic venous pressure gradient are commonly employed to assess portal hypertension before surgery. Postoperative recurrence and hepatic decompensation are frequent challenges following resection. In many low- and middle-income countries (LMICs), where cadaveric organ donation programs are scarce, living donor liver transplantation (LDLT) serves as the only curative option for patients with HCC and advanced cirrhosis. Yet, factors such as limited donor availability, cultural barriers, financial constraints, and resource shortages contribute to high dropout rates among patients awaiting transplantation. Ensuring donor safety through comprehensive preoperative evaluation, implementing stringent legal frameworks to prevent organ trafficking and donor coercion, are essential components of a successful LDLT program.

In several countries, outreach transplant initiatives have been launched with support from international surgical societies and visiting experts. Despite national support schemes, the high cost of postoperative care, particularly immunosuppressive therapy, can impact recipient adherence to follow-up care. Some

H. M. Dabbous (✉)
Tropical Medicine Department, Ain Shams Center for Organ Transplant, Ain Shams University, Cairo, Egypt

M. F. A. Ghaffar
Department of Surgery, Ain Shams Center for Organ Transplant, Ain Shams University, Cairo, Egypt

R. Elwakil et al. (eds.), *Approach to Hepatocellular Carcinoma (HCC) Management in Low/Middle-Income Countries*,
https://doi.org/10.1007/978-981-96-3894-9_6

transplant centers sustain their activities through a combination of government funding, community initiatives, and charitable contributions. Although new hepatopancreatobiliary surgical units and transplant programs are emerging in various LMICs with international collaboration, the substantial economic burden remains a significant barrier to widespread implementation.

Keywords

HCC · Hepatocellular carcinoma · Liver transplantation · Living donor · Liver resection · LMICs

Abbreviations

AALDLT	Adult Living Donor Liver Transplantation
AASLD	American Association for The Study of Liver Diseases
AFP	Alpha-Fetoprotein
AKI	Acute Kidney Injury
ALI	Acute Lung Injury
ALT	Alanine Transaminase
APVB	Anomalous Portal Venous Branches
AR	Acute Rejection
AR	Anatomical Resection
ARDS	Acute Respiratory Distress Syndrome
AST	Aspartate Aminotransferase
BCLC	Barcelona Clinic Liver Cancer
BMI	Body Mass Index
CKD	Chronic Kidney Disease
CR	Chronic Rejection
CSA	Cyclosporine
CT	Computed Tomography
CVP	Venous Pressure
DDLT	Deceased Donor Liver Transplant
EASL	European Association for the Study of the Liver
eGFR	Mean Glomerular Filtration Rate
ELSD	Extra-Corporal Liver Support Devices
PTFE	Polytetrafluorethylene
ERCP	Endoscopic Retrograde Cholangiopancreatography
FDA	Food and Drug Administration
GW/RW	Graft Weight To Recipient Weight
HA	Hepatic Artery
HAS	Hepatic Artery Stenosis
HAT	Hepatic Artery Thrombosis
HBV	Hepatitis B Virus

HCC	Hepatocellular Carcinoma
HCV	Hepatitis C Virus
HOC	Hyperosmolar Citrate
HTK	Histidine, Tryptophan, And Ketoglutarate
HVPG	Hepatic Venous Pressure Gradient
ICG-R15	Indocyanine Green 15-Minute Retention Rate
INR	International Normalized Ratio
ISGLS	International Study Group of Liver Surgery
LDLT	Living Donor Liver Transplantation
LMICs	Low/Middle-Income Countries
LT	Liver Transplantation
MARS	Molecular Adsorbent Recirculating System
MELD	Model for End-Stage Liver Disease
MRCP	Magnetic Resonance Cholangiopancreatography
MRI	Magnetic Resonance Imaging
mTOR	Mammalian Target of Rapamycin
MVI	Microvascular Invasion
NAC	N-Acetylcysteine
NCI	National Cancer Institute
OS	Overall Survival
PHLF	Post-hepatectomy Liver Failure
PTLD	Post-transplantation Lymphoproliferative Disease
PV	Portal Vein
PVS	Portal Vein Stenosis
PVT	Portal Vein Thrombosis
RETREAT	Risk Estimation of Tumor Recurrence After Transplant
RPR	Rapid Plasma Regain
SMV	Superior Mesenteric Vein
TACE	Trans-Arterial Chemoembolization
TNM	Tumor, Node, Metastasis
UAE	United Arab of Emirates
UMHTC	United States Multicenter HCC Transplant Consortium
US	Ultrasonography
UW	University of Wisconsin
VEGF	Vascular Endothelial Growth Factor

6.1 Introduction

Surgical management remains the only potentially curative treatment for hepatocellular carcinoma (HCC). Treatment decisions depend on tumor characteristics, hepatic functional reserve, organ availability, waiting time, and local expertise and resources. Currently, surgical resection, orthotopic liver transplantation (LT), and local ablative therapies are the main potentially curative options (Ziparo et al. 2002).

Liver transplantation is considered the ideal treatment for HCC. However, organ shortage continues to pose a significant challenge (Yao et al. 2002). In low- and middle-income countries (LMICs), financial constraints further limit access to liver transplantation.

This chapter discusses the surgical options available for treating HCC, highlighting the specific challenges of liver transplantation and barriers to surgical treatment of HCC in LMICs.

6.2 Liver Resection

Historically, liver resection (LR) was regarded as a high-risk procedure (Foster and Berman 1977), with mortality rates reaching up to 10% in some centers (Thompson et al. 1983). However, advances in perioperative management and surgical techniques have significantly improved outcomes, with current mortality rates below 3% and five-year survival rates approaching 70% (Lee et al. 2010).

6.2.1 Preoperative Evaluation

HCC in non-cirrhotic livers is an excellent indication for liver resection (Llovet et al. 2005).

In cirrhotic patients, however, resection becomes more complex and requires careful assessment of residual liver volume, portal pressure, and severity of cirrhosis.

6.2.1.1 Child-Pugh Classification

The Child-Pugh score is commonly used to assess hepatic functional reserve preoperatively. Liver resection can be safely performed in patients with Child-Pugh class A cirrhosis, although this classification alone may not be sufficient in all cases (Belghiti et al. 2000).

6.2.1.2 Indocyanine Green 15-Minute Retention Rate (ICG-R15)

The ICG-R15 test has been proposed as a predictor of residual liver function (Makuuchi and Sano 2004).

Indocyanine green (ICG) is a plasma protein-bound dye exclusively metabolized by hepatocytes (Prodeau et al. 2019), and its clearance can now be measured directly using fingertip optical sensors (Giannelli et al. 2020).

Patients with ICG-R15 < 14% are considered suitable candidates for major hepatectomy (Clavien et al. 2007).

The Makuuchi algorithm proposes the following ICG-R15 thresholds:

- **<10%**: Suitable for trisectionectomy or bisegmentectomy
- **10–19%**: Suitable for hemihepatectomy or right-sided sectionectomy
- **20–29%**: Suitable for segmentectomy

- **30–39%**: Suitable for limited resection (e.g., wedge resection)
- **≥40%**: Enucleation only.

A French multicenter study reported that 92% of patients survived 3 months post-resection, highlighting the effectiveness of preoperative assessment (Prodeau et al. 2019).

6.2.1.3 Portal Pressure Assessment

Portal hypertension (PH) and serum bilirubin levels are key factors determining respectability. Signs suggestive of PH include esophageal varices, thrombocytopenia (<100,000/mm^3), and splenomegaly.

The hepatic venous pressure gradient (HVPG) is the gold standard for measuring portal pressure. An HVPG >6 mmHg indicates cirrhosis (Blasco et al. 2006), and HVPG is measured invasively via the transjugular route.

Guidelines from the European Association for the Study of the Liver (EASL) and the American Association for the Study of Liver Diseases (AASLD) recommend using HVPG <10 mmHg and normal bilirubin levels as key criteria for resection.

However, the most recent EASL guidelines (2019) suggest that HVPG >10 mmHg should not automatically contraindicate surgery.

Combining portal pressure assessment with resection extent and MELD score offers better predictive accuracy (Giannelli et al. 2020; Citterio et al. 2016).

6.2.1.4 Functional Remnant Liver Volume (FRLV) Evaluation

CT-based volumetric assessment is standard for evaluating FRLV.

- In a normal liver, a safe residual volume is **25–30%**.
- In cirrhotic livers, it should be **40–50%** (Shindoh et al. 2012).

If FRLV is inadequate, strategies such as portal vein embolization (PVE), transarterial chemoembolization (TACE) followed by PVE, liver venous deprivation (Guiu et al. 2021), radioembolization (Shehta et al. 2020), or the ALPPS procedure (Zhang et al. 2020) can be employed to enhance liver volume (see Fig. 6.1).

The only problem with these retractors is their cost, especially in developing countries with limited budgets for medical facilities. An alternative to this system is to use two simple bars mounted to the operation table connected to a handheld retractor Morrison Retractor by a sterile gauze bandage (see Fig. 6.2).

This gauze could be substituted by a stainless-steel chain hooked to the bar on the one side and a hand retractor on the other side (see Fig. 6.3).

6.2.1.5 The Vessel Sealing Devices

The mode of parenchymal transection in hepatectomy has been a subject of significant debate for decades, and many different technologies and techniques have become available to surgeons. The clamp–crush technique, first reported in 1974,

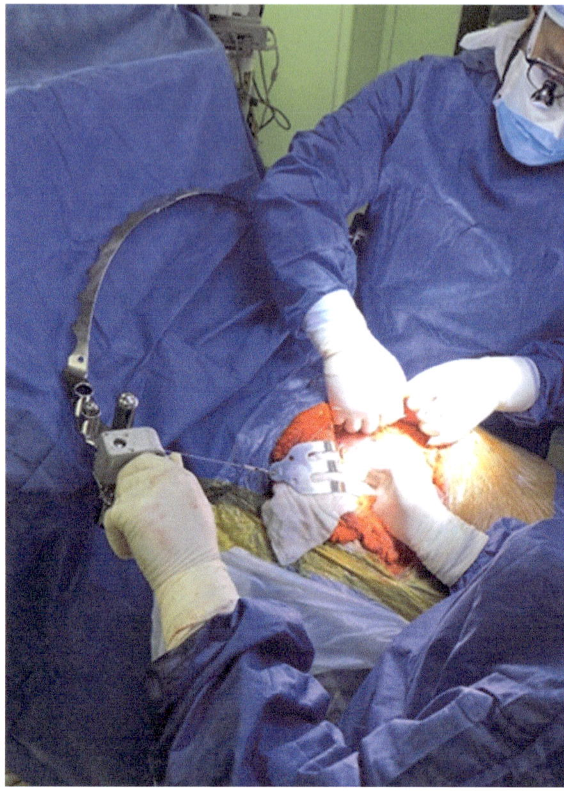

Fig. 6.1 Arm retractor fixed to the operating table (The photo is courtesy of Prof. Mohamed F. Abdel Ghaffar)

was one of the earliest methods and remained the standard technique of parenchymal division for many surgeons (Aldrighetti et al. 2006).

Today, numerous devices are available for the division of liver parenchyma in both open and minimally invasive surgeries. These include the cavitron ultrasonic surgical aspirator (CUSA) (Tyco et al.), harmonic scalpel (Ethicon Endo-Surgery, Cincinnati, Ohio, USA), Ligasure (Valleylab et al.), TissueLink (Salient et al.), water-jet dissection, radiofrequency-assisted resection, microwave-assisted resection, vascular staplers, and others (Poon 2007).

What is the best technique for parenchymal resection?

To date, no single technique has been proven superior; there is no conclusive evidence identifying the ideal method (Yang et al. 2017).

Vessel Sealing Devices:

Vessel sealing devices are commonly used in surgical procedures to seal blood vessels. Their advantages include shorter operative times, decreased blood loss, fewer postoperative complications, and faster patient recovery.

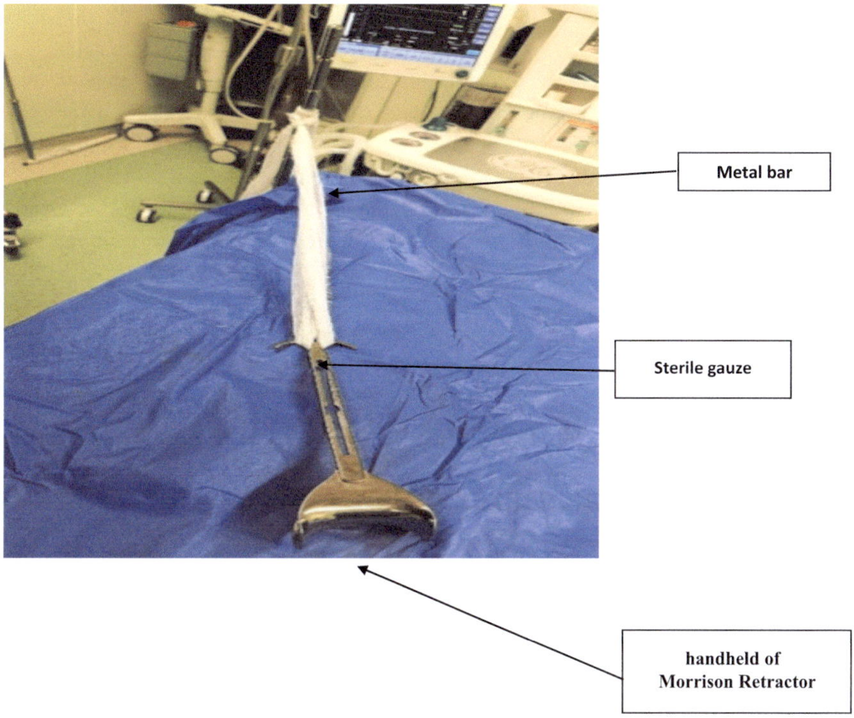

Fig. 6.2 Simple bar mounted to the operation table connected to a handheld retractor Morrison Retractor by a sterile gauze bandage. (The photo is courtesy of Prof. Mohamed F Abdel Ghaffar)

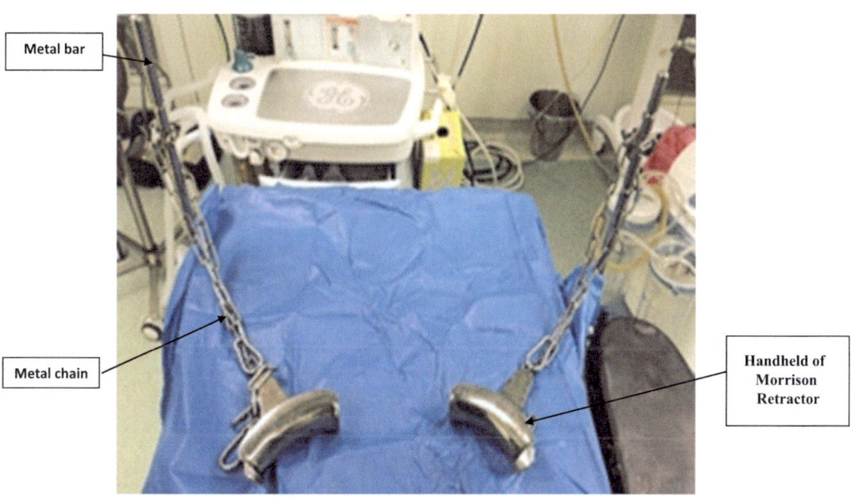

Fig. 6.3 Stainless-steel chain hooked to the bar mounted to the operation table on the one side and a hand retractor on the other side. (The photo is courtesy of Prof. Mohamed F Abdel Ghaffar)

Ultrasonic Vessel Sealing:

Ultrasonic systems operate by vibrating an active component at speeds over 55,000 Hz against a static component, with tissue positioned between the two. Ultrasonic techniques employ piezoelectric ceramics in transducers, eliminating the need for electrical current to pass through the patient. As the vessel is divided, a coagulum forms, achieving effective sealing.

However, a notable drawback of ultrasonic devices is their high running cost, including the expense of the device itself, disposable handles, and the requirement to change the cable approximately every 100 cases.

When ultrasonic vessel sealing devices are not available, simpler methods such as cavitron ultrasonic surgical aspirator (CUSA) combined with bipolar diathermy are also viable options. Bipolar cautery, in particular, offers advantages by reducing blood loss during hepatectomy and shortening operation time (Rocca et al. 2021).

6.3 Liver Transplantation

6.3.1 History of Liver Transplantation

Welch first proposed liver transplantation as a treatment in 1955 (Welch 1955). In 1958, the first orthotopic liver transplantation was described in dogs (Moore et al. 1959). The world's first human liver transplant was performed on March 1, 1963, on a 3-year-old boy. Unfortunately, the patient died due to a coagulation disorder and uncontrollable bleeding (Starzl et al. 1963).

Initially, immunosuppressive medications such as azathioprine and corticosteroids, originally developed for kidney transplantation, were administered to liver transplant recipients. However, the outcomes were disappointing. In the first five cases, no patient survived longer than 23 days due to ischemia-reperfusion injury and acute rejection (Starzl et al. 1963).

In 1967, Starzl performed multiple liver transplants, achieving the first "long-term" survival in a 19-month-old girl with hepatocellular carcinoma who survived for over a year with preserved liver function (Starzl et al. 1968).

In 1968, Roy Calne, a surgeon, and Roger Williams, a hepatologist, initiated the first European liver transplantation program (Calne and Williams 1968).

The history of liver transplantation advanced significantly in 1979 when Calne introduced the use of cyclosporine as an immunosuppressant (Calne et al. 1979). In 1989, Starzl et al. reported 1- and 5-year survival rates of 73% and 64%, respectively, among 1179 liver transplant recipients (Starzl et al. 1989).

The first successful transplantation of a liver graft from a living-related donor was performed by Strong et al. in July 1989 for a 17-month-old recipient (Strong et al. 1990).

Living donor liver transplantation (LDLT) using left-lobe grafts was first attempted in adult recipients in 1993. However, this approach was not widely adopted because the relatively small graft size often failed to meet the metabolic demands of adult recipients (Hashikura et al. 1994). To address this issue, right-lobe liver graft transplantation was introduced for adult recipients in 1996 (Lo et al. 1997).

Tacrolimus, a novel immunosuppressive agent, was successfully used in 1990 for liver transplant recipients who experienced rejection despite conventional therapy. Its success in converting patients from cyclosporine to tacrolimus prompted further clinical studies using tacrolimus as the primary immunosuppressant in liver transplantation (Fung et al. 1990, 1991; Todo et al. 1990).

Regarding organ preservation, the Collins solution was the first effective preservation solution (Collins et al. 1969). In 1980, the Eurotransplant Foundation modified it to develop the Euro-Collins solution (Dreikorn et al. 1980).

Marshall's solution, a hyperosmolar citrate (HOC) solution created by Ross et al. in the late 1970s, continues to be used mainly for renal grafts (Ross et al. 1976).

The University of Wisconsin (UW) solution, developed in 1987, significantly changed transplantation practices by improving graft preservation.

Additionally, the histidine-tryptophan-ketoglutarate (HTK) solution, created in the 1980s, was designed for hypothermic storage during transport and for the perfusion and flushing of liver, kidney, heart, lung, and pancreas grafts (Bretschneider 1980).

6.3.2 Liver Transplantation in Egypt (A LMIC Perspective)

The first successful liver transplantation (LT) in Africa involved the transplantation of the left lateral segment of a mother's liver to her 6-year-old child, who was affected by liver cirrhosis secondary to glycogen storage disease. This procedure marked the 74th reported living donor liver transplantation (LDLT) worldwide (Habib et al. 1993).

In 2001, the Egyptian Medical Syndicate established regulatory frameworks that paved the way for the initiation of LDLT programs, with the first case performed in August of the same year (El-Meteini et al. 2003; Khalaf et al. 2005).

Earlier efforts in 1992 involved two cadaveric liver transplantation procedures; however, both were unsuccessful (unpublished data; Amer and Marwan 2016).

In 2010, the Egyptian Parliament passed legislation recognizing brain death and permitting cadaveric organ transplantation, although the enactment of executive regulations remained pending. One of the principal challenges in expanding cadaveric organ donation continues to be societal acceptance of the brain death concept (Yilmaz 2021).

Currently, the Egyptian Ministry of Health is developing an electronic registry for individuals willing to donate organs post-mortem, and the Ministry of Justice has initiated legal measures to document organ donation processes. Egypt now hosts 17 active liver transplantation centers, performing approximately 370 liver transplants annually across both public and private healthcare sectors.

6.3.3 Experience with Liver Transplantation in Other Middle Eastern Countries

Liver transplantation programs in the Middle East are largely confined to a few countries and rely predominantly on living donors. In several countries, ambiguity regarding the legal definition of brain death has impeded the establishment of deceased donor liver transplantation (DDLT) programs (Al-Hashim and Al-Busaidi 2015).

Currently, Egypt and the Kingdom of Saudi Arabia (KSA) account for more than 90% of all liver transplants performed in the Arab world. Despite KSA conducting the first DDLT in the region in 1990, progress in expanding DDLT services has been slow (Shaheen 2016). By 2013, only seven countries in the region had reported conducting DDLT procedures (Khalaf et al. 2014). Religious and ethical concerns have also hindered the further development of liver transplantation programs (Abaalkhail et al. 2021).

Qatar performed its first liver transplant on December 6, 2011 (Khalaf et al. 2013). In the United Arab Emirates (UAE), brain death was legally recognized in May 2017, with the first DDLT performed in February 2018. However, due to a shortage of deceased donors, LDLT programs were established, including collaborations with the Cleveland Clinic Transplant Center (Kumar et al. 2021).

In Kuwait, the first successful liver transplant was completed on January 17, 2018, for a patient with cirrhosis secondary to non-alcoholic steatohepatitis (NASH) (Jamal et al. 2021).

In Africa, LDLT procedures have been extended through international outreach programs, with an Indian team conducting LDLT in Sudan in 2022 (Tdx Talks, YouTube), and an Egyptian team performing LDLT in Côte d'Ivoire (Medafrica Times).

6.3.4 Selection Criteria for Living Donor Liver Transplantation (LDLT)

Indications and Contraindications

Indications for liver transplantation include acute liver failure, decompensated cirrhosis with associated complications, specific hepatic malignancies, and liver-based metabolic diseases.

Patients presenting with acute liver failure are prioritized for transplantation (Ostapowicz et al. 2002). Candidates with cirrhosis typically become eligible for liver transplantation when their Model for End-Stage Liver Disease sodium-adjusted (MELD-Na) score reaches or exceeds 15 (EASL 2018).

Additional eligibility may arise if patients develop MELD exception conditions, such as hepatocellular carcinoma (HCC), hepatopulmonary syndrome, or portopulmonary hypertension (EASL 2018). Refractory ascites and other cirrhosis-related complications may also prompt consideration for transplantation (EASL 2018).

Patients diagnosed with primary liver neoplasms like HCC may be eligible if they meet defined selection criteria. Liver transplantation may also be considered for selected cases of neuroendocrine tumors with hepatic metastases.

Contraindications include the presence of advanced cardiopulmonary disease, extrahepatic malignancies, metastatic HCC, and intrahepatic cholangiocarcinoma (Martin et al. 2014).

6.3.5 Evaluation of the Recipient

The goal of pre-transplantation evaluation is to assess the patient's ability to tolerate surgery, immunosuppression, and post-transplant care (Mahmud 2020). Specific testing varies depending on the patient's age, medical history, and the transplantation center's practice (Mahmud 2020).

Laboratory tests for evaluation include:

- ABO-Rh blood typing
- Liver biochemical and synthetic function tests (ALT, AST, ALP, bilirubin, INR)
- Complete blood count with differential
- Creatinine clearance
- Serum sodium
- Serum alpha-fetoprotein
- Calcium and vitamin D levels
- Serologies for CMV, EBV, varicella, HIV, hepatitis A, B, C, and RPR
- Urinalysis
- Urine drug screen

Cardiopulmonary evaluation aims to detect coronary artery disease, valvular heart disease, cardiomyopathy, obstructive or restrictive lung disease, hepatopulmonary syndrome, and pulmonary hypertension (Plotkin et al. 1996).

- Noninvasive cardiac testing is advised for patients >40 years old or younger if risk factors are present (Lentine et al. 2012).
- Coronary angiography is recommended for those with CAD, diabetes, or > 2 cardiovascular risk factors (Krill et al. 2017).
- Transthoracic contrast-enhanced echocardiography is advised to detect valvular heart disease, portopulmonary hypertension, or cardiac dysfunction (Fallon et al. 2008).
- Pulse oximetry screening is suggested to detect hepatopulmonary syndrome (Arguedas et al. 2003).

Cancer screening includes:

- Abdominal CT/MRI for HCC
- Skin examination for skin cancer
- Colorectal cancer screening (age ≥ 50 or earlier in high-risk individuals)
- Cervical, breast, and prostate cancer screening based on age and sex

Infectious disease evaluation includes tuberculosis screening. Positive results may require treatment either pre- or post-transplantation. Dental health must be optimized before transplantation.

Vaccinations recommended before transplantation include COVID-19, hepatitis A and B, pneumococcus, influenza, diphtheria, pertussis, and tetanus.

Additional Assessments
- Hepatic imaging to assess vascular anatomy and tumor staging
- Upper endoscopy in patients with cirrhosis or portal hypertension
- Bone density screening for osteoporosis (Guañabens et al. 2013)
- Psychological evaluation and social support assessment (Dick et al. 2009)
- Substance use disorder treatment prior to transplantation

6.3.6 Evaluation of the Donor

Donor evaluation prioritizes donor safety (Manas et al. 2016).

Key Considerations
- No strict age cutoff, but older donors require more rigorous work-up.
- BMI >30 kg/m^2 requires liver biopsy due to risk of steatosis (Lin et al. 2023).
- Donors with controlled hypertension without major end-organ damage may be considered (Chen et al. 2003).
- Cardiovascular disease risk factors should prompt exclusion.

Laboratory and Imaging Evaluation
- Comprehensive liver function tests.
- Imaging for fatty infiltration, biliary, and vascular anatomy.
- Liver biopsy if liver disease is suspected.

Infection Screening
- Active HBV and HCV are contraindications.
- HBV core antibody-positive and HCV antibody-positive (RNA-negative) donors may be considered in exceptional cases.
- CMV or EBV positivity is acceptable but requires counseling.
- HIV infection is an absolute contraindication (Manas et al. 2016).

Cancer Screening
- Detailed clinical examination, particularly in donors >45 years old (Trotter et al. 2007).

Advanced Imaging
- CT or MRI with contrast
- MRCP for biliary anatomy (gold standard)

Graft Volume Calculation
- Adjust for percentage of steatosis.
- Minimum acceptable graft weight/standard liver volume is 40%.
- Donor remnant liver volume should be ≥30% (Ishizaki et al. 2012).
- Small-for-size grafts (GW/RW ratio < 0.8) require caution, especially in decompensated patients (Kiuchi et al. 2003).

Experience in Egypt
- A retrospective study at Ain Shams Center showed the main causes for donor rejection were Factor V Leiden mutation (23%), positive hepatitis markers (19.8%), and drug abuse (12.7%). Anatomical issues like portal vein trifurcation and small liver graft size were also major surgical reasons for rejection (El-Meteini et al. 2014).

6.3.7 Management of Patients with Liver Disease on the Waiting List

The MELD score has been used since 2002 to prioritize access to liver transplantation (Wiesner et al. 2003).

Challenges
- Some patients, such as those with cholestatic diseases, refractory ascites, chronic encephalopathy, and hepatopulmonary syndrome, are poorly represented by MELD and may need exception points (Northup et al. 2015).

Important considerations
- MELD >35: High post-transplant mortality risk and risk of over-indication (Artru et al. 2017).
- MELD 18–25: Long waiting times, risk of acute deterioration.

Suggested strategies

1. Antiviral therapy in HCV cirrhotics (Belli et al. 2016).
2. Regular liver ultrasound for HCC screening.
3. Endoscopy for GI bleeding prevention.

4. Management of refractory ascites (TIPS or repeated paracentesis).
5. Encourage physical activity during waiting time (Debette-Gratien et al. 2015).

For patients with HCC

- Bridge therapies (radiofrequency ablation, surgical resection, transarterial chemoembolization) are crucial for maintaining eligibility during waiting periods exceeding 6 months (EASL 2018).

6.3.8 LDLT in the Absence of a Cadaveric Program (Challenges and Technical Modifications)

Popoola et al. (2018) reported that the low number of living donors remains a significant global challenge. Recent studies have shown that the decision to donate an organ is influenced by personal life issues, family status, and the donor-recipient relationship (Agerskov et al. 2014). The decision-making process is often affected by medical uncertainties, concerns about post-donation recovery, family responsibilities, the health of the recipient, and the future health of the donor (Mishra 2019).

Insufficient donor inquiries, existing health comorbidities, and socioeconomic barriers are among the most significant challenges to living donor liver transplantation (LDLT) (Kaplan et al. 2022).

The rising prevalence of obesity, metabolic syndrome, and fatty liver disease is further limiting the pool of suitable donors. Programs are increasingly offering culturally concordant donor navigators and implementing dietary or weight-loss programs. Some data suggest that a high body mass index (BMI), without associated metabolic syndrome or significant hepatic steatosis (>10%), does not necessarily increase the risk of adverse outcomes (Knaak et al. 2017).

In the absence of a cadaveric program, some centers have adapted by accepting donors with complex vascular variants, using left-lobe grafts (LLG) in adults, and reducing the expected graft volume to 0.8% of the recipient's weight (Amer and Marwan 2016).

Initially, most liver transplant centers rejected donors with trifurcated portal veins, but such variations are now increasingly accepted (Amer et al. 2010). In middle hepatic vein-dominant livers, grafts often contain large segment 5 and/or 8 veins requiring reconstruction. Techniques using natural vascular grafts or synthetic materials like ringed expanded polytetrafluoroethylene (ePTFE) are now employed to prevent anterior segment congestion (Kamel et al. 2015).

In Egypt, the right lobe graft without the middle hepatic vein remains the standard for adult living donor liver transplantation, although a few centers are now using the left-lobe graft to prioritize donor safety (Amer et al. 2014).

6.3.9 Complications of Liver Transplantation

Postoperative complications of liver transplantation can be mechanical or non-mechanical.

6.3.9.1 Vascular Complications

- Hepatic artery thrombosis (HAT)
- Hepatic artery stenosis (HAS)
- Portal vein thrombosis (PVT)
- Portal vein stenosis (PVS)

6.3.9.2 Biliary Complications

- Biliary strictures (anastomotic and non-anastomotic)
- Biliary leaks
- Choledocholithiasis
- Cholangitis

6.3.9.3 Infections and Fever

- Cytomegalovirus (CMV) infection
- Epstein-Barr virus (EBV) infection
- Fungal infections

6.3.9.4 Postoperative Malignancy

- Skin cancer
- Solid organ malignancy
- Recurrence of primary tumor

6.3.9.5 Liver Allograft Rejection

- Acute rejection (AR)
- Chronic rejection (CR)

6.3.9.6 Neurological Complications

- Encephalopathy
- Brain hemorrhage
- Seizures

6.3.9.7 Renal Dysfunction

- Acute kidney injury (AKI)
- Chronic kidney disease (CKD)

6.3.10 Liver Transplantation in Hepatocellular Carcinoma (HCC)

Liver transplantation (LT) remains the best treatment option for patients with decompensated cirrhosis. For hepatocellular carcinoma (HCC), LT addresses both tumor removal and hepatic insufficiency (Mazzaferro et al. 2008).

Living donor liver transplantation (LDLT) is a crucial strategy to address organ shortages, with more than 300 LDLTs performed annually in Egypt. Deceased donor liver transplantation (DDLT) remains rare despite legislative approval in 2010.

6.3.10.1 Indications for Transplantation in HCC Patients

LT is indicated for patients with:

- A single lesion ≤5 cm
- Up to three separate lesions (none >3 cm)
- No gross vascular invasion, regional nodal involvement, or distant metastases

Strict adherence to these criteria can achieve five-year survival rates of 75% or higher, comparable to LT outcomes for cirrhosis without HCC (Mazzaferro et al. 1996; Milan criteria).

6.3.10.2 Expanded Transplant Criteria

Patients beyond Milan criteria may still qualify after successful tumor downstaging. Expanded criteria include:

- UCSF criteria: single nodule ≤6.5 cm or 2–3 nodules ≤4.5 cm each, total diameter ≤ 8 cm (Yao et al. 2007).
- Up-to-7 criteria: sum of the largest tumor size and tumor number ≤ 7 (Mazzaferro et al. 2009).

Candidates meeting OPTN downstaging protocols can receive MELD exception points if the tumor burden can be reduced and AFP remains <1000 ng/mL.

6.3.10.3 Bridging with Neoadjuvant Locoregional Therapy

"Bridging" treatment is recommended for transplant candidates with expected waiting times ≥6 months to prevent tumor progression (Wiesner et al. 2004).

Complete pathological response after locoregional therapy correlates with significantly lower recurrence rates (DiNorcia et al. 2020).

6.3.10.4 Downstaging with Neoadjuvant Locoregional Therapy

Patients initially outside criteria can be "downstaged" into transplant eligibility. A 6-month observation period after successful downstaging is generally recommended, with an AFP level < 1000 ng/mL (Berry and Ioannou 2013; Shaker et al. 2018).

6.3.10.5 Prognostic Factors and Outcomes in HCC Transplantation

LDLT offers the advantage of a faster transplant timeline compared to DDLT, crucial in HCC where waiting may lead to tumor progression (Elkomos et al. 2023).

While survival after LDLT and DDLT is similar in many studies, some suggest slightly better survival with LDLT.

HCC recurrence after LDLT remains controversial; potential causes include liver regeneration and surgical techniques (Vakili et al. 2009; Fisher et al. 2007).

Prognostic factors for recurrence include tumor size, number, vascular invasion, differentiation grade, AFP levels, and TNM staging (Castroagudín et al. 2005).

The RETREAT score, based on microvascular invasion, AFP at transplantation, and viable tumor burden, is used to predict recurrence risks (Houben and McCall 1999).

Minimizing immunosuppression is important due to its association with tumor regrowth. Sirolimus (an mTOR inhibitor) and everolimus have shown promise in reducing recurrence rates while preserving graft function (Rodríguez-Perálvarez et al. 2013; Lee et al. 2021).

6.3.10.6 Portal Vein Thrombosis (PVT)

PVT occurs in 2% to 26% of liver transplantations (Sugawara et al. 2006).

The goal during LT is to ensure adequate graft blood flow and decompress the splanchnic circulation.

Yerdel's classification (2000) grades PVT as:

- **Grade 1:** <50% PV occlusion, minimal SMV extension
- **Grade 2:** >50% PV occlusion, minimal SMV extension
- **Grade 3:** Complete PV and proximal SMV thrombosis
- **Grade 4:** Complete PV and SMV thrombosis

Surgical strategies vary by grade and include thrombectomy, interposition grafts, and use of collateral veins (Fig 6.4).

Grade IV portal vein thrombosis is the most challenging and often requires combined liver-intestine transplantation, feasible mainly in centers with a cadaveric donor program. Cavoportal and reno-portal anastomoses have been considered technical alternatives for graft portal inflow reconstruction (D'Amico et al. 2013).

Portal vein (PV) reconstruction using large, dilated paracholedochal veins offers certain advantages over other surgical options that use systemic blood flow for portal inflow.

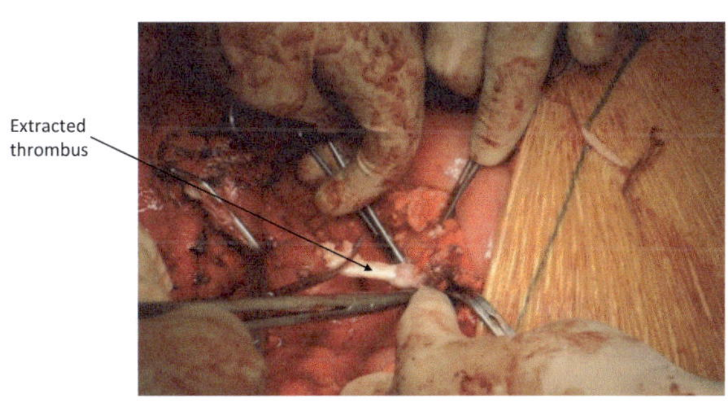

Fig. 6.4 Eversion thrombectomy. (The photo is courtesy of Prof. Mohamed F. Abdelghaffar)

Although liver transplantation theoretically offers a curative option in these cases, in daily practice, many indications for liver resection remain contraindications for liver transplantation, limiting this approach.

Anomalous portal venous branches (APVB) in right lobe graft donors, resulting in two separate openings, present a technical challenge in vascular reconstruction.

Cheng et al. classified portal vein configurations into five types (Cheng et al. 1997):

- **Type I:** The right anterior and posterior branches arise from a short common trunk (normal anatomy).
- **Type II:** Early division of the anterior and posterior sectoral branches (trifurcation).
- **Type III:** Independent posterior sectoral branch arising directly from the main portal vein trunk.
- **Type IV:** Anterior sectoral branch originating from the umbilical portion of the left portal vein.
- **Type V:** Other variations.

Different surgical techniques have been described to manage APVB, depending on the distance between the two portal openings.

If the two openings are close enough, **venoplasty** can be performed on the back table to create a single orifice for anastomosis.

When the openings are too far apart to be joined, each branch can be separately anastomosed to the recipient's right and left portal vein branches.

Alternatively, a **Y-graft** derived from the recipient's portal vein may be used to facilitate reconstruction (Guler et al. 2013).

6.3.10.7 Recipient PV as Interposition Graft Between V8/V5 and Recipient MHV/VFiC (Figs. 6.5 and 6.6)

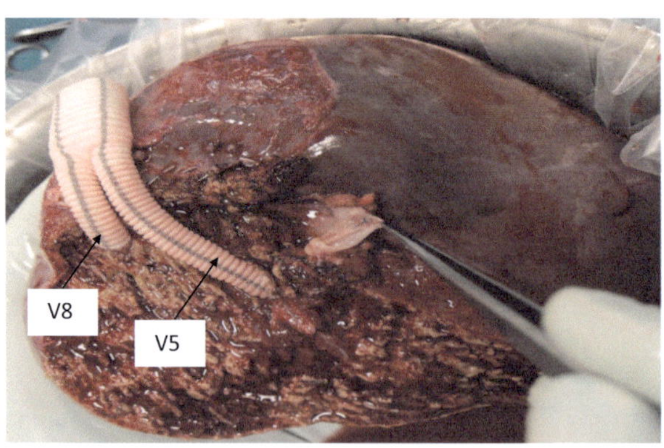

Fig. 6.5 Y-Shaped synthetic graft V5 (Vein of segment 5)—V8 (Vein of segment 8) (The photo is courtesy of Prof. Mohamed F. Abdel Ghaffar)

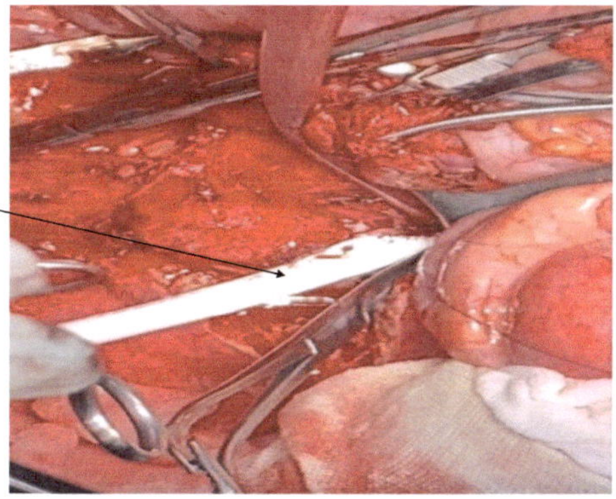

Fig. 6.6 Reno-portal anastomosis. SG: Synthetic graft—PV: Portal vein—LRV: Left renal vein (The photo is courtesy of Prof. Mohamed F. Abdel Ghaffar)

6.3.10.8 Post-Transplantation Surveillance

Following liver transplantation for hepatocellular carcinoma (HCC), patients remain at risk for disease recurrence. However, there is no consensus regarding the optimal surveillance approach.

The 2010 International Consensus Conference guidelines recommend contrast-enhanced computed tomography (CT) or magnetic resonance imaging (MRI) along with alpha-fetoprotein (AFP) measurements every 6–12 months (Clavien et al. 2012a, b).

6.3.10.9 Immunosuppression Protocol and Follow-Up in India

According to a retrospective study by Pamecha et al. (2021), 611 living donor liver transplants (LDLT) were performed in India between June 2011 and October 2019. HCC accounted for 6.5% (n = 53) of transplant activity, with 40 patients having a preoperative diagnosis and 13 detected incidentally. The median Model for End-Stage Liver Disease (MELD) score for patients with HCC was 18.

Only 10 patients (19%) underwent transplantation primarily for HCC, while the majority had indications related to progressive liver decompensation. Thirty-two patients met the "up-to-7" criteria, whereas 21 were outside these criteria. Overall 5-year survival was 85.4%, with recurrence-free survival at 83.3% after a median follow-up of 35 months (range 13–59 months). These outcomes were comparable to LDLT performed for other indications (5-year survival 81.2%).

The Risk Estimation of Tumor Recurrence After Transplant (RETREAT) score most accurately predicted recurrence risk ($p = 0.03$), with an odds ratio of 6.8 (Pamecha et al. 2021).

The immunosuppression protocol typically involves:

- **Intraoperative Phase:** Administration of methylprednisolone (100 mg) during the anhepatic phase, tapered over the next 5 days.
- **Maintenance Phase:** Combination therapy with tacrolimus, mycophenolate mofetil, and prednisolone.
  - Mycophenolate mofetil is avoided in patients with a post-transplant platelet count $<30 \times 10^9$/L.
  - Tacrolimus trough levels are maintained at 5–7 ng/mL during the first week post-transplant.

Patients are discharged once they are fully ambulatory, have stable graft function, all surgical drains are removed (ascitic output <200 mL), and are stabilized on maintenance immunosuppression.

More recently, immunosuppression strategies have shifted toward mammalian target of rapamycin (mTOR)-based regimens in HCC patients, based on emerging evidence.

Follow-up Protocol

- Every 3 months for the first 2 years
- Every 6 months thereafter

Surveillance for Recurrence

- Ultrasound (US) of the abdomen with AFP measurement at every visit
- Annual abdominal contrast-enhanced CT
- If AFP is elevated or a suspicious nodule is detected on US, further evaluation with contrast-enhanced CT is undertaken.

6.4 Special Issues in Liver Transplantation for the Management of HCC in LMICs: A Surgeon's Perspective

Liver transplantation offers the best outcomes for patients with early and select intermediate-stage HCC. However, it presents several limitations in low- and middle-income countries (LMICs).

Although LDLT is available in many LMICs (e.g., Egypt since 2001), it is constrained by donor availability due to cultural reasons and a high prevalence of conditions such as hepatitis C virus (HCV) infection and schistosomiasis (Amer and Marwan 2016).

Additionally, the **cost of the procedure** and the need for **long-term follow-up** are significant barriers. While some insurance systems may cover the transplantation itself, they often do not cover the costs of re-admissions or further interventions.

The financial considerations should also account for:

- Evaluation costs for potential donors who are ultimately deemed unsuitable
- Indirect costs, such as time lost from work for both donors and recipients

Right hepatectomy donors may not return to work for 2–3 months postoperatively, leading to potential income loss depending on employer leave policies (Russo and Brown Jr 2003).

Complications occur in 15–30% of donors, and donors must be informed that insurance may not cover treatment costs for donation-related complications.

Other key challenges include:

- **Biliary complications:** Occurring in up to 40% of LDLT cases (Chok and Lo 2016), often requiring repeated endoscopic retrograde cholangiopancreatography (ERCP) and interventional radiology procedures.
- **Immunosuppression:** Associated with costs, infectious complications, and the necessity for rigorous follow-up.
- **Absence of a cadaveric donor program:** Limits graft availability, especially for complex cases (e.g., high body mass index, high MELD scores), and exposes recipients to greater risk if urgent re-transplantation becomes necessary.

Therefore, when accepting a patient into a liver transplantation program in LMICs, the **availability of financial resources to manage possible late complications** must be considered.

6.5 Conclusion

Surgical management of hepatocellular carcinoma (HCC), through either resection or transplantation, remains the only potentially curative treatment option. The choice of management strategy is influenced by tumor characteristics, hepatic functional reserve, organ availability, wait time, and the expertise and resources available locally.

Over the past few decades, advancements in perioperative care and hepatic surgical techniques have significantly transformed the field of liver resection. However, patients undergoing liver resection for HCC continue to face a high risk of tumor recurrence, approaching 70% within 5 years. Approximately 70% of recurrences occur within the first 2 years post-resection, typically representing local invasion or intrahepatic metastasis.

Conversely, liver transplantation offers the best outcomes for patients with early and select intermediate-stage HCC, yet it is not without limitations. In many low- and middle-income countries (LMICs), including Egypt (where living donor liver transplantation [LDLT] has been available since 2001), the availability of suitable donors remains a major constraint. Although deceased organ donation has been legalized in some LMICs, practical implementation is hindered by cultural and logistical challenges.

The increasing demand for organs, coupled with a limited supply in Arab countries with transplantation programs, has also raised concerns regarding organ trafficking and transplant tourism. Therefore, the decision to accept a patient into a liver transplantation program must consider not only the medical indications but also the availability of financial resources to manage potential long-term postoperative complications.

Addressing these challenges will require enhanced collaboration between liver transplant programs in LMICs and the international transplant community, with the goal of ensuring equitable access to transplantation and improving outcomes for patients with HCC worldwide.

References

Abaalkhail FA, Al Sebayel MI, Shagrani MA, et al. Clinical practice guidelines for liver transplantation in Saudi Arabia. Saudi Med J. 2021;42(9):927–68.
Agerskov H, Bistrup C, Ludvigsen MS, Pedersen BD. Living kidney donation: considerations and decision-making. J Renal Care. 2014;40:88–95.
Al-Hashim AH, Al-Busaidi M. Understanding the concept of brain death in the middle East. Oman Med J. 2015;30(2):75–6.
Aldrighetti L, Pulitano C, Arru M, et al. 'Technological' approach versus clamp crushing technique for hepatic parenchymal transection: a comparative study. J Gastrointest Surg. 2006;10:974–9.
Amer K, El-Balouly A, Inomata Y, et al. Feasibility of left lobe graft in adult living donor liver transplantation. Egypt J Surg. 2014;33:5–13.
Amer K, Wendt N, Bourquain H, et al. Surgical strategies for venous anatomical variations of right lobe graft in Living Donor Liver Transplantation (LDLT); International Medical Center (IMC) experience. Egypt J Vasc Endovasc Surg. 2010;6:43–52.
Amer KE, Marwan I. Living donor liver transplantation in Egypt. Hepatobiliary Surg Nutr. 2016;5(2):98–106.
Arguedas MR, Abrams GA, Krowka MJ, Fallon MB. Prospective evaluation of outcomes and predictors of mortality in patients with hepatopulmonary syndrome undergoing liver transplantation. Hepatology. 2003;37(1):192–7.
Artru F, Louvet A, Ruiz I, Levesque E, Labreuche J, Ursic-Bedoya J, et al. Liver transplantation in the most severely ill cirrhotic patients: a multicenter study in acute-on-chronic liver failure grade 3. J Hepatol. 2017;67:708–15.
Belghiti J, Hiramatsu K, Benoist S, Massault P, Sauvanet A, Farges O. Seven hundred forty-seven hepatectomies in the 1990s: an update to evaluate the actual risk of liver resection. J Am Coll Surg. 2000;191:38–46.
Belli LS, Berenguer M, Cortesi PA, Strazzabosco M, Rockenschaub SR, Martini S, Morelli C, et al. Delisting of liver transplant candidates with chronic hepatitis C after viral eradication: a European study. J Hepatol. 2016;65:524–31.
Berry K, Ioannou GN. Serum alpha-fetoprotein level independently predicts post-transplant survival in patients with hepatocellular carcinoma. Liver Transpl. 2013;19(6):634–45.
Blasco A, Forns X, Carrión JA, et al. Hepatic venous pressure gradient identifies patients at risk of severe hepatitis C recurrence after liver transplantation. Hepatology. 2006;43(3):492–9.
Bretschneider HJ. Myocardial protection. Thorac Cardiovasc Surg. 1980;28:295–302.
Calne RY, Rolles K, White DJ, Thiru S, Evans DB, McMaster P, et al. Cyclosporin A initially as the only immunosuppressant in 34 recipients of cadaveric organs: 32 kidneys, 2 pancreases, and 2 livers. Lancet. 1979;2(8151):1033–6.
Calne RY, Williams R. Liver transplantation in man. I. Observations on technique and organization in five cases. Br Med J. 1968;4:535–40.
Castroagudín JF, Delgado M, Villanueva A, Bustamante M, Martínez J, Otero E, Tomé S, Martínez SM, Segade FR, Conde R, Dominguez-Muñoz E, Varo E. Safety of percutaneous ethanol injection as neoadjuvant therapy for hepatocellular carcinoma in waiting list liver transplant candidates. Transplant Proc. 2005;37(9):3871–3.
Chen YS, Cheng YF, De Villa VH, et al. Evaluation of living liver donors. Transplantation. 2003;75(3):S16–9.
Cheng YF, Huang TL, Chen CL, Sheen-Chen SM, Lui CC, Chen TY, et al. Anatomic dissociation between the intrahepatic bile duct and portal vein: risk factors for left hepatectomy. World J Surg. 1997;21:297–300.
Chok KSH, Lo CM. Biliary complications in right lobe living donor liver transplantation. Hepatol Int. 2016;10:553–8. https://doi.org/10.1007/s12072-016-9710-0.
Citterio D, Facciorusso A, Sposito C, et al. Hierarchic interaction of factors associated with liver decompensation after resection for hepatocellular carcinoma. JAMA Surg. 2016;151(9):846–53.

Clavien PA, Lesurtel M, Bossuyt PM, Gores GJ, Langer B, Perrier A. Recommendations for liver transplantation for hepatocellular carcinoma: an international consensus conference report. Lancet Oncol. 2012a;13(1):e11–22.

Clavien PA, Lesurtel M, Bossuyt PM, Gores GJ, Langer B, Perrier A. Recommendations for liver transplantation for hepatocellular carcinoma: an international consensus conference report. Lancet Oncol. 2012b;13(1):e11–22.

Clavien PA, Petrowsky H, DeOliveira ML, Graf R. Strategies for safer liver surgery and partial liver transplantation. N Engl J Med. 2007;356(15):1545–59.

Collins GM, Bravo-Shugarman M, Terasaki PI. Kidney preservation for transportation. Initial perfusion and 30 hours' ice storage. Lancet. 1969;2:1219–22.

D'Amico G, Tarantino G, Spaggiari M, et al. Multiple ways to manage portal thrombosis during liver transplantation: surgical techniques and outcomes. Transplant Proc. 2013;45(7):2692–9.

Debette-Gratien M, Tabouret T, Antonini M-T, Dalmay F, Carrier P, Legros R, et al. Personalized adapted physical activity before liver transplantation: acceptability and results. Transplantation. 2015;99(1):145–50.

Dick AA, Spitzer AL, Seifert CF, Deckert A, Carithers RL, Reyes JD, et al. Liver transplantation at the extremes of the body mass index. Liver Transpl. 2009;15(8):968–77.

DiNorcia J, Florman SS, Haydel B, Tabrizian P, Ruiz RM, Klintmalm GB, Senguttuvan S, Lee DD, Taner CB, Verna EC, et al. Pathologic response to pretransplant locoregional therapy is predictive of patient outcome after liver transplantation for hepatocellular carcinoma: analysis from the US multicenter HCC transplant consortium. Ann Surg. 2020;271:616–24.

Dreikorn K, Horsch R, Rohl L. 48- to 96-hour preservation of canine kidneys by initial perfusion and hypothermic storage using the Euro-Collins solution. Eur Urol. 1980;6:221–4.

EASL. EASL (European Association for the Study of the Liver) clinical practice guidelines: management of hepatocellular carcinoma. J Hepatol. 2018;69:182–236. Erratum in: J Hepatol. 2019;70(4):817

Elkomos BE, Abdo M, Mamdouh R, Abdelaal A. Can living donor liver transplantation provide similar outcomes to deceased-donor liver transplantation for hepatocellular carcinoma? A systematic review and meta-analysis. Hepatol Int. 2023;17(1):18–37.

El-Meteini M, Dabbous H, Sakr M, Ibrahim A, Fawzy I, Bahaa M, Abdelaal A, Fathy M, Said H, Rady M, El-Dorry A. Donor rejection before living donor liver transplantation: causes and cost effective analysis in an Egyptian transplant center. Hepat Mon. 2014;14(1):e13703.

El-Meteini M, Fayez A, Fathy M, et al. Living related liver transplantation in Egypt: an emerging program. Transplant Proc. 2003;35(7):2783–1786.

Fallon MB, Krowka MJ, Brown RS, Trotter JF, Zacks S, Roberts KE, Shah VH, Kaplowitz N, Forman L, Wille K, Kawut SM. Pulmonary Vascular Complications of Liver Disease Study Group Impact of hepatopulmonary syndrome on quality of life and survival in liver transplant candidates. Gastroenterology. 2008;135(4):1168–75.

Fisher RA, Kulik LM, Freise CE, Lok AS, Shearon TH, Brown RS, et al. Hepatocellular carcinoma recurrence and death following living and deceased donor liver transplantation. Am J Transplant. 2007;7(6):1601–8.

Foster JH, Berman MM. Solid liver tumors. Major Probl Clin Surg. 1977;22:1–342.

Fung JJ, Todo S, Jain A, McCauley J, Alessiani M, Scotti C, et al. Conversion from cyclosporine to FK 506 in liver allograft recipients with cyclosporine-related complications. Transplant Proc. 1990;22(1):6–12.

Fung JJ, Todo S, Tzakis A, Alessiani M, Abu-Elmagd K, Jain A, et al. Current status of FK 506 in liver transplantation. Transplant Proc. 1991;23(3):1902–5.

Giannelli V, Roux O, Laouénan C, et al. Impact of cardiac function, refractory ascites and beta blockers on the outcome of patients with cirrhosis listed for liver transplantation. J Hepatol. 2020;72(3):463–71.

Guañabens N, Monegal A, Cerdá D, Muxí Á, Gifre L, Peris P, Parés A. Randomized trial comparing monthly ibandronate and weekly alendronate for osteoporosis in patients with primary biliary cirrhosis. Hepatology. 2013;58(6):2070–8.

Guiu B, Herrero A, Panaro F. Liver venous deprivation: a bright future for liver metastases: but what about hepatocellular carcinoma. Hepatobiliary Surg Nutr. 2021;10(2):270–2.

Guler N, Dayangac M, Yaprak O, Akyildiz M, Gunay Y, Taskesen F, Tabandeh B, Bulutcu F, Yuzer Y, Tokat Y. Anatomical variations of donor portal vein in right lobe living donor liver transplantation: the safe use of variant portal veins. Transpl Int. 2013;26:1191–7.

Habib NA, Higgs BD, Marwan I, et al. Living-related liver transplantation in Africa. Int Surg. 1993;78(2):121–3.

Hashikura Y, Makuuchi M, Kawasaki S, et al. Successful living-related partial liver transplantation to an adult patient. Lancet. 1994;343:1233–4.

Houben KW, McCall JL. Liver transplantation for hepatocellular carcinoma in patients without underlying liver disease: a systematic review. Liver Transpl Surg. 1999;5(2):91–5.

Ishizaki Y, Kawasaki S, Sugo H, Yoshimoto J, Fujiwara N, Imamura H. Left lobe adult-to-adult living donor liver transplantation: should portal inflow modulation be added? Liver Transpl. 2012;18(3):305–14.

Jamal M, AlMahmeed H, AlGhanem M, AlMatooq M, Sadek A, AlMousawi M, Al-Sabah S, Vilca Melendez H, Rela M, Heaton N, Jassem W. Organ transplantation in Kuwait and the recent initiation of a liver program. Transplantation. 2021;105(10):2125–7.

Kamel R, Hosny K, Amer K, et al. Synthetic graft for reconstruction of middle hepatic vein tributaries in living-donor liver transplant. Exp Clin Transplant. 2015;13(1):318–22.

Kaplan A, Rosenblatt R, Jackson W, Samstein B, Brown RS. Practices and perceptions of living donor liver transplantation, nondirected donation, and liver paired exchange: a national survey. Liver Transpl. 2022;28:774–81.

Khalaf H, Derballa M, Elmasry M, Khalil A, Yakoob R, Almohannadi M, Almaslamani M, Fadhil R, Al-Kaabi S, Al-Ansari A, Almaslamani Y. First liver transplant in Qatar: an evolving program facing many challenges. Exp Clin Transplant. 2013;11(5):423–5.

Khalaf H, El-Meteini M, El-Sefi T, et al. Evolution of living donor liver transplantation in Egypt. Saudi Med J. 2005;26(9):1394–7.

Khalaf H, Marwan I, Al-Sebayel M, El-Meteini M, Hosny A, Abdel-Wahab M, Amer K, El-Shobari M, Kamel R, Al-Qahtani M, Khan I, Bashir A, Hammoudi S, Smadi S, Khalife M, Faraj W, Bentabak K, Khalfallah T, Hassoun A, Bukrah A, Mustafa I. Status of liver transplantation in the Arab world. Transplantation. 2014;97(7):722–4.

Kiuchi T, Tanaka K, Ito T, Oike F, Ogura Y, Fujimoto Y, Ogawa K. Small-for-size graft in living donor liver transplantation: how far should we go? Liver Transpl. 2003;9(9):S29–35.

Knaak M, Goldaracena N, Doyle A, Cattral MS, Greig PD, Lilly L, et al. Donor BMI >30 is not a contraindication for live liver donation. Am J Transplant. 2017;17:754–60.

Krill T, Brown G, Weideman RA, Cipher DJ, Spechler SJ, Brilakis E, Feagins LA. Patients with cirrhosis who have coronary artery disease treated with cardiac stents have high rates of gastrointestinal bleeding, but no increased mortality. Aliment Pharmacol Ther. 2017;46(2):183–92.

Kumar S, Miller CM, Hashimoto K, Quintini C, Kumar A, Balci NC, Pinna AD. Liver transplantation in the United Arab Emirates from deceased and living donors: initial 2-year experience. Transplantation. 2021;105(9):1881–3.

Lee KK, Kim DG, Moon IS, et al. Liver transplantation75.0 versus liver resection for the treatment of hepatocellular carcinoma. J Surg Oncol. 2010;101:47–53.

Lee SG, Jeng LB, Saliba F, Singh Soin A, Lee WC, De Simone P, Nevens F, Suh KS, Fischer L, Jin Joo D, Fung J, Joh JW, Kaido T, Grant D, Meier M, Rauer B, Sips C, Kaneko S, Levy G. Efficacy and safety of Everolimus with reduced tacrolimus in liver transplant recipients: 24-month results from the pooled analysis of 2 randomized controlled trials. Transplantation. 2021;105(7):1564–75.

Lentine KL, Costa SP, Weir MR, Robb JF, Fleisher LA, Kasiske BL, Carithers RL, Ragosta M, Bolton K, Auerbach AD, Eagle KA. American Heart Association Council on the kidney in cardiovascular disease and council on peripheral vascular disease cardiac disease evaluation and management among kidney and liver transplantation candidates: a scientific statement from the American Heart Association and the American College of Cardiology Foundation. J Am Coll Cardiol. 2012;60(5):434–80.

Lin JS, Muhammad H, Lin T, Kamel I, Baghdadi A, Rizkalla N, Ottmann SE, Wesson R, Philosophe B, Gurakar A. Donor BMI and post-living donor liver transplantation outcomes: a preliminary report. Transplant Direct. 2023;9(2):e1431.

Llovet JM, Schwartz M, Mazzaferro V. Resection and liver transplantation for hepatocellular carcinoma. Semin Liver Dis. 2005;25:181–200.

Lo CM, Fan ST, Liu CL, et al. Adult-to-adult living donor liver transplantation using extended right lobe grafts. Ann Surg. 1997;226:261–9.

Mahmud N. Selection for liver transplantation: indications and evaluation. Curr Hepatol Rep. 2020;19(3):203–12.

Makuuchi M, Sano K. The surgical approach to HCC: our progress and results in Japan. Liver Transpl. 2004;10(2):S46–52.

Manas D, Burnapp L, Andrews PA. Summary of the British Transplantation Society UK guidelines for living donor liver transplantation. Transplantation. 2016;100(6):1184–90.

Martin P, DiMartini A, Feng S, Brown R Jr, Fallon M. Evaluation for liver transplantation in adults: 2013 practice guideline by the American Association for the Study of Liver Diseases and the American Society of Transplantation. Hepatology. 2014;59(3):1144–65.

Mazzaferro V, Chun YS, Poon RTP, et al. Liver transplantation for hepatocellular carcinoma. Ann Surg Oncol. 2008;15(4):1001–7.

Mazzaferro V, Llovet JM, Miceli R, et al. Predicting survival after liver transplantation in patients with hepatocellular carcinoma beyond the Milan criteria: a retrospective, exploratory analysis. Lancet Oncol. 2009;10(1):35–43.

Mazzaferro V, Regalia E, Doci R, Andreola S, Pulvirenti A, Bozzetti F, Montalto F, Ammatuna M, Morabito A, Gennari L. Liver transplantation for the treatment of small hepatocellular carcinomas in patients with cirrhosis. N Engl J Med. 1996;334(11):693–9.

Mishra N. 118.8: experiences of living organ donors around organ donation period: a qualitative study. Transplantation. 2019;103:S18.

Moore FD, Smith LL, Burnap TK, Dallenbach FD, Dammin GJ, Gruber UF, et al. One-stage homotransplantation of the liver following total hepatectomy in dogs. Transplantation Bulletin. 1959;6(1):103–7.

Northup PG, Intagliata NM, Shah NL, Pelletier SJ, Berg CL, Argo CK. Mortality on the liver transplant waiting list: unintended policy consequences and model for end stage liver disease (MELD) inflation. Hepatology. 2015;61:285–91.

Ostapowicz G, Fontana RJ, Schiødt FV, Larson A, Davern TJ, Han SH, McCashland TM, Shakil AO, Hay JE, Hynan L, Crippin JS, Blei AT, Samuel G, Reisch J, Lee WM, U.S. Acute Liver Failure Study Group. Results of a prospective study of acute liver failure at 17 tertiary care centers in the United States. Ann Intern Med. 2002;137(12):947–54.

Pamecha V, Sinha PK, Rajendran V, et al. Living donor liver transplantation for hepatocellular carcinoma in Indian patients— is the scenario different? Indian J Gastroenterol. 2021;40:295–302.

Plotkin JS, Scott VL, Pinna A, Dobsch BP, De Wolf AM, Kang Y. Morbidity and mortality in patients with coronary artery disease undergoing orthotopic liver transplantation. Liver Transpl. 1996;2(6):426–30.

Popoola AA, Olanrewaju TO, Bolaji BO, Ajiboye TO. Expanding renal transplantation organ donor pool in Nigeria. Saudi J Kidney Dis Transpl. 2018;29:1181–7.

Poon RT. Current techniques of liver transection. HPB. 2007;9:166e173.

Prodeau M, Drumez E, Duhamel A, et al. An ordinal model to predict the risk of symptomatic liver failure in patients with cirrhosis undergoing hepatectomy. J Hepatol. 2019;71(5):920–9.

Rocca A, Cipriani F, Belli G, et al. The Italian consensus on minimally invasive simultaneous resections for synchronous liver metastasis and primary colorectal cancer: a Delphi methodology. Updat Surg. 2021;73:1247–65.

Rodríguez-Perálvarez M, Tsochatzis E, Naveas MC, et al. Reduced exposure to calcineurin inhibitors early after liver transplantation prevents recurrence of hepatocellular carcinoma. J Hepatol. 2013;59(6):1193–9.

Ross H, Marshall VC, Escott ML. 72-hr canine kidney preservation without continuous perfusion. Transplantation. 1976;21:498–501.

Russo MW, Brown RS Jr. Financial impact of adult living donation. Liver Transpl. 2003;9:S12–5. https://doi.org/10.1053/jlts.2003.50228.

Shaheen FAM. Organ transplantation in Saudi Arabia. Transplantation. 2016;100:1387–95.

Shaker MK, Montasser IF, Sakr M, Elgharib M, Dabbous HM, Ebada H, Dorry AE, Bahaa M, Meteini ME. Efficacy of loco-regional treatment for hepatocellular carcinoma prior to living donor liver transplantation: a report from a single center in Egypt. J Hepatocell Carcinoma. 2018;5:29–36.

Shehta A, Lee JM, Suh KS, et al. Bridging and downstaging role of transarterial radio-embolization for expected small remnant volume before liver resection for hepatocellular carcinoma. Ann Hepatobiliary Pancreat Surg. 2020;24(4):421–30.

Shindoh J, Tzeng D, CW, Vauthey JN. Portal vein embolization for hepatocellular carcinoma. Liver. Cancer. 2012;1(3–4):159–67.

Starzl TE, Groth CG, Brettschneider L, Penn I, Fulginiti VA, Moon JB, et al. Orthotopic homotransplantation of the human liver. Ann Surg. 1968;168(3):392–415.

Starzl TE, Marchioro TL, Vonkaulla KN, Hermann G, Brittain RS, Waddell WR. Homotransplantation of the liver in humans. Surg Gynecol Obstet. 1963;117:659–76.

Starzl TE, Todo S, Tzakis AG, Gordon RD, Makowka L, Stieber A, et al. Liver transplantation: an unfinished product. Pt 2Transplant Proc. 1989;21(1):2197–200.

Strong RW, Lynch SV, Ong TH, et al. Successful liver transplantation from a living donor to her son. N Engl J Med. 1990;322:1505–7.

Sugawara Y, Makuuchi M, Tamura S, et al. Portal vein reconstruction in adult living donor liver transplantation using cryopreserved vein grafts. Liver Transpl. 2006;12:1233.

Thompson HH, Tompkins RK, Longmire WP. Major hepatic resection: a 25-year experience. Ann Surg. 1983;197(4):375–88.

Todo S, Fung JJ, Demetris AJ, Jain A, Venkataramanan R, Starzl TE. Early trials with FK 506 as primary treatment in liver transplantation. Transplant Proc. 1990;22(1):13–6.

Trotter JF, Wisniewski KA, Terrault NA, Everhart JE, Kinkhabwala M, Weinrieb RM, Fair JH, Fisher RA, Koffron AJ, Saab S, Merion RM, A2ALL Study Group. Outcomes of donor evaluation in adult-to-adult living donor liver transplantation. Hepatology. 2007;46(5):1476–84.

Vakili K, Pomposelli JJ, Cheah YL, Akoad M, Lewis WD, Khettry U, et al. Living donor liver transplantation for hepatocellular carcinoma: increased recurrence but improved survival. Liver Transpl. 2009;15(12):1861–6.

Welch CS. Liver graft. Maroc Med. 1955;34(359):514–5.

Wiesner R, Edwards E, Freeman R, Harper A, Kim R, Kamath P, et al. Model for end-stage liver disease score and allocation of donor livers. Gastroenterology. 2003;124:91–6.

Wiesner RH, Freeman RB, Mulligan DC. Liver transplantation for hepatocellular cancer: the impact of the MELD allocation policy. Gastroenterology. 2004;127:S261–7.

Yang X, Chub C, Yang J, et al. Estimation of right-lobe graft weight from computed tomographic volumetry for living donor liver transplantation. Transplant Proc. 2017;49:303–8.

Yao FY, Bass NM, Nikolai B, et al. Liver transplantation for hepatocellular carcinoma: analysis of survival according to the intention-to-treat principle and dropout from the waiting list. Liver Transpl. 2002;8:873–83.

Yao FY, Xiao L, Bass NM, Kerlan R, Ascher NL, Roberts JP. Liver transplantation for hepatocellular carcinoma: validation of the UCSF-expanded criteria based on preoperative imaging. Am J Transplant. 2007;7(11):2587–96.

Yilmaz S. Liver transplantation in the Middle East. In: Carr BI, editor. Liver cancer in the Middle East. Springer; 2021. p. 654.

Zhang J, Huang H, Bian J, et al. Safety, feasibility, and efficacy of associating liver partition and portal vein ligation for staged hepatectomy in treating hepatocellular carcinoma: a systematic review. Ann Transl Med. 2020;8(19):1246.

Ziparo V, Balducci G, Lucandri G, Mercantini P, Di Giacomo G, Fernandes E. Indications and results of resection for hepatocellular carcinoma. EJSO. 2002;28:723–8.

Interventional Radiology for HCC Management

7

Sameh Abdel Wahab, Allam Elsayed Allam, and Ali El Said Abdel Rahman

Abstract

Radiofrequency ablation (RFA) was first introduced into clinical practice in 1993 by Rossi et al. marking a significant advancement in minimally invasive treatments. Since then, a substantial body of literature has emerged evaluating the long-term outcomes of percutaneous interventional radiology (IR) therapies for hepatocellular carcinoma (HCC). Various staging systems have been developed to guide clinical decision-making and treatment selection, factoring in tumor extent, liver function, and patient performance status. Among these, the Barcelona Clinic Liver Cancer (BCLC) staging system remains the most widely endorsed by international hepatic societies.

When managing early and very early-stage HCC (tumors typically between 3 and 5 cm), therapeutic options are relatively limited and primarily include surgical resection, liver transplantation, and percutaneous ablation. In patients classified as BCLC stage A, ablation is particularly valued for preserving healthy liver tissue and minimizing surgical complications. Moreover, IR-based treatments have an important role beyond what is outlined in standard guidelines, offering effective and generally well-tolerated options across different stages of HCC. Procedures such as ablation and embolization, whether used individually or in combination, also serve critical roles in downstaging or bridging patients toward potential curative treatments like surgery or transplantation.

S. A. Wahab (✉) · A. E. Allam
Faculty of Medicine, Ain Shams University, Cairo, Egypt
e-mail: allamelsayed@med.asu.edu.eg

Ali El Said Abdel Rahman
Interventional Radiology Department, National and Tropical Medicine Research Institute, General Organisation of Teaching Hospitals and Institutes (GOTHI), Cairo, Egypt

R. Elwakil et al. (eds.), *Approach to Hepatocellular Carcinoma (HCC) Management in Low/Middle-Income Countries*,
https://doi.org/10.1007/978-981-96-3894-9_7

Although the significance of IR procedures in the management of HCC is well recognized, there is inequality in the use of IR in low/middle-income countries (LMICs) compared to high-income countries (HICs) due to several factors. Most of LMICs experience paucity in the percutaneous IR services for HCC. Most of the causes for lacking such services are the non-availability of IR tools, logistical and affordability issues. Along with the financial issues and insurance obstacles for most of the residents of low-income countries, the lack of IR training and multidisciplinary team experience adds to the delay of getting benefit from such procedures, as it is available to a limited number of patients and confined to a certain modality such as percutaneous ethanol injection. This leads to more deterioration in the results of the patient's management, which is reflected in the patient's survival. The role of IR in the management of HCC is discussed in this chapter.

Keywords

HCC · HCC interventional management · HCC ablation · HCC RFA · TACE · TARE · LMICs

Abbreviations

AEs	Adverse effects
AFP	Alfa fetoprotein
AI	Artificial intelligence
ART	Assessment for Re treatment score
BCLC	Barcelona Clinic of Liver Cancer
B-SIRT	Boosted -selective internal radiation therapy
C	Celsius
c-TACE	Conventional TACE
CT	Computed tomography
CUPI	Chinese University Prognostic index
DEB-TACE	Drug Eluting Beads TACE
FDA	Food and Drug Administration
HAP	Hepatoma Arterial Embolization Prognostic Score
HBV	Hepatitis B virus
HCC	Hepatocellular carcinoma
HCV	Hepatitis C virus
HIFU	High intensity focused ultrasound
HKLC	Hong Kong Liver Cancer Staging System
JIS	Japanese Integrated Staging Scoring System
KHz	Kilo hertz
LSF	Lung Shunt Fraction

LTX	Liver transplantation
LTP	local tumor progression
LMICs	Low/middle-income countries
IGF-I	Insulin growth factor I
MELD	Model of end stage liver
MDT	Multidisciplinary team
MRI	Magnetic resonance imaging
MHz	Mega hertz
MWA	Microwave ablation
NASH	Nonalcoholic steatohepatitis
OS	Overall survival
PEI	Percutaneous ethanol ablation
PFS	Progression free survival
PE	Performance status
PVAs	Polyvinyl Alcohol Particles
RCT	Randomized Controlled Trial
RECIST	Response Evaluation Criteria in Solid Tumors
RFA	Radiofrequency ablation
RL	Radiation lobectomy
RS	Radiation segmentectomy
STATE	Selection for Trans Arterial Treatment Evaluation
TACE	Trans Arterial Chemoembolization
TAE	Trans Arterial Embolization (bland embolization)
TARE	Trans Arterial Radioembolization
TKIs	Tyrosine kinase inhibitors
TOC	Trans arterial Oily Chemoembolization (Chemo-lipiodolization)
TTP	Time to progression
US	Ultrasonography
USA	United States of America
VEGF	Vascular endothelial growth factor
WHO	World Health Organization

7.1 Introduction

Hepatocellular carcinoma (HCC) is the most prevalent type of primary liver cancer and ranks as the sixth most common cancer worldwide as well as the third leading cause of cancer-related deaths (Raoula et al. 2019). The development of HCC is typically linked to underlying cirrhosis, which may result from chronic hepatitis B and C infections (HBV and HCV), nonalcoholic steatohepatitis (NASH), autoimmune or drug-induced hepatitis, type 2 diabetes mellitus, and chronic alcohol use. Among cirrhotic patients, the risk of developing HCC is estimated to be between 1% and 8%, with HCV-associated cirrhosis carrying a higher risk (3–8%) compared to HBV (Ioannou et al. 2007). In Egypt, HCC represents the most common cancer, with its incidence rising significantly with advancing age, peaking around 70 years (Imam Waked et al. 2023).

Locoregional therapies for HCC offer survival outcomes comparable to surgical resection, while minimizing postoperative complications and the need for prolonged recovery. Conceptually, a patient population is considered "cured" when their life expectancy matches that of individuals who have never experienced the disease (Cucchetti et al. 2023).

The Barcelona Clinic Liver Cancer (BCLC) staging system, widely endorsed by international liver disease societies, categorizes HCC into five stages (0, A, B, C, D), incorporating tumor characteristics, liver function, and patient performance status to guide therapeutic decisions (Llovet et al. 1999). In the most recent update, BCLC stage A now encompasses both early and very early-stage HCC, highlighting options such as liver transplantation, surgical resection, and ablation, while recognizing the prolonged waiting periods associated with transplantation (Lucatelli and Guiu 2022).

Although liver transplantation is considered the optimal curative strategy for early-stage HCC, various limitations—including high costs, limited medical infrastructure, and organ shortages—pose significant barriers, particularly in low- and middle-income countries (LMICs). Moreover, many patients present with compromised liver function due to portal hypertension or multifocal disease, complicating surgical resection. Consequently, only about 9–27% of patients qualify for surgery (Vogl et al. 2015).

For individuals unsuitable for surgical intervention, careful evaluation by a multidisciplinary team (MDT) is crucial to balance tumor control with preservation of liver function. In such cases, interventional treatments like radiofrequency ablation (RFA) for very early-stage disease (BCLC 0) and trans-arterial chemoembolization (TACE) for intermediate-stage disease (BCLC B) are strongly recommended.

Currently, interventional radiology (IR) plays a transformative role in the management of HCC, offering minimally invasive options such as ablation and embolization to achieve curative or palliative outcomes. These therapies can also serve as bridging strategies to liver transplantation or downstaging interventions to make patients eligible for surgical resection (Holzwanger and Madoff 2018).

Despite the proven benefits of IR techniques, access to these therapies remains significantly unequal between high-income countries (HICs) and LMICs, largely due to differences in resources and healthcare infrastructure (Jamil et al. 2022).

This chapter explores the role of locoregional therapies provided by IR in the management of HCC, while also shedding light on the disparities in access to these critical interventions in low- and middle-income settings.

7.2 Radiofrequency Ablation Techniques

RF ablation is tailored to Barcelona Clinic Liver Cancer (BCLC) classification stage A HCC patients who are not eligible for either liver resection or liver transplantation. (Vogl et al. 2015).

Ablation has become mainstream management for HCC, in early stages, due to its excellent local control ability and high safety profile (Lucatelli and Guiu 2022).

Although the use of various ablation modalities is considered a relatively young technology, ablation has been treated as a tool in the field of tumor ablation since the last century and was first introduced in the early 1990s for tumor resection. It has been proven as a method cauterization since then.

The effects of radiofrequency on tissues previously explained by Jacques d'Arsonval (1851–1940) who was a French physiology scientist. It did not take long before the thermal ablation needle, the so-called probe, was invented (Mcgahan et al. 1990).

The use of heat to treat tumors comes very early from Egyptian and early Greek descriptions of medical practice when superficial masses were subjected to cautery (Singletary 2003).

Thermal ablation was little known in the 1980s when it emerged as a minimally invasive option for HCC treatment. These techniques aimed to destroy tumor tissue using extreme heat. Two different approaches have been developed:

- Thermal disruption method: temperatures ranging from 60 °C to 100 °C were applied directly to the target tissue. A prominent example of this approach is radiofrequency ablation (RFA).
- Hyperthermia procedures: These maintained the target temperature at approximately 42 °C to 45 °C. Although they were less aggressive, they were still aimed at inducing tumor cell death.

Around 1995, radiofrequency ablation (RFA) gained attention as the primary percutaneous ablation technique for HCC. RFA uses high-frequency electrical current to generate heat within the tumor, causing coagulative necrosis. It gained popularity due to its effectiveness, minimal invasiveness, and relatively low complication rate. The goal of malignant tumor ablation: Primarily, all tumor ablation therapies aim to ensure destruction of all neoplastic cells within a specific area using energy or chemicals.

Studies investigating tumor progression following surgical resection have revealed the presence of viable malignant cells beyond the macroscopic tumor margins. Based on these findings, ablation therapies aim not only to target the visible tumor but also to treat adjacent tissue that may harbor microscopic disease. Efforts are made to create a deliberate "excision margin" around the tumor to ensure comprehensive eradication of potential malignant cells.

Complete destruction of the tumor remains the primary objective; however, the precision and specificity of the intervention are equally critical. A key principle of tumor ablation therapy is to achieve effective tumor control while minimizing collateral injury to surrounding healthy tissues and critical structures (Vansonnenberg et al. 2004).

Various techniques have been developed for tumor ablation, the majority of which are thermal-based. However, percutaneous therapies are not restricted to thermal modalities. Non-thermal approaches, such as percutaneous ethanol injection (an early technique introduced in the 1980s) and irreversible electroporation, have also been employed (Lau et al. 2003).

Currently, the spectrum of ablative therapies includes percutaneous ethanol injection (PEI), radiofrequency ablation (RFA), microwave ablation (MWA), cryoablation, and high-intensity focused ultrasound (HIFU) ablation. Among these, RFA remains the most widely utilized technique worldwide due to its established efficacy and accessibility.

7.2.1 Principles of Ablation

7.2.1.1 Basic Principles of Ablation

The basic principles of ablation are based on interaction of the physical effect of high-frequency alternating current (typically 450–500 kHz) with biological tissues with respect to drag-related (frictional) energy losses.

Therefore, "radio frequency" refers to alternating current that oscillates in the high frequency range of alternating current.

An electric field oscillating at high frequencies is generated across the system electrodes, whether active and reference electrodes or across the two active electrodes in a bipolar system.

The ion vibrational motion caused by this oscillatory field causes frictional heating and subsequent "coagulation" necrosis when sufficient energy is applied.

This allows heat to reach the tissue in the immediate vicinity of the electrode (antenna). Further heat distribution is the result of conduction and convection effects (Mcgahan et al. 1990).

A temperature of 45 °C for several hours causes irreversible damage to the cells The latter cytotoxic effect can be significantly reduced to a few minutes by increasing the temperature to 50–60 °C at temperatures between 60 °C and 100 °C, tissue coagulation occurs almost immediately, resulting in irreversible damage to the cell's mitochondrial and cytosolic enzymes and DNA above 100–110 °C, the tissue evaporates and becomes carbonized (Goldberg et al. 1998). Due to the resistivity of the tissue and the energy distribution between the needle electrode and the distributed grounding adherent to the patient, energy is rapidly lost, resulting in heat generation around the electrode, and the generated temperature is decreasing with increasing the distance from the electrode (inverse relation). Taking that in consideration the destruction may reach a diameter 2.2–2.4 cm around a single needle electrode. This means that heat-related damage away from the heat source (RFA) is much less likely as the energy is delivered very precisely and concentrated in the space around the electrode.

Advanced needle design allows handling of volumes up to 5 cm in diameter. The volume can become even larger if it takes longer to reposition the treatment needle and results in overlapping volumes (Raman et al. 2012).

However, the final amount of ablation that is achieved is also highly dependent on tissue-specific properties such as thermal conductivity and convection, in this context, an important effects need to be mentioned, the heat sink effect.

The heat sink effect is observed when the tumor is near a great vessel increasing heat dissipation, frequently a hepatic vein. A benefit from this effect may be achieved by temporary occlusion of these vessels (e.g., balloon occlusion of the hepatic vein, and in the Pringle maneuver, temporary occlusion of the portal vein) (Dominique et al. 2001).

In summary, the effectiveness of RF energy exposure is dependent on the following (Dominique et al. 2001)

- Probe design.
- Amount and duration, and energy used (watts, hours).
- Inherent tissue factors (thermal coupling and heat conversion).
- Effects of heat sinks.

Many techniques can be applied to improve and enhance the ablation (Dominique et al. 2001)

- Technique to improve heat conduction by the injection of saline increasing the number of ions available and by this process increasing the electric current flow.
- Decreasing tumor heat tolerance by decreasing its blood flow with embolization operations or the use of by prior chemotherapy and/or radiation therapy.
- Increasing energy deposition (Kettenbach et al. 2003), (Lubienski et al. 2005).

7.2.2 RF Generators and Equipment

7.2.2.1 Monopolar and Bipolar Systems

RF electrodes consist of an insulated metal shaft and an uninsulated active tip. The electrical circuit is closed when the needle tip touches the desired tissue connecting the generator to the patient. Modifications were made to the probe design to increase the ablation volume by shape modification as an umbrella or inverted umbrella design or increasing surface area as in cluster design. Also the inner cooling system help to increased tha baltion voume by guarding against charring and heat insulation.

Currently, available electrodes allow ablation volumes of spherical diameters of 2–5 cm. In the technical environment of a monopolar system, the patient is connected to a resistor in a closed circuit consisting of an RF generator, a large dispersive electrode (usually a ground pad placed on the patient's thigh), and a needle electrode (antenna).

Due to the relatively high electrical resistance of the tissue compared to metal electrodes, ions in the tissue move rapidly around the electrode, thereby generating heat by its energy.(Brieger et al. 2003).

In a bipolar system, two active electrodes are placed within the same needle design. They are beneficial in decreasing energy loss between electrodes.

Although a variety of ablation systems is available currently, the commercially available systems for ablation are RF and the most commonly used for use are the internally cooled cluster devices or perfusion-enabled devices to allow for larger coagulation volumes. User experience and selection of needle design with proper handling are factors for enhancing application of the procedure (Lubienski et al. 2005).

Internally Cooled Single and Cluster Electrode System "Cooltip, Valleylab, Tyco Healthcare previously and Covidien RFA system by Medtronic healthcare recently" primarily uses an algorithm in which high pulsed energy is delivered for about (10–15 minutes) with no guided control parameter to feedback the system (Pereira et al. 2004).

A system with impedance control (Boston Scientific) and a bipolar single or multiple electrode system in which a gradually increasing or fixed amount of energy is applied as tissue desiccation progresses guided by tissue resistence.

Another multi-tine system, "Angio Dynamics RITA", the output is controlled by monitoring a parameter which is the temperature and this feedback obtained from thermometers at the tips of the tines (Poon et al. 2004).

7.2.3 Bioeffects of the Ablation Techniques

7.2.3.1 Bioeffects of RFA

The alternating current (300–1000 kHz) generates temperatures of 60–100 °C from the needle tip. This effect causes coagulative necrosis occur almost immediately within the targeted tumor, causing cellular irreversible damage. The ablation zone size achieved reaches 3–5 cm in diameter.

To guard against missing minute satellites or microvascular invasion around the lesion, the process to "completely" treat HCC, the resection zone should include not only the entire target tumor but also 0.5–1.0 cm of peritumoral tissue to ensure safety margins are included. Although the hyperthermia affects the blood flow at the microvascular level, larger caliber blood tubes are not affected, and counter heat propagation is known as the heat sink effect (Kim et al. 2014). Antitumor efficacy is influenced by tumor location, blood flow, and tumor size (Dakua and Nayak 2022) (Fig. 7.1).

7.2.3.2 Bioeffects of Chemical Ablation

Intratumorally administration of chemical ablative agents such as ethanol or acetic acid has proven to be an effective method to destroy local tumors percutaneously.

The success of ethanol infusion in the treatment of localized hepatocellular carcinoma has been widely reported (Vansonnenberg et al. 2004).

The injection of ethanol into the neoplastic mass enhances cellular dehydration and cellular death. Also, it causes small vessel thrombosis and causes tumor ischemia.

Percutaneous ethanol injection therapy (PEIT) is preferably performed with ultrasound guidance, watching ethanol dispersed within the lesion (Lau et al. 2003).

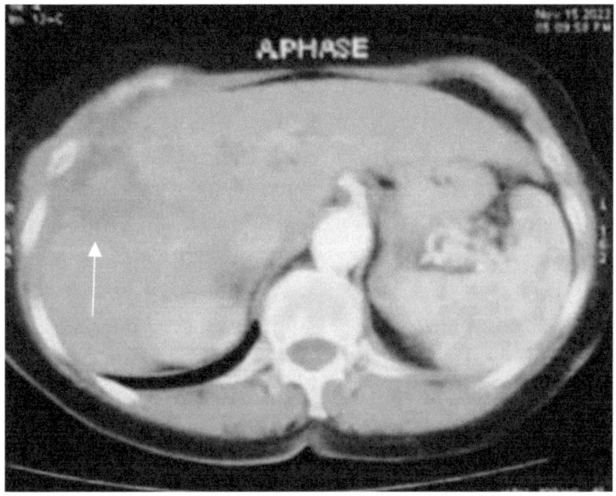

Fig. 7.1 CT revealed central coagulative necrosis (or hematoma) (long thin white arrow) caused by ablation

7.2.3.3 Bioeffects of Microwave Ablation

Microwave ablation (MWA) encompasses electromagnetic techniques that utilize devices operating at frequencies exceeding 900 MHz to achieve tumor destruction. In this process, water molecules, being dipolar and possessing uneven charge distributions—attempt to continuously realign with the oscillating electric field generated by microwave energy.

The intense and rapid oscillation of water molecules, which can occur billions of times per second, generates frictional heat, ultimately leading to coagulative necrosis and subsequent cell death. Additionally, microwave energy induces ion collision within tissues, where kinetic energy is transformed into thermal energy, further contributing to tissue heating. A less dominant mechanism of heat generation involves dipole rotation within biological structures (Liang and Wang 2007).

Currently, the most commonly used frequencies for MWA are 915 MHz and 2450 MHz, with the majority of commercial systems operating at 2450 MHz. Devices utilizing 915-MHz microwaves offer greater tissue penetration than those operating at 2450 MHz, theoretically allowing for the creation of larger ablation zones. However, the extent of tissue ablation is not determined by frequency alone; it is also significantly influenced by the dielectric properties of the target tissue and the specific design of the microwave antenna. Consequently, a device operating at 915 MHz does not necessarily produce a larger ablation area compared to one at 2450 MHz (Liang and Wang 2007).

7.2.3.4 Bioeffects of Cryotherapy Ablation

Cryoablation achieves tumor destruction by applying extremely low temperatures, typically ranging between −20 °C and – 40 °C, to induce cytotoxic effects within the targeted tissue. While traditional cryotherapy systems required open surgical access, advancements in technology have led to the development of smaller cryoprobes that now allow for percutaneous application. Compared to thermal ablation techniques, cryoablation offers advantages such as improved pain tolerance and more precise imaging during follow-up evaluations (Lau et al. 2003).

Tumor destruction via cryotherapy is nonspecific to tissue type and results from multiple physical and biochemical mechanisms. These mechanisms vary depending on factors such as the cooling rate, the achieved low temperature, the rate of rewarming, the number of freeze-thaw cycles performed, and the delayed ischemic injury following thawing. It is well established that cellular structures cannot survive temperatures below −40 °C, and significant cellular damage is evident at temperatures of −20 °C or lower. Repetitive cycles of freezing and thawing enhance the likelihood of complete cellular death. Beyond the immediate physicochemical effects on cells, cryoablation also induces vascular injury, leading to ischemia, which further contributes to extensive tissue necrosis (Lau et al. 2003).

7.2.4 Standards and Guidelines of Percutaneous HCC Management

Choice of treatment for HCC patients with a curative intent has only limited options such as liver transplantation, resection, or ablation, and this is done by collaboration of multiple specialities of surgeons with the internal medicine hepatologist and interventional radiologist, with the oncologist to tailor the specific treatment plan (Dakua and Nayak 2022).

Since ablation has been in use for the last three decades and the preference of ablation by interventional radiologists is sought over other modalities in locoregional treatment. Moreover, it can also be used as a bridge before the liver transplant or as a palliative care method to prevent tumor progression and extend survival. (Dakua and Nayak 2022).

7.2.4.1 Indications and Contraindications

To determine the eligibility of the patient, liver function tests, mainly albumin and bilirubin, as well as the performance status of the patient, is necessary. This is the guidelines set by the Barcelona Clinic Liver Cancer (BCLC) staging system which states that the early and very early stage of HCC (stage 0 and stage A) can benefit from ablation. Regarding the ablation indication in general: in general lesions with 2 cm diameter or less diagnosed as HCC by triphasic CT and elevated alpha feto protein tumor marker (AFP) is considered stage 0 and more than 2 cm HCC lesions are stage A as long as Child Pugh A classification of liver profile is maintained, so if we enumerating the points favoring ablation it will be as follows:

- Single lesion less than 5 cm or maximum 3 lesions each is 3 cm in diameter.
- Lesions away from the blood vessels by about 10 mm to avoid heat sink effect or biliary injury.
- No vascular invasion or extrahepatic spread.
- Nodular pattern of the HCC, no infiltrative type (Dakua and Nayak 2022).

And as regards the contraindications of ablation:

- Lesions near the portal tract and bile ducts by less than 10 mm for fear of biliary injury.
- Exophytic lesions from the liver surface.
- Dilated intrahepatic biliary radicles.
- Proximity to bowel or colon.
- Impaired coagulopathy.

All the mentioned points are crucial to achieve free ablation margin from tumoral cells, therefore few challenges are present when obtaining tumor free safe margin such as:

- Possibility of incomplete necrosis and recurrence.
- Injury of extrahepatic structures.
- Risk of tumor seeding.
- Difficult tumor access.

So decision of RF ablation must be refined to beneficial without increase risk of complications and if so surgical resection or other interventional modality such as TACE may be tailored to achieve better outcome. (Dakua and Nayak 2022; Kim et al. 2014).

7.2.4.2 Optimal Candidates for Ablation

There is some sort of agreement that stage 0 BCLC with less than 2-cm HCC has the best ablation long-term outcome due to its relatively encapsulated nature, fewer microsatellites, and relatively microvascular invasion by histopathological consideration. Also, in considering the short rehabilitation and hospital stay of the RF ablation procedure as it is an easy procedure compared to surgery, the guidelines recommend the ablation before resection compared to the old version of the BCLC guidelines.(Kim et al. 2014).

Regarding the neoplastic hepatic burden, the limit is 3 as regard number of the lesions to be treated as per Milan criteria used with the size limit of each lesion not more than 3 cm and if single lesion it should not exceed 5 cm; however, the patient general condition and operator experience may determine the feasibility of treating multiple lesions by ablation and number of sessions needed to be treated (Kim et al. 2014).

However, variability in these situations depends upon operator experience and use of precision medicine to tailor the appropriate decision for each patient, for example, ablation of more than 3 lesions or ablation of lesions larger than 5 cm.

7.2.5 Technique and Procedure of the Ablation

7.2.5.1 Technique of RFA

Ablation is performed in aseptic conditions, usually under the effect of a combination of sedative and analgesic medication (for example, fentanyl citrate 1 mg per kilogram of body weight) and midazolam hydrochloride (0.010–0.035 mg/kg) or under general anesthesia using a laryngeal mask to make the operation tolerable. Vital cardiovascular and respiratory data must be monitored during the procedure (Vogl et al. 2015).

Ablation can be performed percutaneously, laparoscopically, thoracoscopically, or at laparotomy (Liang and Wang 2007).

7.2.5.2 Procedure of RFA

Radiofrequency ablation (RFA) can be administered using percutaneous, laparoscopic or open surgical (laparotomy) approaches (Mai and Machi 2001; Welling 2020). The percutaneous technique can be carried out under local anesthesia, conscious sedation, or general anesthesia, depending on the clinical scenario. Before the procedure, standard laboratory investigations, including complete blood count and liver function tests, are conducted and repeated 24 hours after the intervention to monitor for complications. Patient positioning is determined by the location of the tumor and the anticipated path of needle insertion, typically placing the patient in either the supine or left lateral position. Based on the equipment used, dispersive electrodes are placed on the patient's back or lower extremities. The procedure follows standard sterile preparation and draping protocols (Piccioni et al. 2019; Shamim et al. 2017).

Local anesthetic is infiltrated along the planned needle trajectory from the skin surface down to the peritoneal layer. A small skin incision is made with a lancet, after which the ablation electrode is advanced carefully under ultrasound guidance to the target within the tumor (Piccioni et al. 2019) (Fig. 7.2).

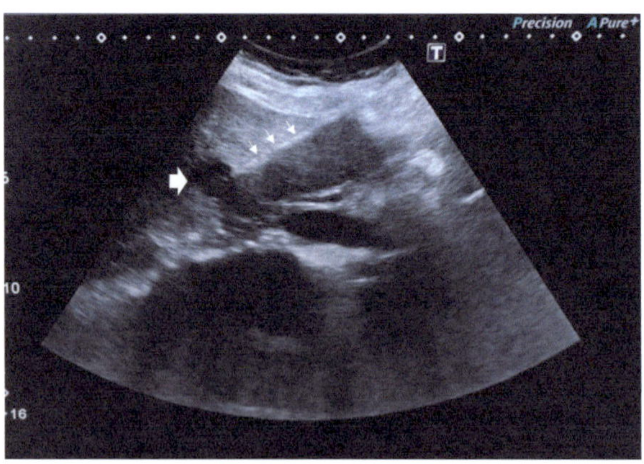

Fig. 7.2 Ultrasound image showing a case of liver cirrhosis and a longitudinally applied needle (short white arrows) with its tip entering the border of the hepatic HCC (thick short white arrow)

When using the cold needle technique, the electrodes are connected to a peristaltic pump, and an RF generator is activated (Lencioni 2010). To achieve the desired value of RF current, the output power of the generator is increased. To maintain this value constant during each treatment session, it may be necessary to manually adjust the generator output to compensate for changes in tissue impedance. The exposure time for each needle puncture is 6–12 minutes.

During thc procedure, adjust the degree of cooling of the needle by changing the speed of the peristaltic pump to maintain the temperature of the liquid in the range of 20–25 °C as indicated by the thermometer attached to the needle tip. When pulsed radiofrequency current is applied to an internally cooled electrode, a larger local current density can accumulate within the tissue in a short time, increasing the amount of coagulative necrosis.

Simultaneously applying groups of three electrodes at 0.5 cm is technically more complex, but results in a larger coagulation area than when using a single needle (Lencioni 2010; Vansonnenberg et al. 2004). While ablation continue the burning outcome of the tumoral tissue results in what called ablation cloud appears hyperechoic in ultrasound as water vapor appears hyperechoic. This gives assumption of the area ablated continuously monitored by the operator during procedure (Fig. 7.3).

The generator output is regulated manually or automatically according to the used device to maintain the temperature between 95 °C and 105 °C (Lencioni 2010; Vansonnenberg et al. 2004; Welling 2020).

For the largest lesions, a "pullback" technique can be used in which the needle tip is inserted deep into the tumor, activating the generator, then the hook is pulled, the needle is withdrawn 1.5 cm, and the generator is activated again. This process can be repeated two to four times, if the lesion is large and in need to achieve safety margin. The RF generator can be connected to a computer and continuously records the temperature curve obtained during the treatment through special software, providing objective documentation of the treatment results (Lencioni 2010).

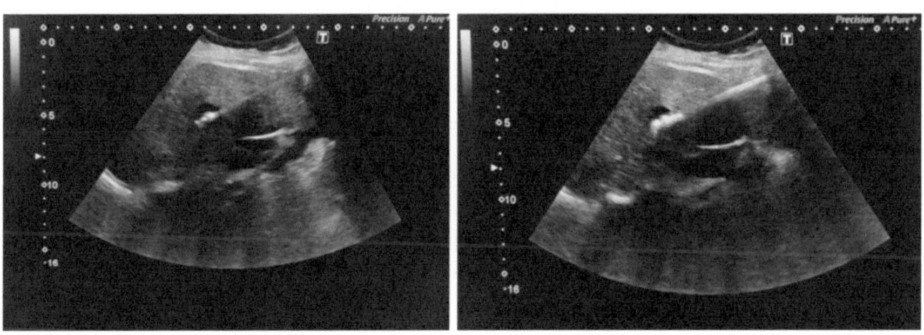

Fig. 7.3 Ultrasound image showing the needle within the tumor, showing an increase in the ablation cloud while the procedure continues

7.2.6 Comparing MWA and RFA

Microwave ablation offers several distinct advantages over radiofrequency ablation. Primarily, microwave heating is an active process, in contrast to the passive nature of RF heating. As a result, microwave ablation provides a broader and more uniform active heating zone and does not depend on electrical conductivity within the tissue. Furthermore, microwave energy is less affected by tissue desiccation or charring, enabling consistent transmission through biological tissues. This characteristic allows intratumorally temperatures to remain elevated throughout the procedure, leading to wider ablation margins, reduced procedural times, and more thorough tumor destruction (Liang and Wang 2007) (Fig. 7.4).

Another advantage of microwave ablation (MWA) is its reduced susceptibility to the perfusion-mediated heat sink effect, a phenomenon where thermal energy is carried away by blood flow in nearby vessels. This heat loss, which predominantly affects the conductive heating zone, poses a significant limitation to radiofrequency ablation (RFA). By mitigating this cooling effect, MWA enables more uniform and effective tumor destruction within and around the target zone (Liang and Wang 2007).

Moreover, MWA allows the simultaneous use of multiple energy sources without the risk of electrical interference that often complicates RF-based procedures. This

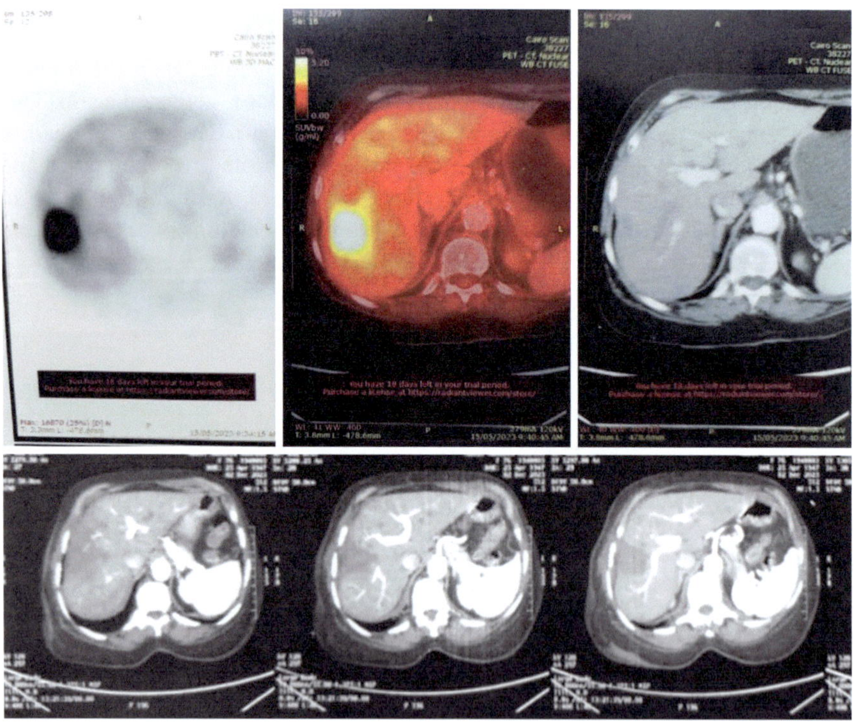

Fig. 7.4 Follow-up of a case of two relatively large hepatic focal lesions (HCC) treated by MWA. The upper three images reveal two lesions in segments VII and VIII. The lower three images revealed triphasic images of the two lesions, showing successful ablation of the lesions by MWA despite their large sizes

synchronized application can create synergistic thermal effects, permitting the treatment of larger tumors within shorter procedural times (Liang and Wang 2007).

Both MWA and RFA are widely utilized in hepatocellular carcinoma (HCC) therapy, differing mainly in their energy sources—MWA uses electromagnetic energy, whereas RFA relies on electrical currents. Despite these technical differences, the therapeutic principle for both methods is similar: inducing high temperatures at targeted sites to achieve coagulative necrosis of the tumor tissue (Tan et al. 2019).

Although MWA theoretically offers several advantages over RFA, such as faster heating and broader ablation zones, clinical evidence has not consistently confirmed its superiority. A recent meta-analysis indicated that MWA might be associated with a slightly higher incidence of major complications compared to RFA, but the difference was not statistically significant (Tan et al. 2019).

7.2.7 Advances in Ablation

7.2.7.1 Technique for Larger Ablation

Given the performance of known RF machines, overlapping ablation techniques, and ablation margins, HCCs larger than 5 cm in diameter should never be treated with ablation alone. In these cases, other treatments or combined treatment strategies should be taken in consideration. It is well-established in some centers in North Africa, East Asia, and especially China. However, this concept may also be inadequate in some centers in North Africa due to a lack of training, and also in Central and West Africa due to a lack of training and inadequate IR services (Hammed et al. 2022; Kim et al. 2014).

For larger HCC, seeking wide safety margin increases the risk of complications, so MDT should be performed based on the patient's liver function reserve, and the appropriate treatment could be delivered. It is also important to consider that when the tumor size increases to 3 cm, the probability of satellite nodules increases to 19%. (Kim et al. 2014).

Various measures have been incorporated to the device aiming to increase the size of the RF zone to 3–4 cm. To overcome that formerly reported inherent limitation, currently available RF techniques include scalable multi-prong designs, internal cooling with cold saline, cluster designs, pulsing of RF energy, and simultaneous injection of saline into the tissue.

The ablation zone can be further enlarged by overlapping multiple ablations or using multiple electrodes simultaneously. Considering these techniques, it becomes possible, at least theoretically, to "technically" ablate HCC up to 4–5 cm in diameter (Kim et al. 2014) (Fig. 7.5).

7.2.7.2 Decreased Blood Flow and Ablation

To address the "heat sink" effect caused by significant blood flow through large vessels within or adjacent to tumors, various strategies have been explored to reduce perfusion either before or during radiofrequency ablation (RFA). One notable method was introduced by Buscarini et al. in 1999, where transcatheter arterial embolization (TAE) was combined with RFA to enhance the treatment of larger

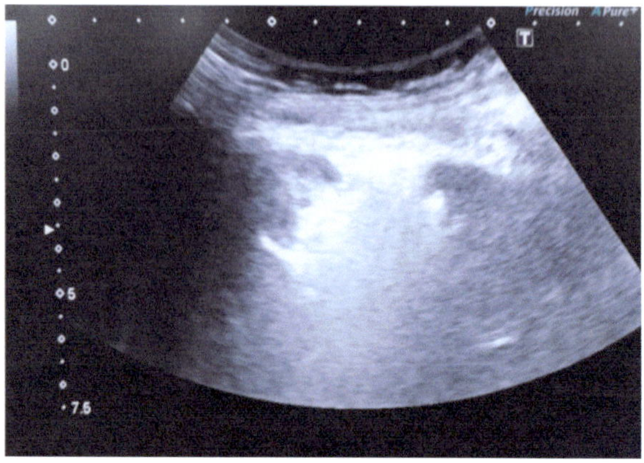

Fig. 7.5 US image of RF ablation with a large ablation using perfusion of saline during ablation

hepatocellular carcinoma (HCC) lesions. Similarly, Rossi and colleagues employed balloon occlusion of the hepatic artery during RFA procedures. In their series involving HCCs with an average size of 4.7 cm, they achieved a local recurrence-free rate of 81% at one year following this combined approach (Garbagnati et al. 2000; Vansonnenberg et al. 2004).

Another technique to diminish hepatic tumor blood flow involves the application of the Pringle maneuver during open surgical RFA. This procedure involves temporarily clamping both the portal vein and hepatic artery after RFA probe placement, thereby minimizing liver perfusion and consequently reducing the "heat sink" phenomenon. Goldberg et al. reported the use of this method in a limited patient cohort in 1998. Their findings indicated a notable enhancement in tumor necrosis volume when the Pringle technique was employed. Specifically, tumors treated without vascular occlusion demonstrated an average necrosis diameter of 2.5 cm, whereas tumors treated with the Pringle maneuver achieved a mean necrosis diameter of 4.1 cm, despite using comparable RFA parameters (Garbagnati et al. 2000; Vansonnenberg et al. 2004).

7.2.7.3 Methods for Precise Localization

Another important limiting factor is that precise targeting is difficult to achieve in some situations. The disturbance of hepatic architecture caused by liver cirrhosis hinders the appropriate ultrasound image, especially is small tumor or macro nodularity of the liver parenchyma. (Kim et al. 2014).

Injection of saline or dextrose 5% into the peritoneal or the pleural spaces are useful to improve the acoustic window in a step called artificial effusion or ascites. It can also be used to protect vital structures such as the colon from thermal damage. Artificial ascites techniques may be a pivotal tool to guard against injury of the intestinal loops or diaphragmatic copula by the heat, never the less facilitating guidance.

Possible improvements in image-guided image fusion as mentioned earlier, it has (1) no radiation hazard, (2) real-time capability, (3) easy access, and (4) low cost. In heterogeneous cirrhotic livers, the edges of lesions are not clearly visible on B-mode ultrasound examination, even after injection of contrast agent, as lesions may develop creating poor sonographic picture and decrease visibility of the target lesion and hindering discrimination of the cirrhotic nodule. Because of these issues, an advanced tool is needed to improve visualization of lesions by combining US images and CT/MR which is the so-called image fusion.

The fusion procedure is explained as follows.

(a) Preoperative CT/MRI acquisition of liver lesions.
(b) Segment the liver to localize the lesion.
(c) Perform intraoperative ultrasound of the liver.
(d) Perform image fusion—convert the images to the same format and spatially align the images.
(e) Overlapping display showing the fusion performed of the US image over the cross-sectional images.
(f) Plane the targeting needle pathway to the lesion.
(g) Ablate liver lesions.
(h) Perform radiofrequency ablation of the lesion with a safety margin of 5–10 mm (Dakua and Nayak 2022; Kim et al. 2014).

Visualization of invisible tumors combining TAE with visually defined beads and lesion ablation guided by CT or catheterization capabilities, improvement. (Dakua and Nayak 2022; Kim et al. 2014).

7.2.7.4 Ablation of Subcapsular Lesions

While subcapsular liver lesions are relatively accessible for ablation, they carry an increased risk of tumor rupture and subsequent hemorrhage. To mitigate these risks, a "no-touch" wedge technique has been developed. This method involves the sequential placement of ablation probes around the lesion under ultrasound (US) guidance, often supplemented by computed tomography (CT) to confirm correct probe positioning (Patel et al. 2013).

During the procedure, probes are strategically inserted tangentially around the tumor margins to fully encase the lesion within the ablation zone. The technique aims to achieve a recommended ablative margin of 5–10 mm, isolating the tumor from the surrounding liver perfusion. This approach is designed to ensure that the regions near the tumor edge—where micrometastases are most likely to occur—are exposed to the active microwave heating zone generated by the probes.

The primary objective of the no-touch technique is to minimize the risk of tumor cell dissemination by preserving the integrity of the tumor capsule during the thermal ablation of small pericapsular tumors (Patel et al. 2013).

7.2.8 Outcome of Ablation

Prognostic factors for HCC were classified into factors related to the tumor itself, factors related to liver function, and factors related to general condition (Osman et al. 2022).

Known risk factors for local tumor progression (LTP) include larger tumor size, inadequate resection margins, large arteriography of HCC, ill-defined tumor margins, poor histopathological grade, and elevated tumor marker levels. However, it is not certain that LTP is frequent in perivascular or subcapsular lesions (Kim et al. 2014).

7.2.8.1 Tumor Recurrence

Recurrence usually occurs in distant parts of the liver other than the primary site. This is caused by an underlying liver disease. The incidence of distant site recurrence typically occurs regardless of locoregional treatment. Shiina et al. and Kim et al. and other studies found that cumulative distant recurrence rates were 10.4% and 26.3% at 1-year follow-up, 52.2% and 57.6% at 3-year follow-up, 68.6% and 77.0% at 5-year follow-up (Kim et al. 2014).

Risk factors for tumor recurrence after ablation therapy include tumor location, tumor size, multiplicity of the tumor, and inadequate margin of safe ablation. The latter is not only a problem for ablation devices, but also for interventional radiologists. Recurrence may also occur due to already existing microcellular neoplastic processes that were not detected by imaging techniques or due to neoplastic tract contamination during the procedure (Vogl et al. 2015).

7.2.8.2 Overall Survival

In the literature, the 3-year overall survival (OS) of hepatocellular carcinoma (HCC) patients treated with radiofrequency ablation (RFA) has been reported to range between 59% and 81%. Siperstein et al. (2007) found a median actuarial survival time of 24 months among 234 HCC patients following RFA. Shuichi Tobinaga et al. demonstrated 1-, 2-, 3-, 4-, and 5-year survival rates of 73.9%, 52.1%, 42.8%, 34.4%, and 26.2%, respectively, with a median estimated survival of 32 months. Their reported cumulative survival rates at 1, 2, and 3 years were 75.6%, 58.5%, and 50.0%, respectively.

Similarly, Vogl et al. (2015) reported 1-, 2-, and 3-year survival rates of 100%, 88%, and 72% for patients treated with RFA, and 100%, 96%, and 79% for those treated with microwave ablation (MWA).

The overarching aim of HCC management is to improve overall survival, and recent therapeutic advances have significantly contributed to better outcomes. Each treatment modality, including resection, RFA, and MWA, offers distinct survival benefits. Interestingly, some studies, such as that by Osman et al. (2022), found no statistically significant difference in overall survival between patients treated with liver resection and those treated with MWA.

Moreover, Shiina et al. reported overall survival rates of 96.6%, 60.2%, and 27.3% at 1, 5, and 10 years, respectively. Similarly, Kim et al. noted cumulative survival estimates of 95.5% at 1 year, 59.7% at 5 years, and 32.3% at 10 years.

7.2.8.3 Poor Prognostic Factors

Many studies discussed that poor prognostic factors include:

- Older age.
- High score Child-Pugh classification.
- Impaired MELD score.
- A non-treated viral disease caused the cirrhosis.
- Development of metastases outside the liver during follow-up.
- Presence of anti-HCV.
- Patients having high tumor burden.

Other poor prognostic factors include markedly elevated tumor marker, damped serum albumin level, portosystemic shunting, large spleen size, markedly altered indocyanine green R15, high serum ferritin level, low serum IGF-I level, high serum VEGF level. (Kim et al. 2014).

7.2.9 Other Methods of Ablation Techniques

7.2.9.1 Percutaneous Ethanol Injection

Percutaneous ethanol injection (PEI) was once a widely used technique for treating small, nodular hepatocellular carcinomas (HCC), demonstrating 5-year survival rates between 32% and 47%. Despite these outcomes, its clinical utility has diminished due to a relatively high rate of tumor recurrence, reaching up to 43%, and the unpredictable extent of ethanol distribution, which may inadvertently damage adjacent healthy liver tissue (Vogl et al. 2015).

The procedure typically involves biweekly sessions throughout four to six treatments. Monitoring of therapeutic efficacy is carried out through serial serum alpha-fetoprotein (AFP) testing, ultrasonography, and computed tomography. In cases where tumor necrosis is incomplete, lesions are large, or new ablation-amenable tumors emerge, additional ethanol sessions may be required (Lau et al. 2003; Shiina et al. 2018).

Although randomized trials are lacking, observational data have shown 3-year survival rates ranging from 47% to 77%. However, the intrahepatic recurrence rate following PEI can exceed 50% (Lau et al. 2003).

Recent developments include using a retractable, tined needle designed to enhance the uniform distribution of ethanol within the tumor, achieving successful ablation in approximately 90% of tumors smaller than 3 cm (Kim et al. 2014). A key advantage of PEI over thermal ablation methods such as radiofrequency ablation is its ability to circumvent the heat-sink effect, thereby minimizing unintended injury to surrounding tissues.

Another benefit of ethanol-based ablation is its diffusion pattern: ethanol penetrates soft tumor tissues more effectively than the surrounding fibrotic or cirrhotic liver parenchyma. This selective infiltration, combined with ethanol-induced microvascular thrombosis and subsequent ischemia, enhances its therapeutic action in hyper-vascular HCCs—a feature not seen in hepatic metastases (Lau et al. 2003).

7.2.9.2 Microwave Ablation

Complete ablation occurred 89–94% using microwave that has been stated in few studies, with low local tumor progression reaching 6–8%.

Also, long-term results revealed 51–57% 5-year survival rate of most of which predominantly Child-Pugh class B cirrhosis. (Vogl et al. 2015) (Fig. 7.6).

The area of complete necrosis is generally the same in RFA and MWA with most studies showing no significant discrepancies in results. Also, survival is better with the complete ablation process and larger ablation area, regardless of the technique used, either RF or MW (Kim et al. 2014).

7.2.9.3 Cryoablation

Cancer was targeted by the cryoablation concept since the mid-nineteenth century when Dr. James Arnott decided to use smashed ice at in a salt solution to freeze breast, cervical, and skin neoplasms at a temperature reaching −18° to −24 °C (Erinjeri and Clark 2010).

It is a spotlight in cryoablation due to the fact that it causes control and shrinkage of the tumors, and the benefit of a significant decrease in pain.

The main advantage of cryoablation over other thermal ablation techniques is the real-time ability to observe the target area during the procedure.

When tissue water is frozen, it transform from liquid to solid, forming ice spheres that can be seen with ultrasound (US), computed tomography (CT), and magnetic resonance imaging (MR). Ice has a slightly lower density than water because it expands slightly during the liquid-to-solid phase transition due to ice's crystal structure.

On CT, a hypodense well delineated area is seen around the cryoprobe or needle forming the ice ball representing the ablation area.

According to the US, the exact area and depth are not assessed due to the echogenic periphery of the ice ball and its resulting sonographic shadowing.

As regard the image appeared in MR it is agreed that T1 and T2 can be helpful sequences to see a well-defined dark signal ice ball. Interestingly, frozen tissue contains a small amount of free water, and its relaxation properties are temperature

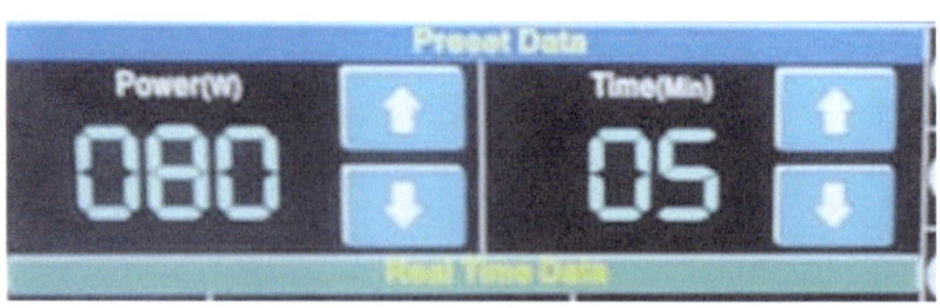

Fig. 7.6 The image demonstrates the increase in the power (watts) of the MW generator that is required for a larger area to be ablated

sensitive, so MR thermography is used to monitor temperature changes (Erinjeri and Clark 2010).

Lacking electronic properties gives the cryoablation advantage that it will not interfere with the CT or MR equipment.

Also, customized ablation area could be achieved by the use of multiple needles, each of which works independently from the other needles (Erinjeri and Clark 2010).

The ice-forming probe produces an anesthetic effect on the nerve and the surrounding tissues, helping in less pain experience (Erinjeri and Clark 2010). So it does not require deep anesthesia and can often be performed on an outpatient basis under moderate sedation.

In contrast to radiofrequency ablation, cryoablation causes a strong inflammatory response. This may be due to the persistent presence of tumor proteins at the site after cryoablation compared to the denaturation of coagulated proteins observed with radiofrequency ablation. In the presence of inflammatory and immunomodulatory mediators, tumor antigens can stimulate immune responses against tumor-specific antigens within the resected tissue, thereby allowing It to attack and kill tumor cells (Erinjeri and Clark 2010).

However, cryoablation has some limitations:

- Each needle produces small ablation area and multiple needles are usually needed for ablation.
- The area showing complete cell death lies a variable distance (4–10 mm or more) inside the ice ball, and so a large safety margin should be frozen to ensure the desired target ablation.
- Some specific complications such as massive hemorrhage and collection due to ice ball fracture, cold injury to adjacent organs, biliary fistula, and cryoshock syndrome (Lau et al. 2003).

7.2.9.4 High Intensity Focused Ultrasound

HIFU can increase tissue temperature by focusing high-energy US waves into a specific, limited focus. Non-invasiveness is the key when comparing HIFU with other ablative procedures. Yet there is a limitation for HIFU, such as very long procedure time and acoustic shadowing of structures like the chest and lung. Rib shadowing causes thermal damage to the overlying soft tissues due to not only attenuation of the US energy but also high absorption of US by the bone cortex, The researchers partially removed a rib to solve this problem in the context of research (Kim et al. 2014).

Wu et al. showed that in patients with advanced HCC, combined HIFU ablation and TACE had improved survival compared to the TACE alone group (1-year survival rate of 42.9% vs. 0%). Also, researchers compared HIFU with other ablation modalities like RFA with no significant difference regarding the survival at 3 years like the Chan et al. study.

Others like Zhang et al. showed that the vascular injury is less likely to occur using HIFU ablation seeking complete tumor necrosis for lesions beside large intrahepatic vessels (Kim et al. 2014).

7.2.9.5 Interstitial Laser Photocoagulation

Laser ablation can be done using US or MRI. The thermocoagulation effect of ILP is caused by the heat generated when light energy is directly or indirectly absorbed by tissue.

The laser light is emitted from the tip of a thin fiber (0.2–0.6 mm in diameter). Absorption of scattered light provides maximum transmission of energy in a uniform distribution, hence heat formation.

The larger the power and exposure time, the more the ablation effect and necrosis. Also wavelength of light and absorption characteristics of the tissue are important determinants.

The neodymium yttrium aluminum garnet laser (Nd: YAG) is the most widely used emitting light at a wavelength of 1064 nm. Smaller tumors up to 1.5 cm can be handled by a single fiber. Yet the larger the lesion the more number of fibers to cover the lesion by proper ablation area.

Bleeding and pain are potential complications as well as effusion and fever (Lau et al. 2003).

7.2.9.6 Irreversible Electroporation

IRE is a non-thermal ablation treatment modality could be beneficial in the control of HCC, it utilizes short electric pulses to induce cell death via apoptosis. The fundamental mechanism of IRE is the creation of holes that are irreversible in cellular membranes by applying them to a series of high-intensity high-voltage electrical pulses (>640 V/cm, >20 A) for a short duration (70–100 μsec) (Shiina et al. 2018).

The tumors near the porta hepatis may take a chance to be treated by IRE as the integrity of the tissue may not be disturbed as compared to the use of others in thermal ablations. However, IRE requires a more invasive setting and is troublesome because of multiple electrodes application and general anesthesia with muscular relaxation necessity. Yet, IRE is not widely used in low- and middle-income countries especially in the setting of HCC treatment (Shiina et al. 2018).

7.2.10 Complications of Thermal Ablation

From a procedural and technical standpoint, RFA is a safe and minimally invasive method. The needles used are typically small (14–17.5 G) compared to biopsy needles, complemented by their inherent ability to cauterize and coagulate (preventing bleeding from the needle guide or tumor dissemination along the guide).

It is worth noting that several complications preclude the use of RFA. Generally, the complications that may happen may be gastrointestinal perforation, hepatic abscess in patients with biliary surgery, hepatic decompensation or liver failure, and heat damage to adjacent organs (Dakua and Nayak 2022).

7.2.10.1 Vascular Complication

Coagulation function as well as the type and location of the target lesion have a direct effect on the risk of bleeding, it also depends on the route to the lesion and intervening structures (Chinnaratha et al. 2016; Chuang et al. 2005).

Direct injuries to the vessel by the needle can cause:

- Bleeding.
- Pseudoaneurysm.
- Arterio-venous and arterioportal fistulas.
- Hepatic and portal vein thrombosis.
- Parenchymal infarction.

The use of real-time image guidance by US, CT or fluoroscopy is generally successful in preventing these injuries and complications (Chuang et al. 2005; Rhim 2005).

At the end of each session or the end of the procedure, the track is ablated by withdrawing the needle (i.e., needle track ablation) to avoid bleeding from the operation site (Chuang et al. 2005; Rhim 2005).

Portal Vein Thrombosis

As the blood flow increases, the degree of heat-sink effect also increases in relation to that blood vessel. Injury to the portal vein may occur even if the vessel is large in caliber due to thermal injury or iatrogenic interruption of the portal venous blood flow as the case in Pringle maneuver (Kim et al. 2014).

Hepatic Vein Thrombosis

It can occur if direct injury by antenna resulting in thrombosis and its best detected by US and dynamic cross-sectional CT and MRI studies during the equilibrium phase and may be associated with perfusional or parenchymal congestion abnormalities, appearing in imaging as wedge-shaped hypoenhancing areas (Kim et al. 2014).

Hepatic Infarction

Dead parenchymal tissue is often recognized as wedge-shaped non-enhancing areas, with branching portal tracts that are easily depicted within the infarcted segments.

It is usually managed by conservative means using antibiotic prophylaxis (Chuang et al. 2005,Akahane et al. 2005).

Subcapsular Hematoma

Bleeding occurs either due direct injury or impaired coagulopathy; however, the cirrhotic parenchyma also aids occurrence of bleeding (Livraghi et al. 2003) Other situations that increase the risk of bleeding are the repeated entry of the needles, and aggressive manipulation near major vessels is a risk factor.

The needle can be manipulated to avoid contact or puncture major vessels as it traverses sufficient normal liver parenchyma. Tract ablation is an effective method to reduce bleeding occurrence (Chuang et al. 2005; Pritchard et al. 2004).

If bleeding occurs, resuscitation is mandatory with vitals monitoring, the hematoma appears as a crescentic or biconvex lesion with attenuation higher than that of water. If conservative management by IV fluids and transfusion could not help control the condition, Transcatheter arterial embolization may be an effective treatment, especially if bleeding is arterial(Akahane et al. 2005).

Hepatic Artery Damage

The damage of the hepatic artery may cause pseudoaneurysms, arterioportal shunts, or bleeding. Small arterioportal shunts are found in 25% of cases in the follow-up triphasic CT (Lencioni et al. 2001). It may cause wedge wedge-shaped area of abnormal attenuation in the hepatic parenchyma (Catalano et al. 2000) Yet most of these shunts disappear spontaneously with no need for further intervention (Lencioni et al. 2001).Embolization of all pseudoaneurysms seems advisable, as they may experience delayed rupture with hemoperitoneum (Bilchik et al. 2001).

7.2.10.2 Infection

Although infections following radiofrequency ablation (RFA) are uncommon, certain predisposing conditions, such as existing infections or immunosuppression, including that associated with diabetes, may increase susceptibility (Elias et al. 2006).

In most cases, infectious complications manifest as hepatic abscesses, often identified when patients present with delayed, persistent, or recurrent fever two to three weeks after undergoing RFA. The likelihood of post-procedural infection may also be elevated in individuals with a history of trans-arterial chemoembolization using lipiodol (Choi et al. 2005).

While prophylactic antibiotic use is common practice, there is currently insufficient evidence to definitively support its effectiveness.

Clinicians should consider the possibility of abscess formation when patients develop fever, leucocytosis, and significant gas accumulation within the ablated lesion (Catalano et al. 2000). It is important to note, however, that the presence of gas within the lesion is not conclusive for infection. Intralesional gas is frequently observed on computed tomography scans immediately following ablation, appearing in up to 63% of cases, and typically resolves in follow-up imaging. Persistent or newly appearing gas on delayed imaging, especially when accompanied by clinical signs of infection, may be more indicative of an abscess.

7.2.10.3 Tumor Seeding

RFA may cause a bothersome issue which is tumor seeding. The neoplastic cells seeding happens when the tumor cells stick to the needle and drop along the antenna pathway (G. Anton Decker et al. 2003). This seeding may be detected 3–12 months after the procedure.

Thirty-two patients were enrolled in a Spanish study after their treatment by RFA, with 12.5% of them having needle track contamination that was proved by biopsy 4 to 18 months after RFA.

Possible risk factors include subcapsular location of the tumor, high tumor density, multiple or large tumors necessitating several needle passes, and poor tumor differentiation (Baert et al. 2008).

Baseline value levels of alpha-fetoprotein, other factors include the fact that cells can be forced into orbit by sudden intratumoral high pressure, which frequently occurs in RFA, and can be heard as a crackling sound. Finally, injecting saline into the tumor during or before RFA may result in cell infiltration. Avoiding risk factors and thermal coagulation of the needle guide during needle withdrawal can possibly eliminate the risk of tumor dissemination. This is especially important when using her RFA in patients awaiting liver transplantation (Llovet et al. 2001).

By proper needle positioning from the first pass the danger of seedling could be avoided, also the care to avoid needle crossing of the tumor to avoid tumor cells push out in its periphery as well as sufficient safety margin around the tumor together with removing the probe by additional ablation of the needle tract will further lower the risk of tumor cell spread.

Again, overlapping technique for large tumors as well as no-touch wedge technique for subcapsular are recommended (Livraghi et al. 2003).

7.2.10.4 Nontarget Damage

Thermal ablation procedures, while generally safe, carry the risk of unintended injury to surrounding structures. Such damage may include burns at grounding pad sites or interference with nearby metallic implants, such as pacemaker leads and implantable cardioverter-defibrillators (Rhim 2005).

In monopolar radiofrequency ablation (RFA) systems, improper placement or inadequate size of the grounding pad can lead to energy concentration at the pad itself, effectively turning it into a secondary electrode. This can result in localized burns, especially when energy output is high. The likelihood of this complication increases with greater power delivery. To mitigate the risk, multiple or larger pads are recommended when higher energy settings are required.

Additionally, insufficient contact between the grounding pad and the patient's skin, caused by factors such as perspiration or hair, can lead to poor energy dispersion. This may create a focal point of high current density, potentially causing thermal injury. Furthermore, defects in insulation along the electrode or coaxial cable can inadvertently act as secondary antennas, leading to burns at the skin entry site (Livraghi et al. 2003).

These specific complications are not seen with microwave ablation systems, as they do not rely on grounding pads for energy dispersion.

To protect adjacent organs from collateral thermal damage during ablation, various displacement techniques can be employed. For example, instilling 5% dextrose solution or air into the peritoneal or retroperitoneal space can create a buffer zone, effectively separating the target lesion from vulnerable structures such as the stomach or colon (Yamakado et al. 2003).

7.2.10.5 Biliary Tract Damage

A large bile duct injury more than 3 mm is less likely to occur. The main bile duct stenosis has been noted only after RFA during a Pringle maneuver. However, in clinical practice, intact blood flow does not guarantee safety from biliary complications.

Many experts recommend the ablation 1 cm distant from the main biliary duct (Elias et al. 2006). However, certain measures could be done to guard against biliary injury, such as prophylactic placement of a biliary stent. And another method by cooling the biliary ducts with chilled saline. While these methods may decrease biliary damage, they may increase the risk of hepatic abscess formation (Mulier et al. 2002).

7.2.10.6 Minor Complications

Patients undergoing radiofrequency ablation (RFA) commonly experience minor adverse effects such as localized pain at the needle insertion site, irritation of the peritoneum, nausea, vomiting, low-grade fever, fatigue, and headaches (Baert et al. 2008). A cluster of these symptoms, known as post-ablation syndrome, occurs in about two-thirds of cases and may persist for several weeks (Baert et al. 2008). Typically, these symptoms are mild and can be effectively managed with supportive care, including the use of simple analgesics and nonsteroidal anti-inflammatory medications (Rhim 2005).

7.2.11 Risk Factors for Complications

The likelihood of complications following radiofrequency ablation (RFA) for hepatocellular carcinoma (HCC) is significantly higher in patients classified as Child-Pugh class C, with an incidence of 27.6%, compared to 8.0% in class A and 6.5% in class B patients (Curley et al. 2000). Tumors located near the liver capsule are particularly prone to complications such as bleeding into the peritoneal cavity, formation of subcapsular hematomas, tumor seeding, and injury to adjacent organs. When ablating centrally located tumors, there is a heightened risk of damage to the bile ducts and central hepatic vessels. Extensive RFA procedures, especially for large or multiple tumors, can increase the chances of serious complications, including liver failure, burns at the dispersive electrode site, muscle breakdown leading to myoglobinemia or myoglobinuria, thrombocytopenia, and severe central hyperthermia. In these complex cases, a staged approach or combination therapies may be necessary to minimize risk (Mulier et al. 2002).

7.2.12 Infrastructures and Their Relation to IR Services

The burden of hepatocellular carcinoma (HCC) in West Africa remains high, largely due to insufficient medical expertise and limited infrastructure needed to provide effective early-stage interventions. A major contributor to the region's elevated rates of morbidity and mortality is the frequent late presentation of HCC, compounded by restricted access and affordability of available treatments for the minority who are diagnosed early (Hammed et al. 2022). In contrast to countries like Germany and the USA, which maintain a sufficient workforce of radiologists, African nations are significantly underserved. For instance, a study by Edzie et al. revealed that as of 2019, Ghana had fewer than two radiologists per million people—a figure approximately 50 times below the recommended standard (Sarkodie et al. 2023). The shortage extends beyond diagnostic radiology to include a lack of specialists in interventional radiology, pediatric radiology, women's imaging, and neuroradiology. Nigeria faces an even starker situation, with only about 250 to 300 radiologists serving a population exceeding 174 million (Sarkodie et al. 2023). Several factors underlie this shortage, including governmental policies, deficiencies in medical education, and broader socio-economic challenges (Sarkodie et al. 2023). Even among the few specialists trained, there is a critical shortage of medical equipment, including basic radiology infrastructure, further discouraging radiologists from specializing in these fields (Sarkodie et al. 2023).

7.3 Trans Arterial Treatment of HCC

Transaretrial treatment of HCC is a non-invasive loco-regional method of treatment that be done in the interventional radiology unit through the arterial supply using specific catheters to block the supplying artery inducing ischemia to the lesion associated with either injection of specific chemotherapy to add cytotoxic effect [transaretrial chemoembolization (TACE)] or radioactive material to destruct the tumor cells [transaretrial radioembolization (TARE)].

7.3.1 Transaretrial Chemoembolization (TACE)

Choosing the most efficient therapy for the HCC patient depends on the patient's three main factors: the performance state (PE), liver function (Child-Pugh score), and tumor stage. Depending on the Barcelona Clinic Liver Cancer (BCLC) staging system, TACE is considered the first line of treatment for intermediate HCC stage, including patients with large or multi-nodular HCC, provided that good liver function with no vascular invasion or extra-hepatic spread evidence (Forner et al. 2018). Also, according to the BCLC, TACE can be used in early HCC stage when surgery and other loco-regional treatment cannot be applied or failed (either due to old age, subcapsular/near main biliary duct or dome location of the HCC). Several studies showed high response rate and outcome with TACE (Baek et al. 2019). It can also be a therapy before liver transplantation (LT) as downstaging therapy, or making the unfit patient fit for LT, as a bridge therapy, keeping the tumor stationary course during waiting time for LT (Galle et al. 2018).

TACE can also be a treatment of HCC with portal vein thrombosis in cases of segmental thrombosis or as part of combination therapy with other systemic treatment, provided that liver function and performance status are good (Raoula et al. 2019).

TACE as a treatment line is also supported by other staging systems rather than BCLC, as the Japanese integrated staging (JIS) scoring system, the Chinese University Prognostic index (CUPI), and the Hang Kong Liver Cancer (HKLC) Staging system (Raoula et al. 2019).

Since the year 2004, two main TACE techniques are widely used: the conventional TACE (c TACE) and the Drug-Eluting Beads TACE (DEB-TACE); however, other TACE techniques are used for the treatment of HCC. Like: chemo-lipiodolization (TOC), in which no embolic agents are used, bland embolization (TAE), in which no cytotoxic drug is used, Trans arterial chemotherapy (TAC), in which no lipiodol or embolic agent is used (no embolization. There are limited uses of them with no enough clinical data on their definite use and their superiority (EASL-EORTC clinical practice guidelines 2012) (Table 7.1).

7.3.1.1 Conventional TACE (cTACE)

It involves the injection of a cytotoxic drug selectively intra-arterially through the tumor-feeding artery, emulsified in an oily radio-opaque agent, followed by embolization of that artery by the embolic agent (Fig. 7.7).

- **Cytotoxic drugs:**

The cytotoxic drugs used involve doxorubicin, epirubicin, idarubicin, mitomycin C, or cisplatin, with doxorubicin the commonest drug used in the Middle East and North Africa, and other contraries, most of which are metabolized in the liver (Raoula et al. 2019).

No evidence of superiority of drug over others on a clinical basis, with wide variations seen between centers and interventional radiologists, also regarding the dose of drug used (some prefer a fixed dose, others based on the body surface area, tumor size, and bilirubin level) (Raoula et al. 2019).

Table 7.1 Different trans arterial techniques for HCC

Procedure	acronym	Cytotoxic agent	Lipiodol	Embolic agent
Transarterial chemoembolization (conventional)	TACE	+	+	+
Transarterial oily chemoembolization (chemo-lipiodolization)	TOCE	+	+	–
Transarterial embolization (bland embolization)	TAE	+	+/–	+
Transarterial chemotherapy	TAC	+	–	–
DEB- Transarterial chemoembolization	DEB-TACE	+	–	+

Adopted and modified from Idée and Guiu (2013)

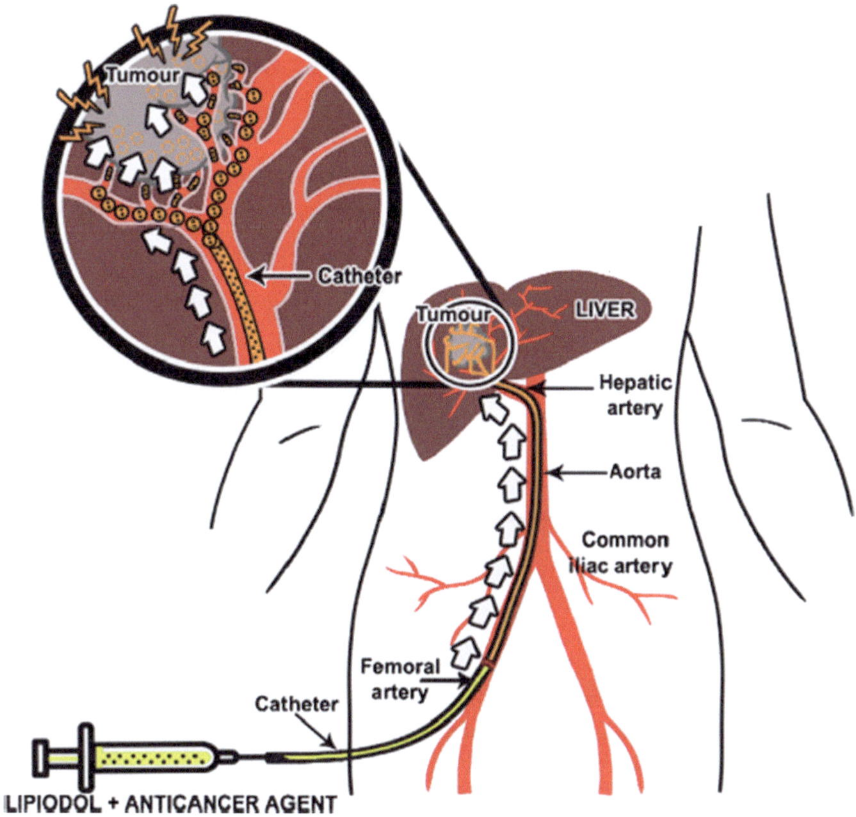

Fig. 7.7 Principle of c TACE (Adopted from Idée and Guiu 2013)

Doxorubicin (Fig. 7.8), which is widely used for the treatment of solid tumor, including HCC and others like lymphoma and leukemia in both children and adult, was discovered in 1969 as a homolog of daunorubicin, isolated from a soil bacterium known as streptomyces peucetius (van der Zanden et al. 2021).

It acts by inhibiting the Topoisomerase IIb (TOP2B) enzyme so prevent the cancer DNA form division and multiplicity, leading to cancer cell death. (Kashifa Fathima et al. 2022). Despite it is highly effective in treatment of HCC, it has some side effects, like fatigue, hair loss, nausea, vomiting, and a decreased appetite. Sometimes, it can affect the heart, so it needs carful follow-up for patient with cardiac problems with HCC (Albrecht et al. 2021). The usual dose used ranges from 50 to 150 mg per session.

- **Lipiodol (Lipiodol® Ultra-Fluid, Guerbet):**

It is an oily contrast media formed of mixture of long chain (C16 and C18) di-iodinated ethyl esters of fatty acids derived from poppy seed oil (Wolff 2001). It is

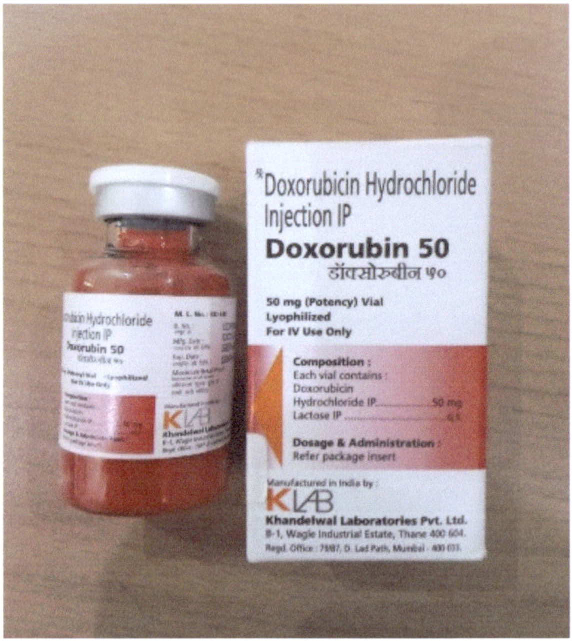

Fig. 7.8 Doxorubicin powder bottle used in TACE

a pale yellow to amber, clear fluid contains 37% iodine (Fig. 7.3). It is found as 10-ml solution for injection. It acts as a carrier of the chemotherapy, also it causes temporary embolization of the tumor microcirculation, helping in the prolongation of the cytotoxic effect of the chemotherapy. That is why retention of the lipiodol at the tumor in the post-treatment CT can be used as a predictor of the overall survival (Idée and Guiu 2013).

- **The embolic agents:**

TACE is commonly ended by transient embolization of the feeding artery to enhance the ischemic necrosis and marinating high dose concentration of the cytotoxic drug, this include gelatin sponge particles, polyvinyl alcohol (PVA) particles, or microspheres (Table 7.2) (Kritzinger et al. 2013).

None of them has a clinical superiority to others. With the gel foam being the most commonly used due to its wide availability and cheap price compared to other (Idée and Guiu 2013).

7.3.1.2 Drug Eluting Beads -TACE (DEB-TACE)

Drug eluting beads (DEBs), they are non-resorbable type of the embolic microspheres that differ from the other microsphere in their ability to load the cytotoxic drug via ion exchange mechanism, so can give more sustained drug release than that in cTACE. Up to 37.5 mg of Doxorubicin /ml of microsphere can be loaded in a time 30–120 minutes. Their diameter range form 40 to 900 μm (Raoula et al. 2019).

Table 7.2 Common embolic agents used in TACE

	Non-spherical		Spherical	
Embolic agent	Gelatin foam	Polyvinyl alcohol	Acrylic	Polyvinyl alcohol
Trade name	Spongel®	Ivalon®	Embosphere®	Bead block®
	Gelfoam®	Contour ®	EmboGold®	Contour SE®
	Curaspon®			
Time of release	1960s	1975	1990s	2000S
Level of occlusion	Proximal	Proximal	Distal	DISTAL
Resorbable	+(day/ week)	+ (month)	No	NO
Size (μm)	Irregular	Variable (45–1180)	Variable (45–1200)	Variable (100–1200)

Adopted and modified from Idée and Guiu (2013)

HepaSphere® microspheres (Merit Medical) are another type of DEBs that have a 30–60 μm that can expand when loaded up to 145–213 μm by doxorubicin solution (Liu et al. 2012). Other examples of DEBs include: Embozene TANDEM® 75-μm microspheres (Boston Scientific) and LifePearl® microspheres (Terumo). Currently, there is not enough clinical data that compare different DEB devices to show superiority of each on another (Raoula et al. 2019).

7.3.1.3 TECHANQUIE of TACE

- **Pre-procedure management:** Patient assessment including [performance status, child-plug scoring, and tumor size, location, behavior (through triphasic CT study of liver or dynamic MRI study) and application of BCLC staging] helps to identify the patient who will undergo TACE treatment (cTACE/ DEB-TACE). Some prefer to give pre-mediation 24 hours before the procedure, including prophylactic antibiotic IM, others start it dearly on the day of the procedure, other medications like pain-killer and gastric protection are also used according to the interventional radiologist.
- **During procedure:** the procedure is done at the interventional unit Cath lab (Fig. 7.9), all the Cath lab involved should have digital subtraction images, newer labs have a cone beam CT, which enables CT images, which improves the technical success (Fig. 7.10). Multiple instruments are involved in the procedure (Fig. 7.11).

Under local anesthesia, a small incision is with insertion of the arterial sheath (either by Seldinger technique, modified Seldinger technique) through a transfemoral approach or transarterial approach, depending of patient condition and pre-imaging vascular anatomy of the hepatic artery. Then, catheterization of the abdominal aorta is done using a specific catheter tube (mostly a cobra catheter 2 or 3), followed by catheterization of the hepatic artery under fluoroscopic imaging. Sometimes a smaller catheter is used (microcatheter) for selective catheterization of the hepatic artery branch to reach feeding arterial supply. HCC is detected by what we call a

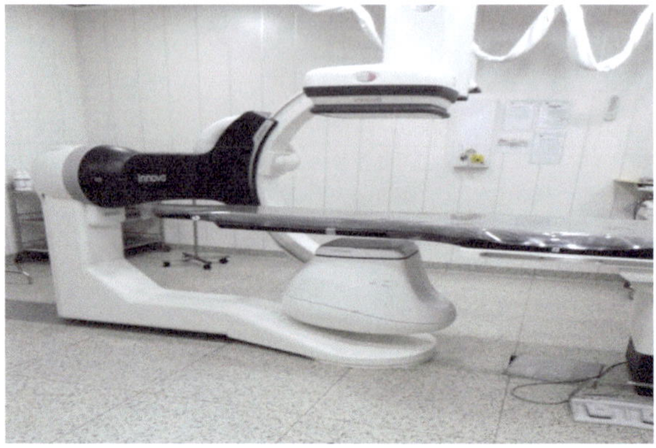

Fig. 7.9 A Cath lab unit in which the procedure is usually done

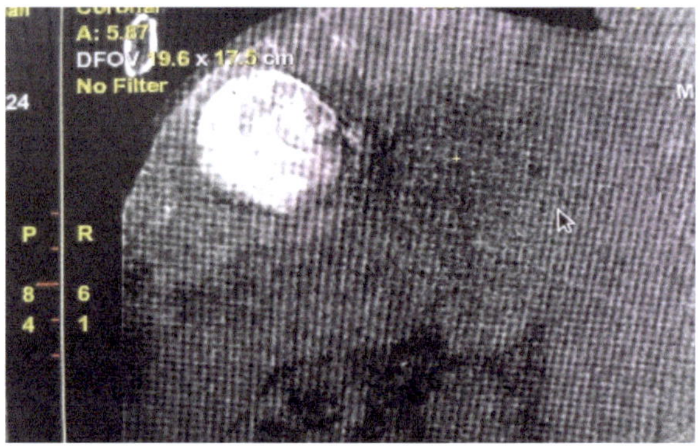

Fig. 7.10 CT image acquired at the end of TACE showing good lipiodol concentration at the lesion

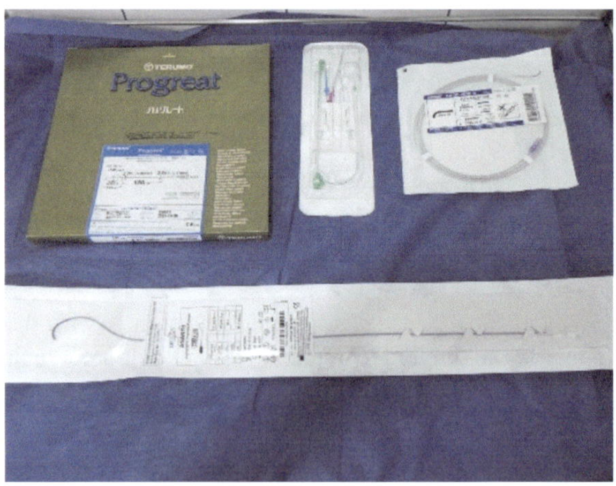

Fig. 7.11 Tools commonly used in TACE

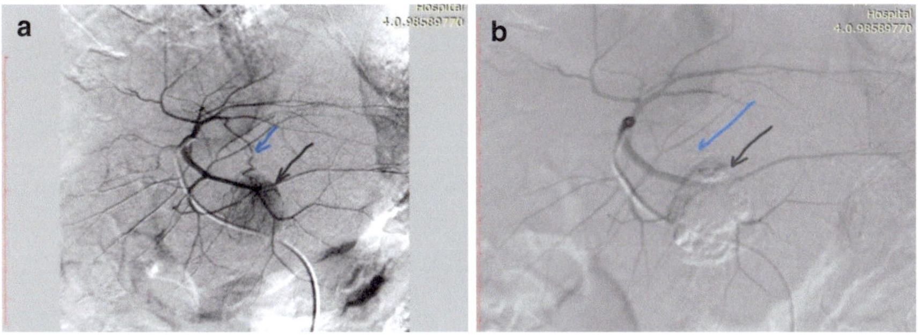

Fig. 7.12 (**a**) The tumoral brush with feeding branch of HCC. (**b**) Post-embolization, no brush is seen

tumoral brush with abnormal tortuous feeding arteries (Fig. 7.12a). In cases of c TACE, mixed emulsion (water in oil) of chemotherapy agent (30–75 mg/m^2 with maximum dose of 150 mg of doxorubicin) with lipiodol in a ratio 1:1 or 1:2) is used, while in DEB-TACE, 50–75 mg of doxorubicin is loaded in 2 ml vial of beads, up to 150 mg can be loaded in 2 vial of beads can be used for large lesion (more than 5 cm) in one session. More sessions can be done, but with a time interval of 2–4 weeks according to patient condition and liver functions. The endpoint of treatment in c TACE, is good lipiodol opacification or the whole amount of W/O emulsion is injected that showed be followed by mechanical embolization till stasis of the second or third lobar arterial branch (Figs. 7.12b and 7.14), while in DEB-TACE, injection should be stopped when feeding arterial stasis is obtained to avoid reflex regarding the amount of beads injected (to avoid non target embolization) (Figs. 7.13 and 7.14).

- **Post-procedure:** Post-procedure medication used (antibiotic, pain killer, and gastric production drugs) for 7–10 weeks to improve the post-procedure side effects as: embolization syndrome with follow-up of hepatic profile, if no another sessions are scheduled. The follow-up response of TACE is done usually after 2 month (with new imaging and laboratory results), if no residual or recurrence is observed, follow-up is scheduled after another 3, 6, and every 6 months.

7.3.1.4 Choosing Between cTACE and DEB-TACE

- **Tumor response and survival:** Most RCTs and observational studies confirmed both are equal with regard to the tumor response and survival. (Facciorusso et al. 2016).
- **Safety:** Both DEBs-TACE and cTACE show the same AEs with no superiority of one over the other, with both showing typical post-embolization syndrome effects with rare doxorubicin systemic complications (Raoula et al. 2019). Non-target embolization is a rare complication; however, it is riskier with DEBs-TACE than cTACE due to the non-resorbability of the microsphere, especially in non-trained hands.

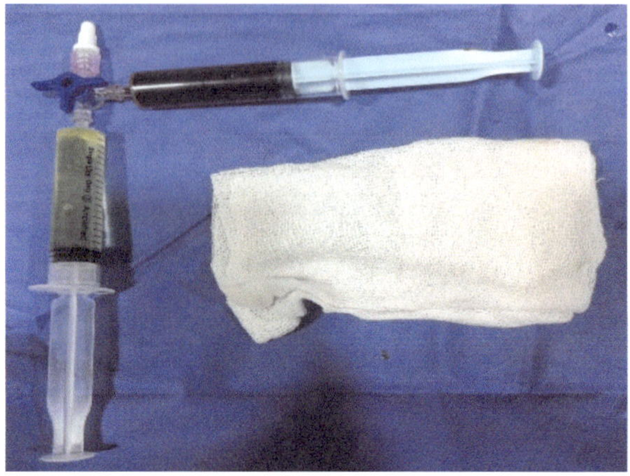

Fig. 7.13 Lipoidal-doxorubicin mixture through 3-way connector

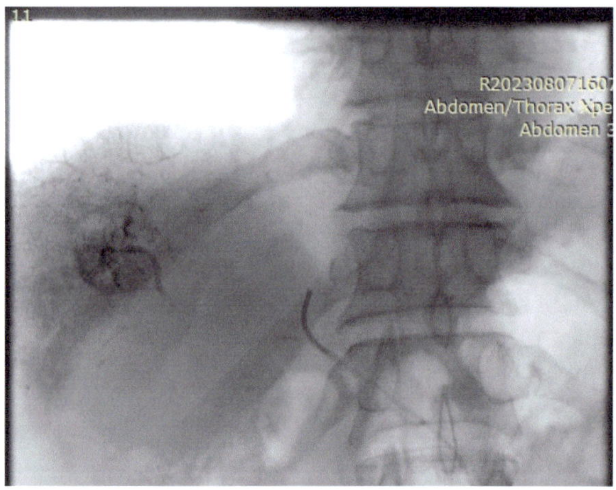

Fig. 7.14 Lipiodol concentration with arterial stasis post-embolization

- **Cost:** Globally, there is no significant cost difference between both techniques but in middle east and Africa, where limited recourses and cost have main impact, cTACE is still cheaper than DEBs-TACE, making the formal is more widely used.

7.3.1.5 Treatment Response of TACE

Up to date, lipiodol concentration with lack of residual contrast enhancement are the main parameter for assessment HCC response, give idea about the overall survival (Raoula et al. 2019).

The Response Evaluation Criteria In Solid Tumor (RECIST), depending on tumor diameter shrunken, and the modified RECIST, depending on contrast enhancement for measures the viable tumor burden, are underestimating the response and do not predict the overall survival of the patient, do cannot replace it as reference of TACE efficacy (Ronot et al. 2014). A lack of lipiodol deposition or partial deposition suggests low lipiodol uptake or missed tumor arterial feeders, so patient can be scheduled for repeat TACE without the need for delayed follow-up (Raoula et al. 2019).

7.3.1.6 When to Repeat or Discontinue TACE?

Transarterial chemoembolization (TACE) remains a cornerstone in the management of intermediate-stage hepatocellular carcinoma (HCC); however, determining when to continue, repeat, or halt treatment is crucial for optimizing outcomes. Several clinical tools have been proposed to aid in these decisions.

Two scoring systems— (Selection for Transarterial Chemoembolization Treatment (**STATE**) and Hepatoma Arterial Embolization Prognostic (**HAP**)— were developed to refine patient selection for initial TACE. Additionally, the Assessment for Re-treatment with TACE (**ART**) and **ABCR** (α-fetoprotein, Barcelona Clinic Liver Cancer stage, Child-Pugh classification, and radiologic Response) scores aim to guide decisions on repeated treatment sessions.

The STATE score incorporates three variables: serum albumin concentration, tumor burden, and C-reactive protein (CRP) levels. In contrast, the HAP score evaluates four parameters: albumin and bilirubin levels, tumor size, and α-fetoprotein concentration. While these scoring systems provide supportive frameworks, they have not yet demonstrated sufficient predictive accuracy to guide clinical decisions independently. Instead, they serve as supplementary tools alongside more established clinical indicators.

In practice, retreatment decisions are more reliably informed by tumor characteristics, liver function (as assessed by the Child-Pugh score), Barcelona Clinic Liver Cancer (BCLC) staging, and radiologic treatment response. According to current recommendations, TACE should be reconsidered or discontinued if there is no radiological evidence of tumor necrosis after two treatment cycles, in cases of continued tumor progression, or if liver function or performance status deteriorates significantly. Other contraindications include the development of portal vein thrombosis or the appearance of extrahepatic metastases, which may necessitate a shift toward systemic or alternative therapies (Raoula et al. 2019; Forner et al. 2014).

7.3.1.7 TACE with Combination Therapy

Many studies showed that combination of TACE with one of the ablation treatments (RF and MW), gives a better response than each alone in both small and large HCC (Seki et al. 2000). The hypoxia effect of TACE can result in increased vascular endothelial growth factor (VEGF) that lead to revascularization of the tumor and its recurrence, so combination with antiangiogenic agents will inhibit the revascularization, delaying the tumor recurrence and progression so improve the overall survival (Chang et al. 2020).

It was found that locoregional treatment as TACE and ablation can cause local inflammation which triggers the release of the tumor antigens that active the host immune system, so combination of TACE with immune Inhibiters can prevent intrahepatic micro metastases which the main cause of recurrence (Kudo 2017).

TACE can be combined with other systemic therapy including sorafenib and immunotherapy for patient with intermediate and advanced HCC with associated vascular invasion as proven with the result of multiple controlled studies with a safety profile and better survival (Meyer et al. 2017).

Problems facing TACE in low/middle-income countries (LMICs)

In the developing countries, inspite of the increased incidence of HCC 2ry to the risk factors, the trans-arterial treatment is not always available as all other newly developed techniques. The cause of this is the cost needed with the lack of governmental coverage to this type of treatment and the absence of non-governmental organizations' (NGOs) financial support for the treatment costs. Hence, cTACE is the most widely accepted line of treatment compared to DEB-TACE and TARE. Another factor affecting is the non-availability of the equipment due to the absence of suppliers.

7.3.2 Trans Arterial Radioembolization (TARE)

It is another transarterial treatment of HCC like TACE, but instead of injection of cytotoxic drugs, microspheres impregnated with radioisotope yttrium-90 (Y90) are selectively injected inside the tumor (Joseph Ralph Kallini et al. 2016).

In 1999, TARE gained the approval of FDA. TARE was typically used for patients with unresectable HCC, not a candidate for TACE, or failed previous TACE, and was used in a lobar or whole liver manner. BCLC is the commonest staging system used for HCC management guide since 2022. The recent BCLC embedded the TARE treatment as one of the main lines of treatment, not only for the intermediate stage only but also in early staging, radiation segmentectomy (RS), and advanced stage with portal vein invasion thrombosis (Reig et al. 2022).

Yttrium 90 (Y90) is the radioactive element used. The idea is that this unstable element undergoes beta decay into a stable element, zirconium-90 at a half-life of 2.67 days (64.2H), emitting a high-speed electron, known as beta particle, with tissue penetration from 2.5 to 11 mm causing cytotoxic destruction of the target tumor (Hickey et al. 2014).

Two types of microspheres are impregnated with Y90: glass and resin type (Table 7.3). Both had gained approval of the Food and Drug Administration (FDA). Resin microspheres have a lower Y90 density per sphere than that of the glass type, meaning more spheres are required and so a higher embolic effect (Piana et al. 2014).

7.3.2.1 Patient Evaluation

The assessment of patient candidate to TARE includes as TACE (performance status and disease burden (Child Pugh score) and tumor stage, in addition to arteriography / macroaggregated albumin (MAA) lung shunting study.

For tumor staging, CT chest and bone scan to exclude extra-hepatic spread. The ideal candidate for patient with HCC compressing less than 70% of the liver volume patient who had single HCC with normal bilirubin level could have lobar or

Table 7.3 Glass and resins impede

	Glass microsphere	Resin microsphere
Diameter of microsphere	20–30 μm	20–60 μm
Activity per sphere	2500 Bq	50 Bq
NO of microsphere for 3 GBq of activity	1.2 million microspheres	40–80 million microspheres
FDA approval	+	+

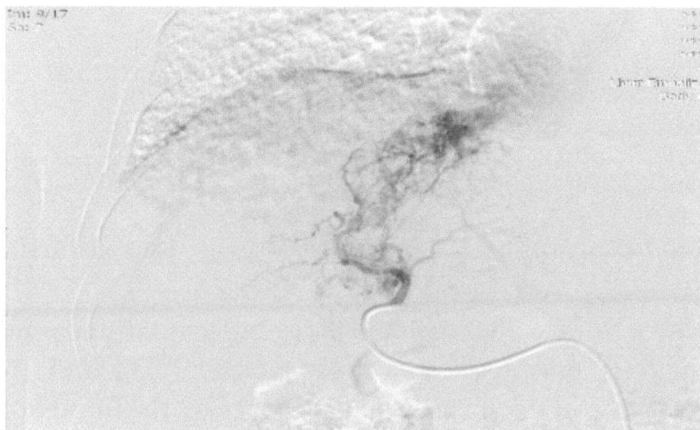

Fig. 7.15 A case of HCC with arterio-venous shunt during pre-treatment angiography. The patient was excluded from TARE treatment

segmental injection but with elevated bilirubin, only segmental injection. Patient with multiple or bi-lobar tumors with normal serum bilirubin, sequential lobar treatment, with abnormal bilirubin, should be excluded from treatment (Joseph Ralph Kallini et al. 2016).

Before TARE, a pre-treatment direct angiogram is done, the value of this is to estimate the anatomical arterial supply of the liver and the selective arterial supply of the tumor. Also, the assessment of the presence of direct arterio-venous shunt, to the lung and other side (Fig. 7.15), which is common with HCC, though complementary injection of 99mTechnetium Macroaggregated Albumin directly into the hepatic artery, followed by scanning the tracer uptake (Fig. 7.16). The problem with this shunt is that it bypasses the tumor capillary bed, so the microsphere can pass directly into the lung, causing fatal radiation pneumonitis. (Salem et al. 2008).

Usually, 4–5 mci of 99mTechnetium Macroaggregated Albumin and the lung shunt fraction (LSF) is calculated using the equation:

$$\text{LSF} = (\text{Total lung count}) / (\text{total lung count} + \text{total abdomen count})$$

LSF of 30 Gy or more /treatment or a cumulative dose of 50 Gy if more than 1 session is needed, excluding the TARE treatment.

TARE can be done on an outpatient basis either on the same day if available or on another day. Up to 170 Gy can be administered. For glass microsphere (Thera Sphere), the goal is to deliver a 120 Gy radiation dose to the liver volume, so the total activity A in GBq is calculated on the basis of the formula:

$$\text{A} = \text{D} \times 50 / \text{m}$$

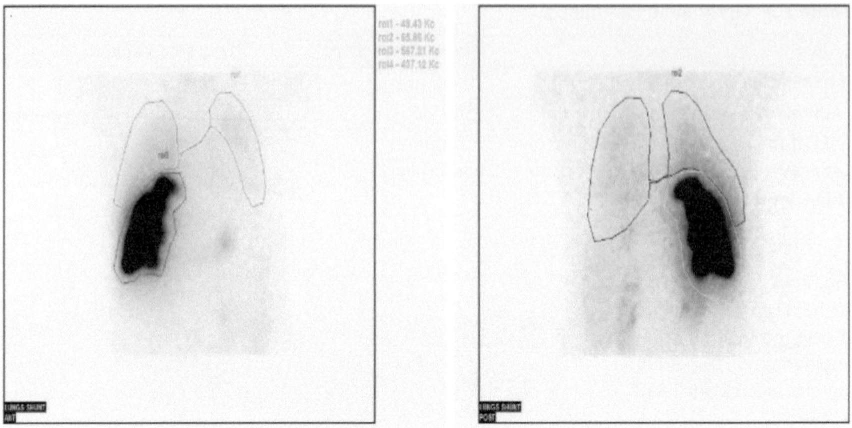

Fig. 7.16 A case of (MAA) lung shunting study before TARE treatment with LSF was only 8.9%

where D is the dose required in Gy and m is the tumor mass calculated from assessed tumor volume in CT converted by factor 1.03 kg/ml.

For resin-microsphere (SIRS-Spheres), the formula commonly used to assess the activity is

$$A = BSA - 0.2 + \left(\%\text{tumor burden} / 100\right)$$

where A is the activity in GBq, BSA is the body surface area in square meters, and the tumor burden% % is the percentage of the liver involved in tumor; however, usually, tumor burden ≥50% requires 3.0 GBq, 25–50% requires 2.5 GBq, ≤ 25% requires 2.0 GBq. This dose is reduced according to LSF (Table 7.4).

7.3.2.2 Post-Treatment Assessment

Is done using either CT or MRI, with varieties in the timing of assessment, with most follow the schedule 2, 4, 6, 8, 11, 14, 18, and 24 months (another follow-up as TACE: 1, 3, 6, 12, 18, and 24 month) (Boas et al. 2015).

Side effect of TARE include abdominal pain, nausea up to vomiting, ascites and pleural effusion, with less commonly seen hepatic abscess, radiation cholecystitis, and radiation pneumonitis (≤ 1%) (Joseph Ralph Kallini et al. 2016).

7.3.2.3 Choosing between TACE and TARE

Overall Survival (OS)

OS most of the RCTs shown no statistically difference between both methods as regard the OS; however, TARE show longer time to progression (TTP) compared to TACE (Brown et al. 2023).

Table 7.4 Dose calculation based on LSF

LSF %	Dose reduction
Less than 10%	No dose reduction
Between 10 and 15%	20% dose reduction
Between 15 and 20%	40% dose reduction
More than 20%	No treatment

Safety

TARE is a well-tolerated outpatient therapy, while TACE typically involves brief hospitalization for symptom management (Kallini et al. 2016).

Cost

Globally, TARE is more expensive than TACE but less expensive than repeated TACE in patients with large HCC, but in the Middle East and Africa, where limited resources and cost have a main impact, TARE is a higher cost than TACE, limiting the application of this method.

7.3.2.4 New Developments in the Practice and Role of TARE

Radiation Segmentectomy (RS)

It was first described in 2011 by Riaz et al. It means delivery of a high dose of Y90 selectively (for a maximum of two segments). So, it maximizes the cytotoxic effect while minimizing the collateral hepatic tissue injury risk. Its goal is ablation of the tumor and adjacent satellite lesion while decreasing the marginal recurrence without risk of needle-tract seeding or hepatic injury. So that provides an alternative therapy to ablation where the percutaneous ablation is not accessible (presence of the focal lesion in the dome, hilum, and caudate lobe). It can be used in early BCLC stage A, as a bridging or downstaging for liver transplant. It gives better response, OS, and TTP than alternative TACE. The best outcome in a patient with Child Pugh class A with a solitary lesion less than 8 cm (Lewandowski et al. 2018).

Radiation Lobectomy (RL)

Beyond the Target: For patient when resection cannot be applied [e.g., due to inadequate future liver remnant (FLR)]. The FLR goal is greater than 20% for patient with normal parenchyma and greater than 40% in liver cirrhosis. Lobar infusion with Y90 (generally 120–150 Gy) has been shown to increase the FLR as portal vein embolization (PVE) but without the fear of tumor progression (atrophy—hypertrophy complex concept), but with longer time than in PVE. The benefit of tumor control making it more suitable in patient when tumor progression beyond resection is highly suggested (Lewandowski et al. 2018).

Boosted -Selective Internal Radiation Therapy (B-SIRT)

It is also called modified RL by others. It combines RS and RL (Fig. 7.15), so it provides an ablative curative-intent high tumor dose that treats the tumor and a lobar parenchymal dose to induce the atrophy-hypertrophy complex and lead to FLR hypertrophy. The higher dose of RS will lead to greater necrosis and effects than the RL alone (Miller et al. 2021).

7.4 Inequality of Access to IR Therapy for HCC in LMICs

The current body of research on the availability of interventional radiology (IR) services in low- and middle-income countries (LMICs) remains very limited, likely reflecting both the underdeveloped IR infrastructure and inadequate reporting systems (Kline et al. 2017). For instance, as of 2017, Tanzania had neither formal IR services nor any officially trained interventional radiologists (Gaupp et al. 2019). In Myanmar, by 2019, only nine specialists across four hospitals were offering IR procedures (Kuo et al. 2021). In contrast, Pakistan has produced 32 IR fellows from five training centers, with graduates practicing both domestically and abroad (Azeemuddin 2020).

Despite global advancements, many LMICs still have limited access to IR compared to high-income countries (HICs) (Shin and Menon 2019). Major barriers include the absence or inadequacy of structured IR training programs, the need for multidisciplinary teamwork, the requirement for highly specialized skills, and the substantial financial investment needed for equipment and operational costs. Furthermore, poor communication between diagnostic radiologists and other healthcare providers often results in low awareness among referring physicians, leaving many patients who could benefit from IR procedures untreated. Additional obstacles include limited professional recognition of the field, staffing shortages, insufficiently developed clinical training pathways, and the inherent complexity of many IR procedures (Jamil et al. 2022).

Addressing these challenges requires comprehensive strategies. Establishing national training initiatives linked with accredited international programs is critical. Engaging medical students and junior doctors through clinical exposure can nurture a new generation of IR specialists. Efforts must also focus on reducing the costs of IR procedures and integrating them into public health insurance schemes. With strategic planning and support, healthcare systems in LMICs can build local IR capacity, enabling access to minimally invasive, life-saving procedures. Moreover, partnerships with international humanitarian organizations and the adaptation of traditional procedural methods to fit local conditions can significantly enhance IR adoption. With sustained commitment, IR can become a more accessible and transformative part of healthcare in LMICs (Jamil et al. 2022).

7.5 Conclusion

Locoregional therapies for hepatocellular carcinoma (HCC) offer outcomes comparable to surgical intervention while being significantly less invasive and associated with fewer postoperative complications and faster recovery times. Radiofrequency (RF) ablation is regarded as the preferred treatment for patients at the early stage of HCC, according to the Barcelona Clinic Liver Cancer (BCLC) classification, particularly for those who are unsuitable candidates for liver resection or transplantation. Conversely, trans-arterial chemoembolization (TACE) is considered the standard of care for patients with intermediate-stage HCC, especially in cases involving large or multiple tumors, provided that liver function is preserved and there is no evidence of vascular invasion or distant metastasis. TACE may also be employed in early-stage HCC when surgical resection or other locoregional therapies are not feasible or have failed, such as in elderly patients or tumors located near critical structures like the biliary ducts or under the diaphragm.

Future research should focus on identifying the patient subgroups most likely to benefit from specific therapies at various disease stages, including the role of minimally invasive ablation in very early and early stages, and exploring optimal therapeutic combinations to improve survival in more advanced stages. However, access to interventional radiology (IR) remains a significant challenge in low- and middle-income countries (LMICs) compared to high-income countries (HICs). Barriers include the lack of structured radiology training programs, the need for multidisciplinary collaboration, the requirement for specialized skills, and the high costs associated with equipment and facility setup. To address these limitations, national-level training initiatives in collaboration with accredited international centers are essential. Moreover, efforts should be made to reduce the costs of IR procedures and incorporate them into public healthcare coverage. Support from international humanitarian organizations and the adaptation of simpler procedural methods can also help expand the availability of IR services in LMICs.

References

Akahane M, Koga H, Kato N, Yamada H, Uozumi K, Tateishi R, Teratani T, Shiina S, Ohtomo K. Complications of percutaneous radiofrequency ablation for hepatocellular carcinoma: imaging spectrum and management. Radiographics. 2005;25(SPEC. ISS):S57. https://doi.org/10.1148/rg.25si055505.

Albrecht KC, Aschenbach R, Diamantis I, et al. Response rate and safety in patients with hepatocellular carcinoma treated with transarterial chemoembolization using 40-mm doxorubicin-eluting microspheres. J Cancer Res Clin Oncol. 2021;147:23–32.

Azeemuddin M. Current status of interventional radiology in Pakistan. Arab J Interv Radiol. 2020;4:1–2.

Baert, A. L., Knauth, L. M., & Sartor, G. K. (2008). Medical radiology diagnostic imaging.

Baek MY, Yoo JJ, Jeong SW, Jang JY, et al. Clinical outcomes of patients with a single hepatocellular carcinoma less than 5 cm treated with transarterial chemoembolization. Kor J Intern Med. 2019;34:1223–32.

Bilchik, A. J., Wood, T. F., & Allegra, D. P. (2001). Radiofrequency ablation of unresectable hepatic malignancies: lessons learned. www.theoncologist.com

Boas FE, Do B, Louie JD, et al. Optimal image in surveillance schedules after liver-directed therapy for hepatocellular carcinoma. J Vasc Intervent Radiol. 2015;26(1):69–73.

Brieger J, Pereira PL, Trübenbach J, Schenk M, Kröber SM, Schmidt D, Aubé C, Claussen CD, Schick F. In vivo efficiency of four commercial monopolar radiofrequency ablation systems: a comparative experimental study in pig liver. Investig Radiol. 2003;38(10):609–16. https://doi.org/10.1097/01.rli.0000077122.70885.94.

Brown AM, Kassab I, Massani M, et al. TACE versus TARE for patients with hepatocellular carcinoma: overall and individual patient level meta-analysis. Cancer Med. 2023;12:2590–9.

Catalano O, Esposito M, Nunziata A, Siani A. Multiphase helical CT findings after percutaneous ablation procedures for hepatocellular carcinoma. Abdom Imaging. 2000;25(6):607–14. https://doi.org/10.1007/s002610000076.

Chang Y, Won Jeong S, Young Jang J, et al. Recent updates of Transarterial chemoembolization in hepatocellular carcinoma. Int J Mol Sci. 2020;21:8165.

Chinnaratha MA, Chuang MYA, Fraser RJ, Woodman RJ, Wigg AJ. Percutaneous thermal ablation for primary hepatocellular carcinoma: a systematic review and meta-analysis. J Gastroenterol Hepatol (Australia). 2016;31(2):294–301. https://doi.org/10.1111/jgh.13028.

Choi, D., Lim, H. K., Ju Kim, M., Jung Kim, S., Hoon Kim, S., Jae Lee, W., Hoon Lim, J., Woon Paik, S., Chul Yoo, B., Seok Choi, M., & Kim, S. (2005). Liver abscess after percutaneous radiofrequency ablation for hepatocellular carcinomas: frequency and risk factors. www.ajronline.org

Chuang C-H, Chen C-Y, Tsai H-M. Image of the month hepatic infarction and hepatic artery pseudoaneurysm with peritoneal bleeding after radiofrequency ablation for hepatoma; 2005. https://doi.org/10.1053/S1542-3565(05)00159-X.

Cucchetti A, Elshaarawy O, Han G, et al. 'Potentially curative therapies' for hepatocellular carcinoma: how many patients can actually be cured? Br J Cancer. 2023;128(9):1665–71. https://doi.org/10.1038/s41416-023-02188-z.

Curley, S. A., Izzo, F., Ellis, L. M. et al. (2000). Radiofrequency ablation of hepatocellular cancer in 110 patients with cirrhosis

Dakua SP, Nayak A. A review on treatments of hepatocellular carcinoma—role of radio wave ablation and possible improvements. Egypt Liver J. 2022;12(1) https://doi.org/10.1186/s43066-022-00191-2.

Decker GA, Gores GJ, Roberts LR. Tumor seeding complicating radiofrequency ablation of hepatocellular carcinoma. J Hepatol. 2003;38(5):692. https://doi.org/10.1016/s0168-8278(03)00028-x.

Dominique E, El Otmany A, Goharin A, et al. How I do it intraductal cooling of the main bile ducts during intraoperative radiofrequency ablation. J Surg Oncol. 2001;76:297.

Elias D, Pietroantonio DD, Gachot B, et al. Liver abscess after radiofrequency ablation of tumors in patients with a biliary tract procedure. Gastroenterol Clin Biol. 2006;30:823.

Erinjeri JP, Clark TWI. Cryoablation: mechanism of action and devices. J Vasc Interv Radiol. 2010;21(SUPPL. 8):S187. https://doi.org/10.1016/j.jvir.2009.12.403.

European Association for the Study of the Liver. European Organization for Research and Treatment of Cancer. EASL-EORTC clinical practice guidelines: management of hepatocellular carcinoma. J Hepatol. 2012;56:908–43.

Facciorusso A, Di Maso M, Muscatiello N. Drug-eluting beads versus conventional chemoembolization for the treatment of unresectable hepatocellular carcinoma: a meta-analysis. Dig Liver Dis. 2016;48:571–7.

Forner A, Gilabert M, Bruix J, et al. Treatment of intermediate-stage hepatocellular carcinoma. Nat Rev Clin Oncol. 2014;11:525–35.

Forner A, Reig M, Bruix J. Hepatocellular carcinoma. Lancet. 2018;391:1301–14.

Galle PR, Forner A, Llovet JM, et al. EASL clinical practice guidelines: management of hepatocellular carcinoma. J Hepatol. 2018;69:182–236.

Garbagnati F, Lencioni R, Allgaier H-P, et al. Percutaneous radio-frequency thermal ablation of Nonresectable hepatocellular carcinoma after occlusion of tumor blood supply 1. Radiology. 2000;217

Gaupp FML, Solomon N, Rukundo I, et al. Tanzania IR initiative: training the first generation of interventional radiologists. J Vasc Intervent Radiol. 2019;30:2036–40.

Goldberg SN, Hahn PF, Tanabe KK, et al. Percutaneous radiofrequency tissue ablation: does perfusion-mediated tissue cooling limit coagulation necrosis? J Vasc Interv Radiol. 1998;9(1 I):101–11. https://doi.org/10.1016/S1051-0443(98)70491-9.

Hammed N, Aderemi O, Babatunde B. Transarterial chemoembolization and microwave ablation for early hepatocellular carcinoma in a Nigerian. Ann Afr Surg. 2022;19(1):58–61. https://doi.org/10.4314/AAS.V19I1.11.

Hickey R, Mulcahy MF, Lewandowski RJ, et al. Chemoradiation of hepatic malignancies: prospective, phase 1 study of full-dose capecitabine with escalating doses of yttrium-90 radioembolization. Int J Radiat Oncol Biol Phys. 2014;88(5):1025–31.

Holzwanger DJ, Madoff DC. Role of interventional radiology in the management of hepatocellular carcinoma: status. Chin Clin Oncol. 2018;7(5):49. https://doi.org/10.21037/cco.2018.07.04.

Ioannou GN, Splan MF, Weiss NS, et al. Incidence and predictors of hepatocellular carcinoma in patients with cirrhosis. Clin Gastroenterol Hepatol. 2007;5(8):938–45.

Jamil H, Tariq W, Ameer MA, et al. Interventional radiology in low- and middle-income countries. Ann Med Surg (Lond). 2022;77:103594. https://doi.org/10.1016/j.amsu.2022.103594.

Idée J-M, Guiu B. Use of Lipiodol as a drug-delivery system for transcatheter arterial chemoembolization of hepatocellular carcinoma: a review. Crit Rev Oncol Hematol. 2013;88:530–49.

Kallini JR, Gabr A, Salem R, et al. Transarterial Radioembolization with Yttrium-90 for the treatment of hepatocellular carcinoma. Adv Ther. 2016;33:699–714.

Kashifa Fathima J, Lavanya V, et al. The effectiveness of various chemotherapeutic agents in cancer treatment. Curr Pharmacol Rep. 2022;8:236–52.

Kettenbach J, Köstler W, Rücklinger E, Gustorff B, Hüpfl M, Wolf F, Peer K, Weigner M, Lammer J, Müller W, Goldberg SN, Kettenbach J. Percutaneous saline-enhanced radiofrequency ablation of Unresectable hepatic tumors: initial experience in 26 patients E. AJR. 2003;180:180. www.ajronline.org

Kim YS, Lim HK, Rhim H, Lee MW. Ablation of hepatocellular carcinoma. In: Best practice and research: clinical gastroenterology, vol. 28. Bailliere Tindall Ltd.; 2014. p. 897–908. https://doi.org/10.1016/j.bpg.2014.08.011.

Kline AD, Dixon RG, Brown MK, Culp MP. Interventional radiology readiness assessment tool for global health. J Glob Radiol. 2017;3:2.

Kritzinger J, Klass D, Ho S, et al. Hepatic embolotherapy in interventional oncology: technology, techniques, and applications. Clin Radiol. 2013;68:1–15.

Kudo M. Immune checkpoint inhibition in hepatocellular carcinoma: basics and ongoing clinical trials. Oncology. 2017;92(1):50–62.

Kuo BJ, Aung MO, Hnin NP, et al. The state of interventional radiology in Myanmar: a national report. J Glob Radiol. 2021;7:1.

Lau WY, Leung TWT, Yu SCH, Ho SKW. Percutaneous local ablative therapy for hepatocellular carcinoma a review and look into the future, vol. 237; 2003. p. 171.

Lencioni R. Loco-regional treatment of hepatocellular carcinoma. Hepatology. 2010;52(2):762–73. https://doi.org/10.1002/hep.23725.

Lencioni R, Cioni D, Bartolozzi C. Percutaneous radiofrequency thermal ablation of liver malignancies: techniques, indications, imaging findings, and clinical results. Abdominal Imaging. 2001;26(4):345–60. https://doi.org/10.1007/s002610000194.

Lewandowski RJ, Gabr A, Abouchaleh N, et al. Radiation segmentectomy: potential curative therapy for early hepatocellular carcinoma. Radiology. 2018;287(3):1050–8.

Liang P, Wang Y. Microwave ablation of hepatocellular carcinoma. Oncology. 2007;72(SUPPL. 1):124–31. https://doi.org/10.1159/000111718.

Livraghi T, Solbiati L, Meloni MF, et al. Treatment of focal liver tumors with percutaneous radio-frequency ablation: complications encountered in a multicenter study. Radiology. 2003;226(2):441–51. https://doi.org/10.1148/radiol.2262012198.

Llovet JM, Vilana R, Brú C, et al. Increased risk of tumor seeding after percutaneous radiofrequency ablation for single hepatocellular carcinoma. Hepatology. 2001;33(5):1124–9. https://doi.org/10.1053/jhep.2001.24233.

Llovet JM, Brú C, Bruix J. Prognosis of hepatocellular carcinoma: the BCLC staging classification. Semin Liver Dis. 1999;19:329–38.

Liu DM, Kos S, Buczkowski A, et al. Optimization of doxorubicin loading for superabsorbent polymer microspheres: in vitro analysis. Cardiovasc Interv Radiol. 2012;35:391–8.

Lubienski, A., Düx, M., Lubienski, K. et al. G. (2005). Radiofrequency thermal ablation: increase in lesion diameter with continuous acetic acid infusion. Cardiovasc Intervent Radiol, 28(6), 789–794. https://doi.org/10.1007/s00270-005-0022-3.

Lucatelli P, Guiu B. 2022 update of BCLC treatment algorithm of HCC: what's new for interventional radiologists? In: Cardio vascular and interventional radiology, vol. 45. Springer; 2022. p. 275–6. https://doi.org/10.1007/s00270-021-03047-1.

Mai J, Machi J. Ultrasound-guided radiofrequency thermal ablation of liver tumors: percutaneous, laparoscopic, and open surgical approaches, vol. 5; 2001. p. 477.

McGahan JP, Browning PD, Brock JM, et al. Hepatic ablation using radiofrequency electrocautery. Investig Radiol. 1990;25(3):267–70. https://doi.org/10.1097/00004424-199003000-00011.

Meyer T, Fox R, Ma YT, et al. Sorafenib in combination with transarterial chemoembolization in patients with unresectable hepatocellular carcinoma (TACE 2): a randomized placebo-controlled, double-blind, phase 3 trial. Lancet Gastroenterol Hepatol. 2017;2(8):565–75.

Miller FH, Vendrami CL, Gaber A, et al. Evolution of radioembolization in treatment of hepatocellular carcinoma: a pictorial review. Radiographics. 2021;41(6):1802–18.

Mulier, S., Mulier, P., Ni, Y et al. (2002). Complications of radiofrequency coagulation of liver tumours. www.bjs.co.uk

Osman AMA, Abdelaziz AO, Deweir M, et al. Hepatic resection versus microwave ablation for the treatment of early hepatocellular carcinoma: a comparative analysis of treatment outcomes and survival predictors. Egypt Liver J. 2022;12(1) https://doi.org/10.1186/s43066-022-00210-2.

Patel PA, Ingram L, Wilson IDC, et al. No-touch wedge ablation technique of microwave ablation for the treatment of subcapsular tumors in the liver. J Vasc Interv Radiol. 2013;24(8):1257–62. https://doi.org/10.1016/j.jvir.2013.04.014.

Pereira PL, Tübenbach J, Schenk M, et al. Radiofreqency ablation: in vivo comparison of four commercially available devices in pig livers. Radiology. 2004;232(2):482–90. https://doi.org/10.1148/radiol.2322030184.

Piana PM, Bar V, Doyle L, et al. Early arterial stasis during resin-based yttrium-90 radioembolization: incidence and preliminary outcomes. HPB (Oxford). 2014;16(4):336–41.

Piccioni F, Poli A, Templeton LC, et al. Anesthesia for percutaneous radiofrequency tumor ablation (PRFA): a review of current practice and techniques. In: Local and regional anesthesia, vol. 12. Dove Medical Press Ltd.; 2019. p. 127–37. https://doi.org/10.2147/LRA.S185765.

Poon RTP, Ng KKC, Lam CM, et al. Radiofrequency ablation for subcapsular hepatocellular carcinoma. Ann Surg Oncol. 2004;11(3):281–9. https://doi.org/10.1245/ASO.2004.08.018.

Pritchard WF, Wray-Cahen D, Karanian JW, et al. Radiofrequency cauterization with biopsy introducer needle. J Vasc Interv Radiol. 2004;15(2 I):183–7. https://doi.org/10.1097/01.RVI.000019398.74740.69.

Raman SS et al. (2012). Creation of radiofrequency lesions in a porcine model: correlation with sonography, CT, and histopathology

Raoula JL, Alejandro Fornerb A, Bolondi L, et al. Updated use of TACE for hepatocellular carcinoma treatment: how and when to use it based on clinical evidence. Cancer Treat Rev. 2019;72:28–36.

Reig M, Forner A, Rimola J, et al. BCLC strategy for prognosis prediction and treatment recommendation: the 2022 update. J Hepatol. 2022;76:681–93.

Rhim H. Complications of radiofrequency ablation in hepatocellular carcinoma. Abdom Imag. 2005;30:409–18. https://doi.org/10.1007/s00261-004-0255-7.

Ronot M, Bouattour M, Wassermann J, et al. Alternative response criteria (Choi, European association for the study of the liver, and modified response evaluation criteria in solid tumors [RECIST]) versus RECIST 1.1 in patients with advanced hepatocellular carcinoma treated with sorafenib. Oncologist. 2014;19:394–402.

Salem R, Parikh P, Atassi B, et al. Incidence of radiation pneumonitis after hepatic intra-arterial radiotherapy with yttrium-90 microspheres assuming uniform lung distribution. Am J Clin Oncol. 2008;31(5):431–8.

Sarkodie BD, Ohene-Botwe B, Mensah YB, et al. Density and regional distribution of radiologists in a low-income country: the Ghana situation. Chin J Acad Radiol. 2023;6(4):188–95. https://doi.org/10.1007/s42058-023-00130-z.

Seki T, Tamai T, Nakagawa T, et al. Combination therapy with transcatheter arterial chemoembolization and percutaneous microwave coagulation therapy for hepatocellular carcinoma. Cancer. 2000;89:1245–51.

Shamim F, Asghar A, Tauheed S, et al. Radiofrequency ablation of hepatocellular carcinomas: a new spectrum of anesthetic experience at a tertiary care hospital in Pakistan. Saudi J Anaesth. 2017;11(1):21–5. https://doi.org/10.4103/1658-354X.197367.

Shiina S, Sato K, Tateishi R, et al. Percutaneous ablation for hepatocellular carcinoma: comparison of various ablation techniques and surgery. Canadian J Gastroenterol Hepatol. 2018;2018 https://doi.org/10.1155/2018/4756147.

Shin DS, Menon BE. Global IR. Interventional radiology in developing countries. J Clin Interven Radiol ISVIR. 2019;3:3–6.

Singletary SE. Radiofrequency ablation of breast cancer. Am Surg. 2003;69(1):37–40.

Siperstein AE, Berber E, Ballem N, et al. Survival after radiofrequency ablation of colorectal liver metastases: 10-year experience. Ann Surg. 2007;246(4):559–67. https://doi.org/10.1097/SLA.0b013e318155a7b6.

Tan W, Deng Q, Lin S, et al. Comparison of microwave ablation and radiofrequency ablation for hepatocellular carcinoma: a systematic review and meta-analysis. Int J Hyperth. 2019;36(1):264–72. https://doi.org/10.1080/02656736.2018.1562571.

Van der Zanden SY, et al. New insights into the activities and toxicities of the old anticancer drug doxorubicin. FEBS J. 2021;288:6095–111.

Vansonnenberg, E., Mcmullen, W., & Solbiati, L. (2004). Tumor ablation.

Vogl TJ, Farshid P, Naguib NNN, et al. Ablation therapy of hepatocellular carcinoma: a comparative study between radiofrequency and microwave ablation. Abdom Imaging. 2015;40(6):1829–37. https://doi.org/10.1007/s00261-015-0355-6.

Waked I, Alsammany S, Tirmazy SH, et al. Multidisciplinary consensus recommendations for management of hepatocellular carcinoma in Middle East and North Africa region. Liver Int. 2023;43:2062–77.

Welling TH. Laparoscopic radiofrequency ablation (RFA) of liver tumors. Laparosc Surg. 2020;4 https://doi.org/10.21037/ls.2019.10.05.

Wolff J. Physiology and pharmacology of iodized oil in goiter pro-phylaxis. Medicine. 2001;80:20–36.

Yamakado K, Nakatsuka A, Akeboshi M, et al. Percutaneous radiofrequency ablation of liver neoplasms adjacent to the gastrointestinal tract after balloon catheter interposition. J Vasc Interv Radiol. 2003;14(9 I):1183–6. https://doi.org/10.1097/01.RVI.0000086530.86489.05.

Systemic Therapy for HCC

8

Mohamed Kamal Shaker, Ashraf Omar, Hesham Elghazaly, and Ghassan Aboualfa

Abstract

Hepatocellular carcinoma (HCC) ranks as the second cause of death related to cancer. The main cause for HCC is liver cirrhosis whatever the cause. The highest rates are seen in Asia and Africa due to higher incidence of hepatitis B, though it is increasing in developed countries due to hepatitis C. Unfortunately, most of cases present in an advanced stage having only option of systemic therapy. HCC continues to be a challenge to treatment due to chemoresistance, liver dysfunction which hinders the delivery of the drugs. HCC is poorly chemo sensitive. In the past years, no single treatment have shown to be superior to another treatment. Until recently patients in need for systemic therapy had nothing except tyrosine kinase inhibitors (TKI) as an option for treatment. In the last decade, immunotherapy introduced in many cancers seems promising in HCC since all HCC develop in cirrhotic patients that have an immunosuppressive environment that might be modulated. Although new systemic therapies provide hope for advanced non-respectable HCC cases yet, the adverse effects related to these drugs should be highly anticipated and considered. This chapter will discuss the evolution of systemic therapy for HCC and highlight the adverse effects associ-

M. K. Shaker (✉)
Tropical Medicine Department, Ain Shams University, Cairo, Egypt

A. Omar
Departments of Hepatology and Tropical Medicine, Cairo University, Cairo, Egypt

H. Elghazaly
Medical Oncology Department Faculty of Medicine, Ain Shams University, Cairo, Egypt

G. Aboualfa
Memorial Sloan Kettering Cancer Centre and Weill Cornell Medical College, New York, NY, USA
e-mail: abou-alg@mskcc.org

R. Elwakil et al. (eds.), *Approach to Hepatocellular Carcinoma (HCC) Management in Low/Middle-Income Countries*,
https://doi.org/10.1007/978-981-96-3894-9_8

ated with the use of systemic therapy in HCC management the chapter will discuss causes of inequality in access to HCC systemic and ways to address this inequality.

Keywords

Combination Therapy · Hepatocellular carcinoma · Immunotherapy · Monotherapy · Systemic Therapy · Tyrosine Kinase Inhibitors

Abbreviations

ACEIs	Angiotensin-converting enzyme inhibitors
AEs	Adverse events
ALT	Alanine transaminase
ARBs	Angiotensin receptor blockers
AST	Aspartate transaminase
CCBs	Calcium channel blockers
CrCl	Creatinine clearance
EASL-EORTIC	European Association for The Study of The Liver-European Organization for Research and Treatment of Cancer.
GI	Gastrointestinal
GERD	Gastroesophageal reflux disease
HBV	Hepatitis B virus
HCV	Hepatitis C virus
HCC	Hepatocellular carcinoma
HIC	High-income countries
HTN	Hypertension
INR	International normalized ratio
Ir AES	Immune-related adverse events
LMICs	Low/middle-income countries
OS	Overall survival
TTP	Time to progression
TKI	Tyrosine kinase inhibitor
NGO	Non-governmental organization
PD	Programmed death
PDL	Programmed death legend
PFS	Progression free survival
SHARP	Sorafenib hepatocellular carcinoma assessment randomized protocol
UFT	Tegafur-uracil
ULN	Upper limit of normal

8.1 Introduction

Hepatocellular carcinoma (HCC) ranks as the second cause of death related to cancer (Jemal et al. 2011). The main trigger for this is liver cirrhosis whatever the cause (Bosch et al. 2004). The highest rates are seen in Asia and Africa due to higher incidence of hepatitis B, though it is increasing in developed countries due to hepatitis C (Venook et al. 2010). Unfortunately, most of cases present in an advanced stage having only option of systemic therapy (Llovet et al. 2008a, b). HCC continues to be a challenge to treatment due to chemoresistance, liver dysfunction which hinders the delivery of the drugs (Thomas 2008). HCC is poorly chemo sensitive, in the past years no single treatment have shown to be superior to another treatment (Lopez et al. 2006). Until recently patients in need for systemic therapy had nothing except tyrosine kinase inhibitors (TKI) as an option for treatment. Immunotherapy introduced in many cancers seems promising in HCC since almost all HCC develop in cirrhotic patients that have an immunosuppressive environment that might be modulated (Ringelhan et al. 2018). Systemic treatment is considered the main line of treatment in advanced HCC cases (Leowattana et al. 2023). Systemic treatments started with conventional chemotherapy treatment; however, HCC is chemo-resistant disease, till the development of tyrosine kinase inhibitors (TKIs) which started to show survival benefit compared to placebo and chemotherapy (Llovet et al. 2008a, b). Then new era evolved in HCC treatment with immunotherapy single or combined modalities with overall survival benefit and better tolerability, opening new options responding to unmet clinical needs in hepatocellular cancer patients (Mandlik et al. 2023). Each category of these lines of systemic treatment has different limitations based on hepatic functions and different reported side effects. The best way to sequence these drugs is not defined yet. So, defining the toxicity profile for each will help the clinicians a lot to select the best candidate for each line for better outcomes. Through this chapter, we will discuss the most common reported side effects to each line in a chronological manner starting with the first developed lines of treatment.

8.2 Cytotoxic Chemotherapy

8.2.1 Monotherapy

Hepatocellular carcinoma is chemo-resistant due to the expression of drug resistance genes also due the liver dysfunction which might hinder the delivery of drugs, till recent years no single treatment have shown superiority on another (Lopez et al. 2006). Doxorubicin has been used since 1970s with different results in a study it showed 79% response (Olweny et al. 1957); however, other studies showed less response rate (10–20%) (Sciarrino et al. 1985). It is not clear whether doxorubicin can prolong survival. A study on 60 patients randomized to doxorubicin versus no treatment showed a significant extension in survival (Lai et al. 1988). Later on, a meta-analysis comparing doxorubicin and no treatment or any other treatment failed to elicit any survival benefit (Mathurin et al. 1988). 5 Fluorouracil (5FU) has undergone extensive evaluation and it showed response range of 10% (Tatef et al. 1995). Capecitabine which is a prodrug that is converted at the site of tumor to 5FU showed very low response rate (Patt et al. 2004). A retrospective study by Patt et al. in 2004 investigating the role of capecitabine showed a response rate of 1% with an overall survival of around 10 months. Gemcitabine another chemotherapy which appeared to be very active in vitro (HCC cell line) showed limited activity in several clinical studies (Matsumoto et al. 2008).

8.2.2 Combination Therapy

Several lines of chemotherapy regimens have been studied for the treatment of HCC (Qin et al. 2013). Shin et al. (2005) reported a trial of cisplatin combined with capecitabine and doxorubicin with a response rate of 25%. In 2013, a study performed by Abdel-Rahman et al. compared the difference between capecitabine and sorafenib (Fig. 8.1).

8.2.2.1 GEMOX Protocol

Doses Per Protocol: Gemcitabine (1000 mg/m^2 by fixed dose rate infusion) on day 1 was followed by oxaliplatin (100 mg/m^2) on day 2, with both drugs repeated every 2 weeks. Grade 3 or 4 toxicities included thrombocytopenia (27%), neutropenia (24%, with two cases of febrile neutropenia), anemia (9%), and neuropathy (9%) (Louafi et al. 2007).

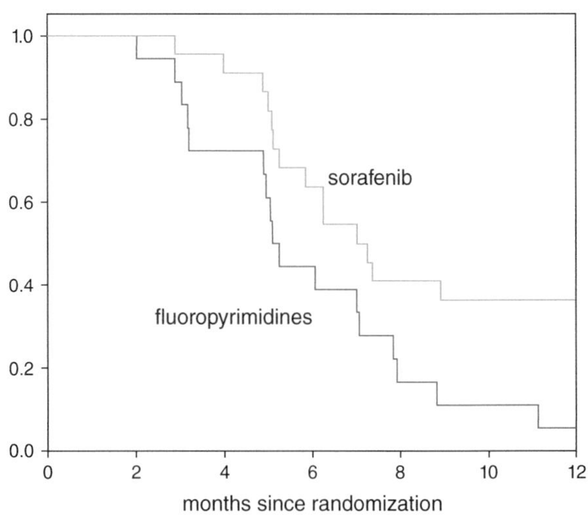

Fig. 8.1 Kaplan Meier analysis of overall survival according to the type of treatment (Abdel-Rahman et al. 2013)

Gemcitabine Plus Cisplatin Combination

Another phase II trial studied the combination of gemcitabine (1250 mg/m^2 on days 1 and 8) and cisplatin (70 mg/m^2 on day 1 of every 21-day cycle). Grade 3 to 4 toxicities included anemia (37%), neutropenia (13%), thrombocytopenia (7%), transaminitis, and mucositis (3% each). Reported most common toxicities for that protocol included in phase II study. Observed grade 3 to 4 toxicities were anemia (44%), neutropenia (26%), and thrombocytopenia (14%) (Parikh et al. 2005).

8.2.2.2 Modified FOLFOX4

Dose per protocol: modified FOLFOX 4

- Oxaliplatin 85 mg/m^2 day 1.
- Leucovorin 400 mg/m^2 over 2 hours days 1 and 2 before fluorouracil.
- Fluorouracil 400 mg/m^2 bolus, then 600 mg/m^2 over 22 hours days 1 and 2 cycle every 2 weeks.

Although the rate of sensory neuropathy was higher in the FOLFOX group (15% versus 0.6%) compared to doxorubicin single age, most cases showed mild neuropathy and there were no significant differences in the rate of grade 3 or 4 toxicities (either hematologic or nonhematologic) between the groups. Neutropenia (30.6%), leukocytopenia (8.7%), thrombocytopenia (7.7%), and anemia (4.9%) were the most frequent grade 3 to 4 adverse events associated with FOLFOX in the study. But because the trial was carried out in Asia, where hepatitis B is the primary cause of liver cirrhosis, it is challenging to interpret the results (Qin et al. 2013).

8.2.3 Hormonal Therapy

As there is a significant male predominance in morbidity and mortality in HCC, it has been postulated that sex hormones might play a role in the development of the tumor. Tamoxifen, a competitive antagonist of estrogen receptors, have been studied showing only little benefit (Perrone et al. 2002).

8.3 Molecular Targeted Therapy

8.3.1 First Line Systemic Therapy

8.3.1.1 Tyrosine Kinase Inhibitors

Tyrosine kinase inhibitors were the mainstay of treatment for advanced hepatocellular carcinoma before immunotherapy was introduced. Patients with incurable hepatocellular carcinoma had higher survival rates while using tyrosine kinase inhibitors; nonetheless, these patients' reported toxicity limited their use, which had a negative impact on their quality of life and frequently resulted in treatment suspension or termination.

Sorafenib

Sorafenib as a tyrosine kinase inhibitor (TKI) acts by inhibiting the growth of multiple kinase enzymes related to angiogenesis, cell proliferation and differentiation Sorafenib blocks tyrosine kinases and pathways essential for angiogenesis and cell proliferation (Liu et al. 2006). In 2008, the **S**orafinib **H**epatocellular carcinoma **A**ssessment **R**andomized **P**rotocol (**SHARP**) trial established sorafenib as the standard treatment for systemic treatment in advanced HCC (Llovet et al. 2008a, b). The sharp trial assessed the efficacy and safety of sorafenib against placebo as a first line treatment in advanced HCC with Child class A patients who are not eligible for surgical or locoregional treatment. The results showed significant increase in the median survival of 10.7 months compared to 7.9 months in placebo arm, progression-free survival (PFS) was also significantly longer (5.8 vs. 2.8 months) (Llovet et al. 2008a, b) (Fig. 8.2).

Similar results were reported from the Asian Pacific trial (Cheng et al. 2009) since that time many other compounds were tried including erlotinib (Zhu et al. 2015a, b), brivanib (Johnson et al. 2013), sunitinib (Chang et al. 2013) as a first line treatment in advanced HCC showing no superiority or even non-inferiority to sorafenib, so sorafenib stayed as a sole player in the field of first line treatment of advanced HCC (Fig. 8.3).

Prior to the introduction of lenvatinib (Kudo et al. 2018), sorafenib was the standard first-line treatment for advanced hepatocellular carcinoma (HCC) that was not eligible for surgery or locoregional therapy. The REFLECT trial demonstrated that lenvatinib was non-inferior to sorafenib, leading to updated guidelines recommending both sorafenib and lenvatinib as first-line treatments for such cases (EASL Clinical Practice Guidelines 2018) (Fig. 8.4).

In 2018, Abdel Azim et al. conducted a phase II trial comparing sorafenib monotherapy to sorafenib combined with tegafur-uracil (UFT) as a first-line treatment for advanced stage hepatocellular carcinoma (HCC). The study concluded that the combination therapy did not demonstrate superiority over sorafenib alone. Moreover, there was a trend toward poorer survival and greater deterioration in quality of life among patients receiving the combination treatment (Fig. 8.5).

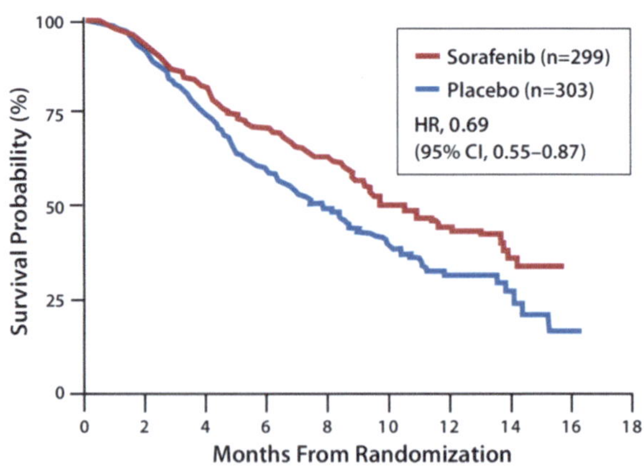

Fig. 8.2 SHARP trial results (Llovet et al. 2008b)

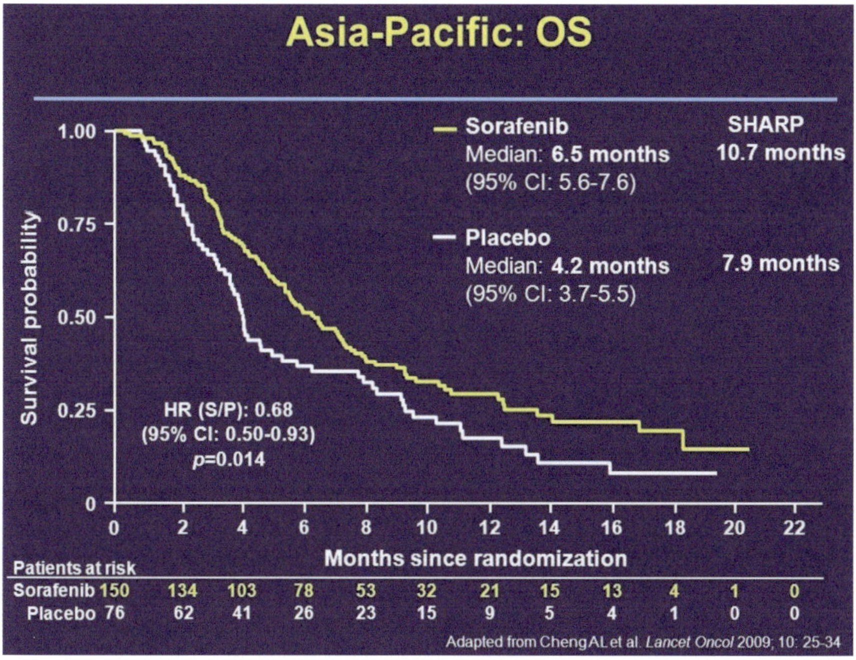

Fig. 8.3 Kaplan-Meier analysis of overall survival in the asian pacific trial (Cheng et al. 2009)

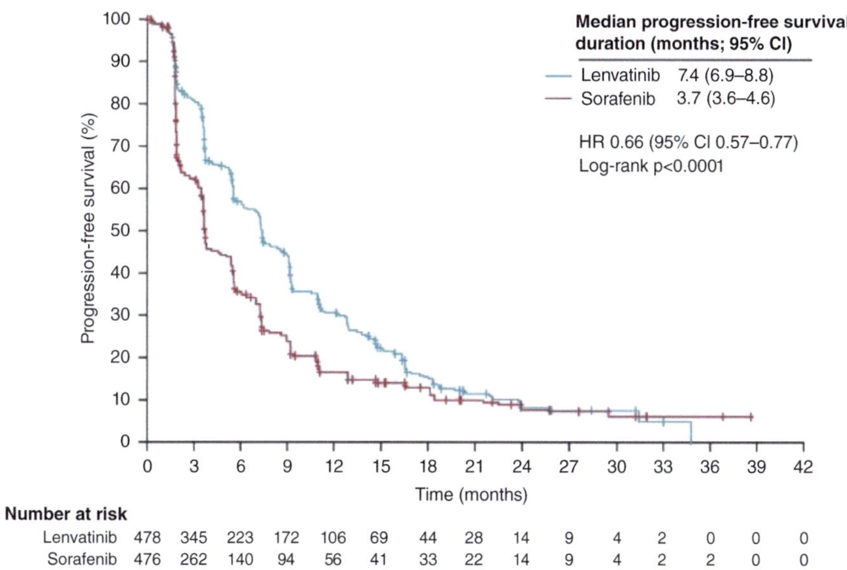

Fig. 8.4 Lenvatinib versus sorafenib in first-line treatment for patients with unresectable hepatocellular carcinoma (Kudo et al. 2018)

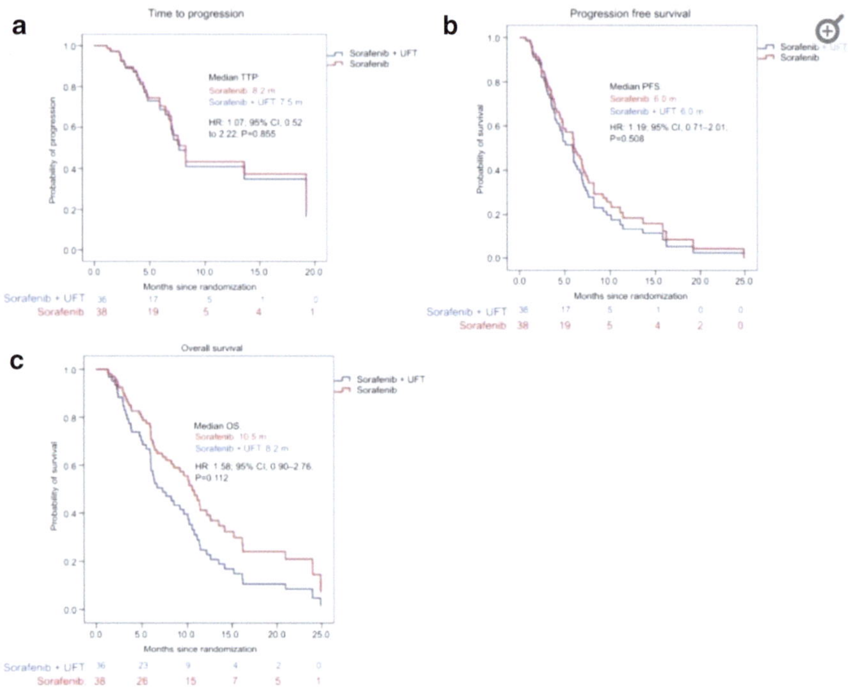

Fig. 8.5 Kaplan-Meier curves for TTP (**a**), PFS (**b**), and OS (**c**) across the two treatment arms (combination arm in blue vs. sorafenib alone in red). OS, overall survival; PFS, progression-free survival; TTP, time to progression; UFT, tegafur-uracil (Azim et al. 2018)

8.3.2 Second-Line Systemic Therapy

8.3.2.1 Regorafenib: RESORCE Trial (Bruix et al. 2017)

Mechanism of Action Regorafenib is an orally active inhibitor of angiogenic (including VEGFR-1, VEGFR-2, and VEGFR-3), stromal, and oncogenic receptor tyrosine kinases.

The toxicity profile of regorafenib is similar to that of other TKIs. Compared to placebo, grade 3 or 4 adverse events occurred more often with regorafenib, including hypertension (15% vs. 5%), hand-foot skin reaction (13% vs. 1%), fatigue (9% vs. 5%), and diarrhea (3% vs. 0%).

In the regorafenib-treatment arm, 6% of patients experienced grade 3 or higher adverse events compared to 8% in the placebo arm. Additionally, 255 (68%) of the 374 patients in the regorafenib arm required dose interruptions or reductions due to adverse events, compared with 60 (31%) of the 193 patients in the placebo arm.

The most common adverse events leading to treatment discontinuation with regorafenib were:

- Increased aspartate transaminase (AST) [8 (2%) of 374 patients vs. 3 (2%) in the placebo group].
- Hand-foot skin reaction (HFSR) [7 (2%) vs. none].
- Increased alanine transaminase (ALT) [4 (1%) vs. none in the placebo arm].

Recommended Dose in HCC Patients 160 mg daily for the first 21 days of a 28-day cycle.

Dosing and Hepatic Impairment

- **Mild Impairment:** (Total bilirubin ≤ ULN and AST > ULN or total bilirubin > ULN to ≤1.5 times ULN) No dosage adjustment necessary; closely monitor for adverse effects.
- **Moderate Impairment:** (Total bilirubin >1.5 times to ≤3 times ULN and any AST) No dosage adjustment necessary; closely monitor for adverse effects.
- **Severe Impairment:** (Total bilirubin >3 times ULN) Use is not recommended as it has not been studied.

8.3.2.2 Lenvatinib: REFLECT Trial (Yamashita et al. 2020)

Mechanism of Action Lenvatinib is a multi-targeted kinase inhibitor (MTKI) that targets VEGFR-1, VEGFR-2, VEGFR-3, PDGFR-β, FGFR-1, FGFR-2, FGFR-3, FGFR-4, KIT, and RET.

Dose Adjusted to Body Weight Patients weighing 60 kg or more should take 12 mg daily, while those weighing less than 60 kg should take 8 mg daily.

Recommended lenvatinib dose reduction for adverse event: First dose reduction: 8 mg once daily. Second dose reduction: 4 mg once daily. Third dose reduction: 4 mg once every other day.

8.3.3 TKIs Adverse Effects

Adverse reactions seen in the class of tyrosine kinase inhibitors (TKIs) are hypertension, diarrhea, asthenia, and hand–foot skin reaction. When patients use this medication for HCC, the majority of the adverse effects are mild.

However, more than 10% of individuals experienced more serious side effects, such as hand-foot skin response or hypertension. In fact, grade 3 hypertension was recorded in up to 23% of lenvatinib-treated patients. Up to 13% of patients treated with regorafenib experienced a grade 3 hand-foot cutaneous response (Rimassa et al. 2019; Kudo et al. 2018).

Regarding when to anticipate experiencing those side effects, the majority of tyrosine kinase inhibitor side effects happen during the first month of treatment. Hand-foot skin response, diarrhea, and hypertension are possible side effects during the first month of oral medication treatment. The skin toxicities, or hand–foot skin response, may also appear several months after therapy initiation. Retrospective data, however, intriguingly suggests that diarrhea and skin toxicity early on may imply a therapeutic benefit from the treatment (Rimassa et al. 2019). The keys of managing toxicity in this patient receiving this kind of agent is education of the patient and monitoring the frequency of the patient's symptoms. If patients have severe side effects, withhold therapy, and, when all the side effects have resolved, consider either restarting the treatment at the same dosage or reducing the dose of treatments. The most common reported side effects with tyrosine kinase inhibitors included hand–foot skin reaction and Stomatitis which will be discussed at the beginning in detail:

Hand and Foot Skin Reaction (HFSR)

The incidence of hand–foot skin reaction (HFSR) is reported to range from ≥1% to approximately 50% of all patients treated with multikinase inhibitors, depending on the specific drug and tumor type. Initial symptoms of HFSR usually appear within the first 2–6 weeks of treatment and include tenderness, paraesthesia, dysesthesia, and intolerance to contact with hot objects. After several weeks of treatment, blisters followed by thickened or hyperkeratotic skin may develop in frictional areas. These skin changes are often painful and can impair range of motion, function, and weight bearing (Lacouture et al. 2008).

Stomatitis and Mucositis

Stomatitis is a general term for inflammation of the oral mucosa, encompassing conditions such as mucositis, dry mouth, dysgeusia, dysphagia, and oral dysesthesia (De Wit et al. 2014). There is limited data on the onset of stomatitis, dry mouth, and dysgeusia with multikinase inhibitors. However, it has been reported that regorafenib-associated stomatitis typically occurs between 5 and 14 days after the start of a treatment cycle, resolves during drug holidays, and may reappear in subsequent treatment cycles (De Wit et al. 2014). Symptomatic relief for stomatitis can be achieved using a mouthwash made of equal parts of 2% viscous lidocaine, diphenhydramine, and bismuth subsalicylate or aluminum/magnesium hydroxide, or alternative mouthwashes. If mouthwash use is painful, pain medication such as viscous lidocaine 2% may be taken first. Aggressive pain relief, including the use of opioids for persistent severe pain, should be administered. As discussed before these two symptoms the most common reported toxicities with TKIs. The following discuss how to manage side effects and dose reduction needed if applicable (Fig. 8.6).

8.3.3.1 Sorafenib Adverse Effects (The GIDEON Research) (Marrero et al. 2016)

Sorafenib-related adverse events (AEs) occurred in 64.9% of patients, with 9.8% of these events being classified as severe. The most frequent serious adverse event was diarrhea (5.2%), occurring in 46% of patients. Other common AEs included

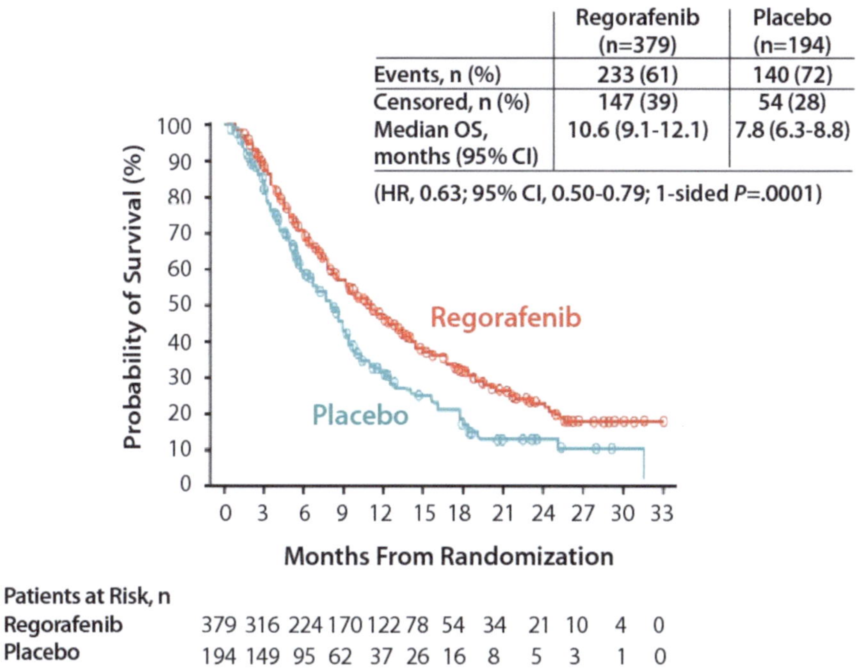

Fig. 8.6 Regorafenib vs. placebo median overall survival results (Bruix et al. 2017)

hand–foot syndrome (HFS) in 16.5% of patients, alopecia in 25%, nausea in 8.0%, and exhaustion in 7.9%.

Dose reductions due to adverse events were common in both the SHARP trial (26%) and the Asia Pacific trial (30.9%). The rates of AEs varied according to Child-Pugh class: 69% in class A, 64% in class B, and 39% in class C. Serious medication responses occurred in 9% of class A, 14% of class B, and 3% of class C patients. The most frequent AEs were:

- HFS: 32% in class A, 17% in class B, and 5% in class C.
- Diarrhea: 28% in class A, 26% in class B, and 11% in class C.
- Exhaustion: 16% in class A, 14% in class B, and 14% in class C.

Hand and foot skin reaction is common side effect induced by sorafenib with reported incidence up to 60% in cases with hepatocellular carcinoma and even similar incidence in cases with renal cell carcinoma. Precautions against hand and foot skin reaction, as previously mentioned, representing the corner stone to tolerate this type of toxicity and to maintain effective dose of sorafenib with decreased incidence of drug interruption and enhanced quality of life.

Common Terminology Criteria for Adverse Events (CTCAE 2006) toxicity grading was used to assess reported degree induced by sorafenib as follows:

HFSR Grades

1. **Mild:** Minimal skin changes or dermatitis (e.g., erythema) without pain.
2. **Moderate:** Skin changes (e.g., peeling, blisters, bleeding, and edema) or pain, not interfering with function.
3. **Severe:** Ulcerative dermatitis or skin changes with pain that interferes with function.

For grade 1 or 2 HFSR, there is no need to change the dose regimen. However, intolerable grade 2 HFSR that does not improve after one or two dose holidays, or a grade 3 episode (e.g., patient unable to walk), may require a dose reduction.

The INSIGHT study (Ganten et al. 2017) reported that sorafenib-related adverse events occurred in 64.9% of patients, with 9.8% classified as severe. The most frequent serious adverse event was diarrhea (5.2%). Other notable medication side effects included HFS (16.5%), nausea (8.0%), and exhaustion (7.9%).

Epigastric Pain

Upper gastrointestinal manifestations as reflux or dyspepsia symptoms commonly occur in patients treated with sorafenib.

Management Approach

Management of Dyspepsia and Gastroesophageal Reflux Disease (GERD)

Symptoms of dyspepsia and GERD can be managed through dietary adjustments, such as a low-fiber diet, changing the timing of sorafenib dosing to be taken before a meal, and the use of supplements like probiotics and digestive enzymes. If these approaches are ineffective, adding a proton pump inhibitor and sucralfate suspension may be beneficial. Sucralfate is indicated for the treatment of peptic ulcers and has shown effectiveness in patients with GERD. There is no reported incidence necessitating dose modifications for sorafenib-induced epigastric pain (Maton, 2003; Katz et al. 2013).

Diarrhea

Diarrhea is commonly associated with sorafenib therapy, usually presenting as CTCAE grade 1 or 2. The concurrent use of the disaccharide lactose for treating hepatic encephalopathy in patients with HCC may exacerbate GI distress, as it is often a source of diarrhea (Blei and Córdoba 2001). Uncontrolled diarrhea can cause dehydration and electrolyte imbalance, significantly impacting patients' quality of life (QOL) and their ability to tolerate cancer treatment (Benson 3rd et al. 2004).

Management Approach

The treatment approach for diarrhea generally includes dietary adjustments, symptomatic control, and monitoring/managing electrolytes. Usually, there is no need to reduce or interrupt the sorafenib dose for grade 1 or 2 events.

Hypertension and Cardiovascular Toxicity

Compared to other types of tyrosine kinase inhibitors, Sorafenib has less incidence of reported induced hypertension and cardiovascular toxicities compared to other types as lenvatininb.

Hypertension should be managed according to basic medical practice and rarely needs dose adjustment for sorafenib.

Myelosuppression

The incidences of sorafenib-associated high-grade anemia, neutropenia, and thrombocytopenia in a meta-analysis were 2.0, 5.1, and 4.0%, respectively (Schutz et al. 2011).

Recommended Dose for Hepatocellular Carcinoma: 400 mg BID daily Recommended Dose reduction Levels according to toxicity:

- Dose Reduction in case of reported hematological toxicity:
  - First Dose Reduction 400 mg orally once daily.
  - Second Dose Reduction 200 mg orally once daily or 400 mg every other day.
  - Third Dose Reduction None
- Dose reduction in case of dermatologic toxicities:
- Grade 1.
  - Continue treatment and consider topical therapy for symptomatic relief.
- Grade 2.
  - First occurrence: Continue treatment and use topical therapy for symptomatic relief; if no improvement within 7 days, interrupt treatment and decrease dose (400 mg daily).
  - No improvement within 7 days or second or third occurrence: Stop drug until toxicity resolves to grade 0–1, then decrease dose by 1 level (400 mg daily).
  - Fourth occurrence: Discontinue drug use.
- Grade 3.
  - First or second occurrence: Stop drug until toxicity resolves to grade 0–1, then decrease dose by 1 level (400 mg daily).
  - Third occurrence: Discontinue drug use.
- **Dose adjustment in case of renal impairment:**
  - **CrCl 40 to 59 mL/minute**: 400 mg twice daily
  - **CrCl 20 to 39 mL/minute**: 200 mg twice daily
  - **CrCl < 20 mL/minute**: Dose not well defined

Hemodialysis (any CrCl): 200 mg once daily (Miller et al. 2009)

- **Dose adjustment in case of hepatic impairment:**
  - **Mild Hepatic Dysfunction:** (bilirubin >1 to ≤1.5 times ULN and/or AST > ULN) 400 mg twice daily.
  - **Moderate Hepatic Dysfunction:** (bilirubin >1.5 to ≤3 times ULN; any AST) 200 mg twice daily.
  - Severe Hepatic Dysfunction:

Albumin < 2.5 g/dL (any bilirubin and any AST): 200 mg once daily.

Bilirubin > 3 to 10 times ULN (any AST): A dose of 200 mg every 3 days was not tolerated; therefore, no dosage has been established for these patients in this pharmacokinetic study.

Drug-Induced Liver Injury During Treatment:

ALT Elevation: Grade 3 or higher (without another cause)—Permanently discontinue sorafenib.

ALT or AST > 3 times ULN with Bilirubin > 2 times ULN: (without another cause)—Permanently discontinue sorafenib.

Alkaline Phosphatase Increase: Any grade, in the absence of known bone pathology, and bilirubin increase (grade 2 or higher)—Permanently discontinue sorafenib.

INR ≥ 1.5: If attributed to drug-induced liver injury—Permanently discontinue sorafenib (Miller et al. 2009).

8.3.3.2 Regorafenib Adverse Effects during Treatment

- **Hepatotoxicity.**

Management of Adverse Reactions

- **Grade 3 AST and/or ALT Elevation:** Withhold the dose until recovery. If the benefit of treatment outweighs the risk of toxicity, resume therapy at a reduced dose of 120 mg once daily.
- **AST or ALT > 20 Times ULN:** Permanently discontinue the medication.
- **AST or ALT > 3 Times ULN with Bilirubin > 2 Times ULN:** Permanently discontinue the medication.
- **Recurrence of AST or ALT > 5 Times ULN Despite Dose Reduction to 120 mg:** Permanently discontinue the medication.
- **Dose Reduction:** If necessary, reduce in 40 mg increments, with the lowest recommended dose being 80 mg/day.

Dermatologic Adverse Events (AE)

- **Grade 2 Hand-Foot Skin Reaction (HFSR; Palmar-Plantar Erythrodysesthesia Syndrome [PPES]):** For the first occurrence, reduce the dose to 120 mg once daily. If grade 2 HFSR recurs at this dose, further reduce to 80 mg once daily. Interrupt therapy if grade 2 HFSR recurs or does not improve within 7 days despite dose reduction.
- **Grade 3 HFSR:** Interrupt therapy for at least 7 days. Upon recovery, reduce the dose to 120 mg once daily. If grade 2 or 3 toxicity recurs at this dose, further reduce to 80 mg once daily upon recovery. Interrupt therapy if grade 2 or 3 HFSR recurs or does not improve within 7 days despite dose reduction.
- **Recurrent or Persistent HFSR at 80 mg Once Daily:** Permanently discontinue treatment.

Other Toxicities

- **Any Grade 3 or 4 Adverse Reaction (excluding hepatotoxicity or infection):** Interrupt therapy. Upon recovery, reduce the dose to 120 mg once daily (except in cases of infection). If any grade 3 or 4 adverse reaction occurs while on this reduced dose (excluding hepatotoxicity or infection), further reduce the dose to 80 mg once daily upon recovery. For any grade 4 adverse reaction, resume therapy only if the benefit outweighs the risk. Permanently discontinue therapy if the patient cannot tolerate 80 mg once daily.

The following adverse drug reactions and incidences are derived from FDA HIGHLIGHTS OF PRESCRIBING INFORMATION for STIVARGA (regorafenib) tablets (FDA, 2012).

>10% AE

- **Cardiovascular:** Hypertension (30% to 59%; hypertensive crisis: <1%).
- **Dermatologic:**
  Alopecia (7% to 24%).
  Palmar-plantar erythrodysesthesia (45% to 67%).
  Skin rash (26% to 30%)
- **Endocrine & Metabolic:**
  Hypocalcemia (17% to 59%).
  Hypokalemia (21% to 31%).
  Hyponatremia (30%).
  Hypophosphatemia (55% to 70%).
  Hypothyroidism (6% to 18%).
  Increased amylase (23% to 26%).
  Weight loss (13% to 32%)
- **Gastrointestinal:**
  Decreased appetite (31% to 47%).
  Diarrhea (41% to 47%).
  Gastrointestinal pain (60%).
  Increased serum lipase (14% to 46%).
  Nausea (17% to 20%).
  Stomatitis (13% to 40%; grades ≥3: 1% to 4%).
  Vomiting (13% to 17%)
- **Genitourinary:** Proteinuria (51% to 84%).
- **Hematologic and Oncologic:**
  Anemia (79%; grade 3: 5%; grade 4: 1%).
  Hemorrhage (11% to 21%; grades ≥3: 2% to 5%).
  Increased INR (24% to 44%; grade 3: ≤4%).
  Lymphocytopenia (30% to 68%; grade 3: 8% to 16%; grade 4: 2%).
  Neutropenia (3% to 16%; grade 3: 1% to 3%; grade 4: 1%).
  Thrombocytopenia (13% to 63%; grade 3: 1% to 5%; grade 4: <1%)
- **Hepatic:**
  Hyperbilirubinemia (33% to 78%).
  Increased serum alanine aminotransferase (45% to 70%).
  Increased serum aspartate aminotransferase (58% to 93%)

- **Infection:** Infection (31% to 32%).
- **Nervous System:**
  Fatigue (≤64%).
  Headache (10% to 16%).
  Pain (55% to 59%).
  Voice disorder (18% to 39%)
- **Neuromuscular and Skeletal:**
  Asthenia (≤64%).
  Muscle spasm (10% to 14%)
- **Miscellaneous:** Fever (20% to 28%).

Adverse Events (AE) by Frequency (1% to 10% AE)
- **Dermatologic:** Exfoliative dermatitis (1%).
- **Gastrointestinal:**
  Mucocutaneous candidiasis (≤3%).
  Pancreatitis (2%)
- **Genitourinary:** Urinary tract infection (6%).
- **Infection:** Fungal infection (≤3%).
- **Neuromuscular & Skeletal:** Tremor (1%).
- **Respiratory:**
  Nasopharyngitis (4%).
  Pneumonia (3%).

<1% AE
- **Cardiovascular:**
  Acute myocardial infarction.
  Ischemic heart disease
- **Dermatologic:**
  Erythema multiforme.
  Stevens-Johnson syndrome.
  Toxic epidermal necrolysis
- **Gastrointestinal:**
  Gastrointestinal fistula.
  Gastrointestinal perforation
- **Nervous System:** Reversible posterior leukoencephalopathy syndrome.
- **Frequency Not Defined:**
  Hepatic: Hepatic failure, hepatotoxicity.

Clinical trials have reported severe and occasionally fatal hepatotoxicity. Hepatic function should be monitored at baseline and during treatment. Dose reductions or discontinuation may be necessary depending on the severity and persistence of hepatic toxicity. Hepatic dysfunction, typically presenting with a hepatocellular injury pattern, often occurred within the first 2 months of treatment. Close monitoring is advised for patients with mild or moderate hepatic impairment; use is not recommended for those with severe impairment. A higher incidence of hepatotoxicity has been noted in Asian patients, particularly Japanese, compared to Caucasians.

After failure of sorafenib as a first line treatment two drugs were evaluated for the treatment of HCC Regorafinib and Cabozantinib based on data from the RESORCE and CELESTIAL study (Bruix et al. 2017; Abou-Alfa et al. 2018).

The RESORCE study evaluated the efficacy of regorafenib compared to placebo in patients who had previously failed sorafenib treatment. The primary endpoint was overall survival (OS), with secondary endpoints including progression-free survival (PFS), objective response rate (ORR), and safety profile. The study demonstrated positive outcomes for the primary endpoint, with OS of 10.6 months for regorafenib versus 7.8 months for placebo.

8.3.3.3 Lenvatinib Side Effects

Due to the high risk of adverse events (AEs) associated with lenvatinib, prophylactic measures and regular monitoring are recommended (Kim et al. 2022). According to the REFLECT trial, hypertension was the most common treatment-related AE in patients with hepatocellular carcinoma receiving lenvatinib, affecting 42% of patients, with most cases being grade ≥ 3 (23%). Other frequently occurring side effects with an incidence over 30% included diarrhea (39%), decreased appetite (34%), and weight loss (31%). The most commonly reported grade ≥ 3 adverse effects were increased blood bilirubin (7%) and proteinuria (6%). Treatment-related toxicity led to dose interruptions in 40% of lenvatinib recipients, dose reductions in 37%, and treatment withdrawal in 9% (Kudo et al. 2018). Clinical studies indicate that the majority of these side effects typically occur within the first 1 to 2 months of initiating lenvatinib therapy.

Management of most of these side effects similar to previously discussed management plan for the reported toxicity with Tyrosine Kinase inhibitors in general, as hypertension and decreased appetite have increased incidence with Lenvatinib, it will be detailed later.

Hypertension Management with Lenvatinib

Given the early onset and high incidence of hypertension associated with lenvatinib, and to prevent complications related to sustained elevated blood pressure (BP), it is essential to manage hypertension proactively. Before starting lenvatinib therapy, it is recommended to perform a formal risk assessment for potential cardiovascular complications (Ikeda et al. 2018).

For patients with systolic blood pressure (SBP) ≥ 140 mmHg to <160 mmHg or diastolic blood pressure (DBP) ≥ 90 mmHg to <100 mmHg (grade 2 hypertension), lenvatinib treatment should continue. In these cases, antihypertensive therapy should be started if the patient is not already on it, or the dose of existing antihypertensive medication should be increased, or an additional antihypertensive agent should be added (Agarwal et al. 2018).

In patients with systolic blood pressure (SBP) ≥ 160 mmHg or diastolic blood pressure (DBP) ≥ 100 mmHg (grade 3 hypertension) despite optimal antihypertensive therapy, lenvatinib treatment should be temporarily paused. Treatment with lenvatinib can be resumed at a lower dose once SBP is reduced to ≤150 mmHg and DBP to ≤95 mmHg, and the patient has maintained a stable dose of antihypertensive medication for at least 48 hours (Lenvima 2020).

There is no strong evidence to guide the selection of antihypertensive agents for patients on lenvatinib. Angiotensin-converting enzyme inhibitors (ACEIs), angiotensin receptor blockers (ARBs), calcium channel blockers (CCBs), and beta blockers are all viable options. However, diuretics are not recommended as first-line treatments because they may exacerbate dehydration and electrolyte imbalances, especially in the presence of diarrhea, which is a common side effect of lenvatinib (Patel et al. 2020).

Decreased Appetite with Lenvatinib

In the REFLECT study, 34% of patients receiving lenvatinib reported a decreased appetite, with grade ≥ 3 adverse events occurring in 5% of these patients. Additionally, 31% of patients experienced a decrease in body weight, with grade ≥ 3 adverse events in 8% of cases. A decrease in body weight led to dose interruption or reduction in 4.2% of lenvatinib recipients (Kudo et al. 2018). To manage these issues, patients can be given antiemetic agents or oral nutrition. Clinical experience suggests that appetite-stimulating drugs, such as megestrol acetate, may also be beneficial (Kim et al. 2022).

8.4 Immunotherapy

Tumor-associated antigens bound to major histocompatibility complex (MHC) molecules are presented on the surface of antigen-presenting cells. These cells display the antigens to immature T cells, leading to their activation and a cascade of events that ultimately result in the T cells inducing tumor cell death. However, this process is negatively regulated by checkpoint proteins such as PD-1, which is expressed on activated T and B cells. When PD-1 is activated by its ligands, PD-L1 and PD-L2, T cell activity is inhibited, leading to immunosuppression. Antibodies targeting PD-1/PD-L1 have demonstrated efficacy across various tumors (Kudo 2019). Hepatocellular carcinoma (HCC) often develops in an immunosuppressive microenvironment, which may be modulated by immunotherapy (Ringelhan et al. 2018). Checkpoint inhibitors have emerged as a new class of therapy for solid tumors (Chen and Han 2015).

These inhibitors work by overcoming tumor-induced immunotolerance, targeting molecules such as PD-1, its ligand PD-L1, or CTLA-4. While the exact rationale for immune-related adverse events remains unclear, blocking these inhibitory checkpoint molecules can lead to a range of adverse effects, typically attributed to an overactive immune response (Passat et al. 2018). These immune-related adverse events generally occur less frequently than those associated with tyrosine kinase inhibitors (TKIs) and often present with a delayed onset, typically emerging beyond week 8 of treatment (Pennock and Chow, 2015).

The REACH study in 2015 demonstrated that patients with elevated alpha-fetoprotein levels above 400 ng/ml who had failed sorafenib as a first-line treatment could benefit from ramucirumab, a VEGF antibody, showing a median overall survival of 7.8 months compared to 4.2 months with placebo (Zhu et al. 2015a, b). In HCC, the CheckMate 040 study, a nonrandomized phase 1/2 trial involving 56 treatment-naïve patients, suggested that nivolumab, a checkpoint inhibitor, might be effective as a first-line therapy in advanced HCC, with an objective response rate (ORR) of 13% and 6- and 9-month survival rates of 89% and 82%, respectively (El-Khoueiry et al. 2017).

The CELESTIAL study compared cabozantinib with placebo in patients who had failed sorafenib, demonstrating a significant improvement in overall survival (10.2 months vs. 8 months) with an acceptable toxicity profile (Abou-Alfa et al. 2018). The IMbrave150 study investigated the combination of bevacizumab (a VEGF antibody) and atezolizumab (a PD-L1 antibody) as a first-line treatment for treatment-naïve HCC. This study found that the combination significantly improved overall survival (6-month survival rate of 85% vs. 72% with sorafenib) and progression-free survival (PFS) (6.8 months vs. 4.3 months with sorafenib) (Cheng et al. 2022) furthermore the subgroup analysis revealed the superiority of combination therapy in all the subgroups (Cheng et al. 2022).

In 2022 the HIMALAYA study conducted by Abou-Alfa et al found that a single, high priming dose of tremelimumab (an anti-cytotoxic T lymphocyte-associated antigen 4) plus durvalumab (an anti-programmed cell death ligand-1), an infusion regimen termed STRIDE, in this global phase 3 trial patients with unresectable naïve HCC patients were randomly assigned to receive one of three regimens: tremelimumab (300 mg one dose) plus durvalumab (1500 mg every 4 weeks; STRIDE), durvalumab (1500 mg every 4 weeks), or sorafenib. They concluded that STRIDE significantly improved overall survival versus sorafenib. Durvalumab monotherapy was non-inferior to sorafenib for patients with unrespectable hepatocellular carcinoma.

8.4.1 Atezolizumab Plus Bevacizumab

Atezolizumab is a humanized monoclonal antibody that targets programmed cell death ligand 1 (PD-L1), while bevacizumab is a monoclonal antibody that inhibits vascular endothelial growth factor (VEGF). In the combination therapy, atezolizumab is administered at 1200 mg intravenously (IV) every 3 weeks, followed by bevacizumab at 15 mg/kg IV every 3 weeks.

According to the IMbrave150 clinical trial, the frequency of all-grade and high-grade adverse events (AEs) in patients receiving the atezolizumab–bevacizumab combination is similar to those observed with anti-PD-1 monotherapy and combinations of PD-1 and CTLA-4 inhibitors. The incidence of grade 3 or 4 treatment-related AEs was comparable between the combination therapy and sorafenib groups (43% vs. 46%), although hypertension, transaminase elevation, and proteinuria were more frequent with the combination therapy, whereas diarrhea was more common with sorafenib (Finn et al. 2020).

Untreated esophageal varices at risk of bleeding are a contraindication for this treatment until they are controlled. Cardiovascular conditions that contraindicate the use of antiangiogenic agents include cerebrovascular accidents (transient or otherwise), ischemic heart disease (especially following acute myocardial infarction or unstable angina), moderate to severe congestive heart failure (NYHA class 2 or higher), poorly controlled arterial hypertension (particularly with a history of hypertensive crisis or encephalopathy), peripheral arterial thrombosis, and significant arrhythmias. Additionally, the need for therapeutic antiaggregation or anticoagulation due to recent thrombotic or cardiovascular events represents a substantial contraindication (Bruix et al. 2021).

Management of varices should follow local practice guidelines. While the IMbrave150 trial did not provide specific recommendations for varices management, general guidelines suggest that patients with small varices might be treated with beta-blockers or not treated at all. For those with medium to large varices, the decision between beta-blockers or endoscopic band ligation should be based on local resources, patient preferences, characteristics, contraindications, and adverse effects.

8.4.2 Tremelimumab Plus Durvalumab

The combination of durvalumab, an anti-PD-L1 monoclonal antibody, with a single priming dose of tremelimumab, an anti-cytotoxic T-lymphocyte-associated protein 4 (CTLA-4) monoclonal antibody, involves administering tremelimumab at 300 mg followed by durvalumab at 1500 mg every 4 weeks.

This combination appears to be tolerable and clinically active in patients who have progressed on, were intolerant to, or refused sorafenib. In clinical trials, grade 3/4 immune-related adverse effects (irAEs) occurred in 50.5% of patients receiving the T300+D regimen, 37.1% in the durvalumab-only group, and 52.4% in the sorafenib group. Grade 3/4 treatment-related AEs (TRAEs) were observed in 25.8%, 12.9%, and 36.9% of patients, respectively. TRAEs leading to death were reported in 2.3% of the T300+D group, 0.0% in the durvalumab group, and 0.8% in the sorafenib group, while TRAEs leading to treatment discontinuation occurred in 8.2%, 4.1%, and 11.0% of patients, respectively (Abou-Alfa et al. 2022).

In terms of treatment-related hematologic AEs, grade 3 or higher in the T300 + D group included increases in AST (2.3%), ALT (1.0%), blood bilirubin (0.3%), and INR (0.3%). For the durvalumab group, the most common were increases in ALT (1.3%) and AST (2.3%). Frequent toxicities in the sorafenib group included increases in AST (1.6%) and ALT (0.8%), blood bilirubin increase (0.5%), and hepatic encephalopathy (0.3%) (Fig. 8.7).

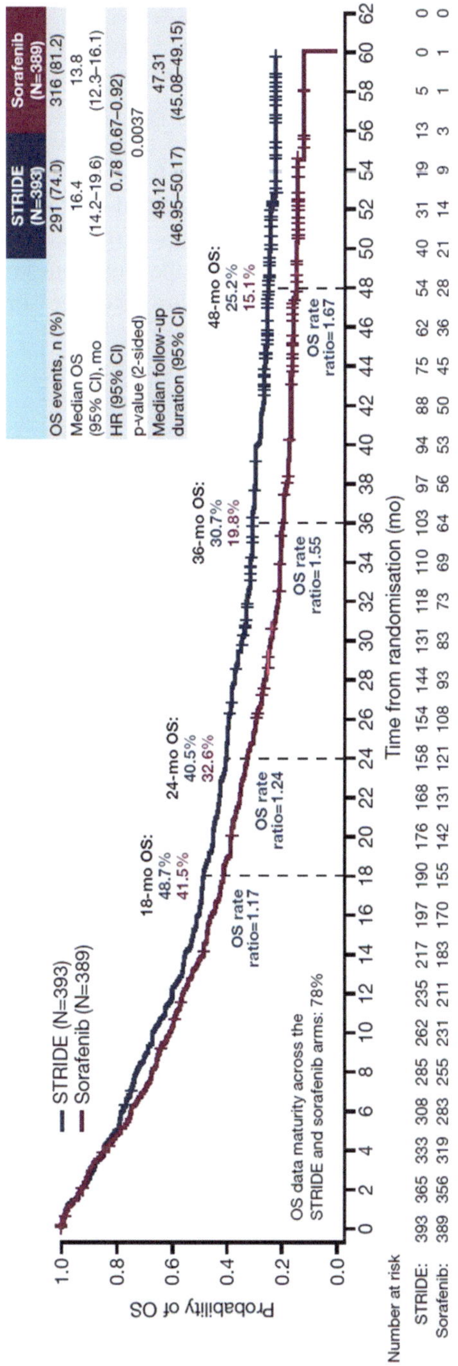

Fig. 8.7 Stride vs. sorafenib results (Abou-Alfa et al. 2022)

8.4.3 Adjuvant Therapy

The IMbrave050 aimed to assess the efficacy of atezolizumab plus bevacizumab as an adjuvant treatment in patients with high-risk hepatocellular carcinoma versus surveillance after curative-intent resection or ablation. In 2023, a phase 3 open-label study was launched by recruiting 668 patients with treated hepatocellular carcinoma either by resection or ablation from 134 hospitals and medical centers from26 countries. All patients were allocated randomly in a 1:1 ratio for receiving atezolizumab plus bevacizumab versus surveillance. Findings showed that the recurrence free survival improved in the treatment arm versus surveillance, however, longer follow up for both recurrence free survival and overall survival is needed (Qin et al. 2023).

8.4.4 Immunotherapy Induced Toxicity

Immune-Related Adverse Events (IrAEs) Immune checkpoint inhibitors (ICIs) targeting PD-1 or CTLA-4 can lead to a range of immune-related adverse events (IrAEs) by enhancing self-immunity. These events can affect any organ system, varying from minor rashes to life-threatening conditions. Unlike PD-1/PD-L1 inhibitors, where IrAEs are not dose-dependent, the adverse effects associated with CTLA-4 inhibitors are dose-dependent. The gastrointestinal tract and skin are frequently affected by both anti-CTLA-4 and PD-1/PD-L1 inhibitors, while the endocrine system and liver are less commonly involved (Wang et al. 2018; Bertrand et al. 2015).

CTLA-4 inhibitors are associated with a higher incidence of IrAEs, with 72% of patients experiencing all-grade IrAEs and 24% experiencing grade 3 or higher IrAEs. Meta-analyzes reveal that during anti-CTLA-4 monotherapy, the most affected organs are the skin (44%), gastrointestinal tract (35%), endocrine glands (6%), and liver (5%), with rash and colitis being the most common. Other organ systems, including the circulatory, ocular, nervous, and musculoskeletal systems, have a very low incidence of IrAEs (Bertrand et al. 2015).

For PD-1 or PD-L1 inhibitors, the incidence of IrAEs is not dose-dependent, with 66% of patients developing at least one IrAE of any grade and 14% developing at least one IrAE of grade 3 or higher. A large meta-analysis of anti-PD-L1 monotherapy identified the skin, gastrointestinal tract, and thyroid gland as common targets for IrAEs. The most severe IrAEs reported include pneumonitis, hepatitis, and neurotoxic effects (Wang et al. 2018).

In phase 2/3 trials, rash was the most common all-grade IrAE, with colitis and elevated aspartate aminotransferase levels being the most frequent high-grade IrAEs. Ipilimumab was associated with a significantly higher incidence of rash and colitis compared to anti-PD-1/PD-L1 agents (De Velasco et al. 2017). For HCC patients, the overall incidence of IrAEs does not significantly differ from other tumor types. The incidence of severe IrAEs in patients treated with PD-1 inhibitors like nivolumab and pembrolizumab is about 10–20%, which is lower compared to the >30% seen in other cancers (Sangro et al. 2020).

8.4.4.1 Cutaneous Toxicity

Cutaneous toxicity is a common adverse effect of ICI therapy, typically manifesting within 2 weeks of starting treatment. Rash and pruritus are the most frequent symptoms. The incidence of grade 3 or higher skin toxicities is less than 1% for monotherapy and around 4% for combination therapies.

When diagnosing and managing skin complications, it is essential to rule out other potential causes such as infections, effects of other drugs (e.g., TKIs), autoimmune diseases, and skin conditions related to chronic liver dysfunction. A thorough assessment and consultation with a dermatologist are recommended. Mild grade 1 or 2 reactions can be managed with topical emollients, mild-strength corticosteroids (e.g., triamcinolone 0.1%), and oral antihistamines. For more severe reactions (grade 2 or 3), systemic corticosteroids at a dose of 0.5–1 mg/kg may be required, and ICI treatment should be paused until symptoms improve to grade 1. For life-threatening reactions, ICI therapy should be permanently discontinued, and patients should receive intravenous methylprednisolone (1–2 mg/kg), with dose tapering based on response (Haanen et al. 2018).

8.4.4.2 Diarrhea

Diarrhea is another prevalent adverse effect during ICI therapy. Incidence rates vary: 11% with pembrolizumab, 10% with nivolumab, 12–24% with nivolumab and ipilimumab combination therapy, 12% with durvalumab and tremelimumab, and 18.8% with atezolizumab–bevacizumab combination therapy. Tremelimumab is associated with a higher incidence, with 30% experiencing grade 1–2 diarrhea and 5% experiencing grade 3 or higher diarrhea. For PD-L1 inhibitors and combination therapies in HCC patients, ≥ grade 3 diarrhea rates are 1% and 2–4%, respectively.

Before initiating ICI therapy, a comprehensive evaluation of gastrointestinal health is recommended. Regular monitoring for diarrhea and colitis during treatment is essential for effective management. New onset or worsening diarrhea should be assessed for gastrointestinal infections, tumor progression, or other causes. Blood tests and stool analysis can help identify thyroid abnormalities, infections, or autoimmune diseases. Biopsy and endoscopy are crucial for diagnosing and assessing colitis (Abu-Sbeih et al. 2018).

For mild diarrhea, ICI treatment can continue while managing symptoms and maintaining internal balance. Persistent grade 2 or higher diarrhea may warrant discontinuation of CTLA-4 agents and possible temporary cessation of PD-1 and PD-L1 agents. Systemic corticosteroids (1–2 mg/kg/day intravenously) should be administered, with reintroduction of PD-1/PD-L1 agents if diarrhea improves to grade 1 or less. If symptoms persist for 2–5 days, immunosuppressive therapy with infliximab (5 mg/kg) should be considered (Cheng et al. 2022). For grade 4 diarrhea or colitis, permanent discontinuation of ICI therapy is necessary, and emergency surgery is indicated if colon perforation occurs. Early use of selective immunosuppressive treatment, such as infliximab, has been shown to improve prognosis in patients with ICI-related colitis (Abu-Sbeih et al. 2019).

8.4.4.3 Hepatotoxicity

Liver-related adverse events (AEs) typically emerge 4–12 weeks after the initiation of immunotherapy. Delayed hepatotoxicity can also arise after the discontinuation of treatment or following management of hepatotoxicity. To diagnose immune-related hepatitis, it is essential to rule out other causes of hepatitis, such as hepatitis flare-ups, biliary tract obstruction, bacterial infections, tumor progression, and the use of hepatotoxic drugs. Steroid therapy is commonly used to manage ICI-induced hepatotoxicity. For grade 2 hepatotoxicity, ICI treatment should be suspended and can be resumed once the condition improves to grade 1. Routine use of corticosteroids is not recommended for grade 2 hepatotoxicity. For grade 3 or higher hepatotoxicity, ICI treatment should be put on hold, and resumption can be considered only when the condition improves to grade 2. If grade 3 hepatotoxicity does not improve during the suspension of ICI treatment, oral prednisone at a dose of 0.5–1 mg/kg/day is recommended. For grade 4 hepatotoxicity, intravenous methylprednisolone at 1–2 mg/kg/day should be administered, and ICI treatment should be permanently discontinued. Reintroduction of ICI treatment may not necessarily lead to a relapse of hepatitis. In cases of steroid-refractory hepatotoxicity, additional immunosuppressive agents such as mycophenolate mofetil, azathioprine, budesonide, cyclosporine, tacrolimus, ursodeoxycholic acid (UDCA), anti-thymocyte globulin (ATG), tocilizumab (an IL-6 receptor antagonist), and plasma exchange may be considered.(Peeraphatdit et al. 2020).

8.4.4.4 Thyroid Dysfunction

Thyroid dysfunction is the most common endocrine irAE in ICI treatment. The rationale of immune-related thyroid dysfunction is not completely known but involves that anti-PD-(L)1 therapy can enhance preexisting antithyroid antibodies through modulating humoral immunity, thereby causes silent inflammatory thyroiditis (Osorio et al. 2017).

Immunotherapy does not need to be discontinued if immune-related thyroid function abnormalities occur. For symptomatic hyperthyroidism, β-blockers can be used to manage the heart rate. If Graves' disease is diagnosed, treatment should follow the EUGOGO group guidelines. In cases where TSH levels exceed 10 mIU/L or symptomatic hypothyroidism is present, and if TSH levels between 5–10 mIU/L are consistently observed, the use of levothyroxine should be considered. Early consultation with an endocrinologist to develop a personalized treatment plan is recommended (Cui et al. 2020).

8.4.5 Virologic Breakthrough Induced by Immunotherapy

Virologic breakthrough, defined as a one-log increase in HBV DNA or HCV RNA from baseline, is a potential concern in patients with hepatocellular carcinoma (HCC), particularly those with preexisting liver disease, such as hepatitis B virus (HBV) or hepatitis C virus (HCV) infections. These patients may be at increased risk of viral reactivation during systemic therapies, including immune checkpoint inhibitors. The American Society of Clinical Oncology recommends universal HBV screening for all patients initiating systemic anti-cancer therapies (cytotoxic chemotherapy, immunotherapy, or targeted therapies). This screening involves three tests: hepatitis B surface antigen (HBsAg), hepatitis B core antibody (anti-HBc), and antibodies to hepatitis B surface antigen (anti-HBs) (Hwang et al. 2020).

While some case reports have highlighted the issue, large studies have shown varied results. In the Keynote-224 and Keynote-240 trials involving pembrolizumab, no cases of HBV flare were reported. Similarly, the Checkmate-040 study with nivolumab did not document any HBV reactivation. The IMbrave-150 study with atezolizumab did not provide specific safety data on HBV DNA changes.

However, it is worth noting that a phase I/II clinical trial of nivolumab combined with ipilimumab reported a 9% rate of HBV virologic breakthrough and a 10% rate for HCV virologic breakthrough (Wang et al. 2021).

For patients with HBV reactivation, antiviral therapy should be started as soon as possible with the goal to prevent hepatitis flare. However, the need to interrupt immunosuppressive therapy should be considered on a case-by-case basis (Lau 2008).

Additionally, clinicians should consider testing for chronic HCV infection before starting potentially immunosuppressive chemotherapy.

8.4.6 Impact of Immunotherapy on Transplantation Outcome

A systematic review of published cases involving organ transplant recipients treated with immune checkpoint inhibitors (ICIs) such as programmed cell death protein 1 (PD-1) inhibitors, programmed death-ligand 1 (PD-L1) inhibitors, or cytotoxic T-lymphocyte antigen 4 (CTLA-4) inhibitors revealed graft rejection rates of 44% for renal transplants, 39% for liver transplants, and 20% for cardiac transplants. The highest rejection rates were observed in patients treated with PD-1 inhibitors, with a 54% incidence reported for nivolumab and 39% for pembrolizumab. The lowest rejection rate was associated with ipilimumab at 23% (Kumar et al. 2020).

Data on the safety of immunotherapy following liver transplantation are limited, but allograft rejection rates can reach up to 39% due to the stimulation of the host immune response by these agents. Given these findings, immunotherapy should generally be avoided in patients who experience recurrence after transplantation.

8.5 Inequality of Access to HCC Systemic Therapy in LMICs

Reports indicate that approximately 70% of cancer-related deaths occur in low- and middle-income countries (LMICs) (World Health Organization, 2018a). Despite bearing nearly 80% of the global cancer burden, LMICs receive less than 5% of the world's resources dedicated to combating cancer. In these regions, many people face limited access to medications, primarily due to poor availability and the necessity to pay for prescriptions out-of-pocket. Without government reimbursement, insurance, or specialized access schemes, patients often bear the full cost of their treatment, leading to financial strain, deprivation, poverty, or premature death.

Access to medicines in LMICs is further restricted by inadequate government funding and weaknesses in the pharmaceutical sector, such as poor procurement and inventory control. These issues contribute to inefficient utilization of medicines and significant price variability both within and between countries (World Health Organization, 2018b).

The lack of comprehensive data on pricing and affordability is a major obstacle to developing effective and transparent pricing policies. Establishing reliable systems to generate quality data is essential for determining the most suitable pricing models for cancer medications (Mattila et al. 2021).

According to a World Health Organization (2018b) report, countries with lower national incomes have reduced availability of anti-cancer medicines or require higher out-of-pocket payments, especially for expensive treatments like targeted therapies. The report noted that 32% of cancer medicines on the essential medicines list (EML) were available in lower-middle-income countries and 57.7% in low-income countries, but only if patients could cover the full cost. The challenge of accessing medicines is compounded by unreliable supply chains and limited commercial motivation in countries such as Bangladesh, Ghana, India, Kenya, Myanmar, Pakistan, Afghanistan, and Burkina Faso (Cherny et al. 2017; Farooqui et al. 2019). In these regions, even generic anti-cancer medicines on the WHO EML are often available only at full cost, and many are not available at all due to unreliable supply. Studies have highlighted significant disparities in the availability of anti-cancer medicines, with newer, more expensive targeted therapies being less accessible. Barriers include unreliable suppliers, budget constraints, and high costs (Cherny et al. 2017). Research by Barr and Robertson (2016) and Moye-Holz et al. (2018) underscores that limited public insurance coverage, non-inclusion in the EML, and outdated clinical guidelines contribute to inequalities in access to innovative cancer treatments. Many families with monthly incomes between 70 and 285 USD cannot afford the high cost of treatment, leading to abandonment of care (Islam et al. 2015). The high cost of generic medicines on the WHO EML further exacerbates these accessibility issues (Eden et al. 2019).

To address these challenges, there is a need to develop policies that ensure equitable access to cancer treatments, improve procurement and supply systems, and enhance affordability for families in LMICs. The poor affordability highlights the need to formulate policies to ensure equitable affordability, streamline public and private sector procurement and supply systems to reduce the cost to families in LMICs.

Another study explored the policy and programmatic strategies employed by various health system stakeholders to improve access to targeted cancer therapies. These efforts led to a notable increase in the number of patients receiving cancer treatments. Pharmaceutical companies played a key role by establishing partnerships and launching access initiatives, such as expanded patient assistance programs (PAPs) and reduced pricing. These initiatives often included discounts or donations directly benefiting patients enrolled in the programs.

Governments also contributed by implementing diverse coverage requirements and social security schemes for payers. They issued compulsory licenses (CLs), facilitated special marketing arrangements, and engaged in price negotiations with manufacturers. Additionally, governments supported pooled procurement strategies to enhance affordability and accessibility of cancer medicines (Sruamsiri et al. 2015).

Egypt as a LMIC provided a model for availability of HCC systemic therapy which started in the beginning of 2022 after the presidential initiative for the early detection of hepatocellular carcinoma. The systemic therapy is distributed in centers of control of viral hepatitis through a multidisciplinary approach also through the health insurance organization all over Egypt for free. According to the Egyptian Minister of Health and Population, Medicines for liver cancer are available at 22 centers affiliated with the National Committee for Control of Viral Hepatitis (NCCVH) at the hospitals of the ministry and universities (Egypt today 2022). This could be a model for the low- and middle-income countries also the non-governmental organizations (NGOs) can play a part in this by initiatives for the treatment of advanced HCC.

In a recent open forum survey study by Abou-Alfa et al. (2023) to assess the real-life access to treatment in Africa showed significant regional variation in the provision of different treatments. The stark disparities in the availability and access to curative treatments are vividly demonstrated in East, West, and Central Africa. In these regions, sorafenib remains the predominant first-line therapy for advanced HCC, despite the availability of several superior options. This issue is exacerbated by reports from Central Africa, where a quarter of patients have no access to any treatments for advanced HCC.

While clinical and translational scientists have made significant strides in developing and utilizing novel therapies, including immune checkpoint inhibitors, primarily in the Western Hemisphere, Africa—home to one of the highest incidences of HCC globally—lacks access to these advanced treatments. Within Africa itself, there is a notable disparity: only a small proportion of patients in most regions receive any HCC treatment compared to Egypt (3% vs. 76%; $P < 0.0001$). Additionally, median survival rates are markedly different, with 2.5 months in most of Africa versus 10.9 months in Egypt ($P < 0.000$). These figures underscore that improved access to care is crucial for enhancing survival rates and highlights the urgent need for equitable access to advanced HCC treatments across the continent (Teaima et al. 2021).

8.6 Conclusion

In conclusion, HCC is a fatal disease. The best way to protect patients from this is to perform surveillance large randomized controlled trial for surveillance revealed that biannual screening reduced mortality by 37%. In advanced cases, the only option will be the systemic therapy. Evolution of systemic therapy for HCC resulted in the emergence of several TKIs and immunotherapies that carry a new hope for advanced HCC cases. Unfortunately, these new drugs are linked to a long list of AE of several grades. This requires a good selection of HCC patients who will be subjected to this kind of therapy, whether in clinical trials or in real-life practice.

Another obstacle that prevents wide use of new systemic therapies for HCC is hindered by several barriers in low- and middle-income countries (LMICs). These barriers include the high cost of drugs, limited public insurance coverage, exclusion from essential medicine lists (EMLs), unavailability at medical facilities, outdated clinical guidelines, and discrepancies within National Essential Medicine Lists (NEMLs) across different income groups.

To address these challenges, it is essential for government and private sector healthcare providers, along with other stakeholders in LMICs, to explore and implement effective policy and program strategies to improve access to targeted cancer therapies. Successful initiatives have included partnerships with pharmaceutical companies to expand PAPs and lower drug prices. These programs typically offer discounts or donations directly to patients enrolled, thereby improving access to necessary cancer treatments for a significant number of patients.

Acknowledgement The authors thank Dr. Rdwa Azeem Assistant lecture, Medical Oncology Department, Faculty of Medicine, Ain Shams University for helping in preparing the early draft of the chapter.

References

Abdel-Rahman O, Abdel-Wahab M, Shaker M, et al. Sorafenib versus capecitabine in the management of advanced hepatocellular carcinoma. Med Oncol. 2013;30:655.

Abou-Alfa GK, Afihene M, Capanu M, et al. Africa guidelines for hepatocellular carcinoma buildup process. JCO Glob Oncol. 2023;

Abou-Alfa GK, Lau G, Kud M, et al. Tremelimumab plus Durvalumab in unresectable hepatocellular carcinoma. NEJM Evid. 2022;1

Abou-Alfa GK, Meyer T, Cheng AL, et al. Cabzozantinib in patients with advanced and progressing hepatocellular carcinoma. N Engl J Med. 2018;379(1):54–63.

Abu-Sbeih H, Ali FS, Qiao W, et al. Immune checkpoint inhibitor-induced colitis as a predictor of survival in metastatic melanoma. Cancer Immunol Immunother. 2019;68(4):553–61. https://doi.org/10.1007/s00262-019-02303-1.

Abu-Sbeih H, Ali FS, Alsaadi D, et al. Outcomes of vedolizumab therapy in patients with immune checkpoint inhibitor-induced colitis: a multi-center study. J Immunother Cancer. 2018;6(1):142. https://doi.org/10.1186/s40425-018-0461-4.

Agarwal M, Thareja N, Benjamin M, Akhondi A, Mitchell GD. Tyrosine kinase inhibitor-induced hypertension. Curr Oncol Rep. 2018;20:65.

Azim HA, Omar A, Atef H, et al. Sorafenib plus tegafur-uracil (UFT) versus sorafenib as first line systemic treatment for patients with advanced stage HCC: a phase II trial (ESLC01 study). J Hepatocell Carcinoma. 2018;19(5):109–19. https://doi.org/10.2147/JHC.S169285.
Barr R, Robertson J. Access to cytotoxic medicines by children with cancer: a focus on low- and middle-income countries. Pediatr Blood Cancer. 2016;63:287–91. https://doi.org/10.1002/pbc.25722.
Benson AB 3rd, Ajani JA, Catalano RB, et al. Recommended guidelines for the treatment of cancer treatment-induced diarrhea. J Clin Oncol. 2004;22(14):2918–26. https://doi.org/10.1200/JCO.2004.04.132.
Bertrand A, Kostine M, Barnetche T, Truchetet M-E, Schaeverbeke T. Immune related adverse events associated with anti-CTLA-4 antibodies: systematic review and meta-analysis. BMC Med. 2015;13:211. https://doi.org/10.1186/s12916-015-0455-8.
Blei AT, Córdoba J. Practice parameters Committee of the American College of Gastroenterology. Hepatic encephalopathy. Am J Gastroenterol. 2001;96:1968–76.
Bosch FX, Ribes T, Diaz M, et al. Primary liver cancer : worldwide incidence and trends. Gastroenterology. 2004;127:S5–S16.
Bruix J, Chan SL, Galle PR, Rimassa L, Sangro B. Systemic treatment of hepatocellular carcinoma: an EASL position paper. J Hepatol. 2021;75(4):960–74. https://doi.org/10.1016/j.jhep.2021.07.004.
Bruix J, Qin S, Merle P, et al. Regorafenib foe patients with hepatocellular carcinoma who progressed on sorafenib treatment (RESORCE): a randomized, double-blind, placebo- controlled, Phase III trial. Lancet. 2017;389(10064):56–66.
Chang AL, Kang YK, Lin DY, et al. Sutinib versus sorafenib in advanced hepatocellular carcinoma: results of a randomized phase III trial. J Clin Oncol. 2013;31(32):4067–75.
Chen L, Han X. Anti-PD-1/PD-L1 therapy of human cancer: past, present, and future. J Clin Invest. 2015;125(9):3384–91. https://doi.org/10.1172/JCI80011.
Cheng AL, Kang YK, Chen Z, et al. Efficacy and safety of sorafenib in patients in the Asia Pacific region with advanced hepatocellular carcinoma: a phase III randomized, double-blind placebo-controlled trial. Lancet Oncol. 2009;10(1):25–34.
Cheng AL, Qin S, Ikada M, et al. Updated efficacy and safety data from IMbrave 150: Atezolizumab plus bevacizumab vs. sorafenib for unresectable hepatocellular carcinoma. J Hepatol. 2022;76:862.
Cherny NI, Sullivan R, Torode J, Saar M, Eniu A. The European Society for Medical Oncology (ESMO) international consortium study on the availability, out-of-pocket costs and accessibility of antineoplastic medicines in countries outside of Europe. Ann Oncol. 2017;28:2633–47. https://doi.org/10.1093/annonc/mdx521.2017.
Common Terminology Criteria for Adverse Events v3.0 (CTCAE) Publish Date: August 9, 2006. Source: https://ctep.cancer.gov/protocoldevelopment/electronic_applications/docs/ctcaev3.pdf
Cui TM, Liu Y, Wang JB, Liu LX. Adverse effects of immune-checkpoint inhibitors in hepatocellular carcinoma. Onco Targets Ther. 2020;13:11725–40. https://doi.org/10.2147/OTT.S279858. PMID: 33235462; PMCID: PMC7678689
De Velasco G, Je Y, Bossé D, et al. Comprehensive meta-analysis of key immune-related adverse events from CTLA-4 and PD-1/PD-L1 inhibitors in cancer patients. Cancer Immunol Res. 2017;5(4):312–8. https://doi.org/10.1158/2326-6066.CIR-16-0237.
De Wit M, Boers-Doets CB, Saettini A, Vermeersch K, de Juan CR, Ouwerkerk J, Raynard SS, Bazin A, Cremolini C. Prevention and management of adverse events related to regorafenib. Support Care Cancer. 2014;22(3):837–46. https://doi.org/10.1007/s00520-013-2085-z.
Eden TOB, Burns E, Chunda-Liyoka C, et al. Are essential medicines available, reliable and affordable in low-middle income countries? J Cancer Policy. 2019;19:100180. https://doi.org/10.1016/j.jcpo.2018.12.001.
EASL. EASL clinical practice guidelines: management of hepatocellular carcinoma. J Hepatol. 2018;69(1):182–236.

Egypt Today. Egypt's Health Ministry launches initiative to treat hepatocellular carcinoma patients. 28 Mar 2022. https://www.egypttoday.com/Article/1/114269/Egypt-s-Health-Ministry-launches-initiative-to-treat-Hepatocellular-carcinoma. accessed in March 2024.

El-Khoueiry AB, Sangro B, Yau T, et al. Nivolumab in patients with advanced hepatocellular carcinoma (CheckMate 040): an open-label, non- comparative, phase 1/2 dose escalation and expansion trial. Lancet. 2017;389(10088):2492–502. https://doi.org/10.1016/S0140-6736(17)31046-2.

Farooqui N, Martiniuk A, Sharma A, Sharma C, Rathore B, Arora RS, et al. Evaluating access to essential medicines for treating childhood cancers: a medicines availability, price and affordability study in New Delhi, India. BMJ Glob Health. 2019;4:e001379. https://doi.org/10.1136/bmjgh-2018-001379.

FDA, HIGHLIGHTS OF PRESCRIBING INFORMATION STIVARGA (regorafenib) tablets. Initial U.S. Approval: 2012.: https://www.accessdata.fda.gov/drugsatfda_docs/label/2012/203085lbl.pdf. Accessed April 2024.

Finn R, Qin S, Ikeda M. Atezolizumab plus Bevacizumab in Unresectable Hepatocellular Carcinoman. Engl J Med. 2020;382:20.

Ganten TM, Stauber RE, Schott E, et al. Sorafenib in patients with hepatocellular carcinoma – results of the observational INSIGHT study. Clin Cancer Res. 2017;

Haanen J, Carbonnel F, Robert C, et al. Management of toxicities from immunotherapy: ESMO Clinical Practice Guidelines for diagnosis, treatment and follow-up. Ann Oncol. 2018;29:iv264. https://doi.org/10.1093/annonc/mdy162.

Hwang JP, Feld JJ, Hammond SP, et al. Hepatitis B virus screening and Management for Patients with cancer prior to therapy: ASCO provisional clinical opinion update. J Clin Oncol. 2020;38(31):3698–715. https://doi.org/10.1200/JCO.20.01757.

Ikeda M, Kobayashi M, Tahara M, Kaneko S. Optimal management of patients with hepatocellular carcinoma treated with lenvatinib. Expert Opin Drug Saf. 2018;17:1095–105.

Islam A, Akhter A, Eden T. Cost of treatment for children with acutelymphoblastic leukemia in Bangladesh. J Cancer Policy. 2015;6:37–43. https://doi.org/10.1016/j.jcpo.2015.10.002.

Jemal A, Bray F, Center MM, et al. Global cancer statistics. CA Cancer J Clin. 2011;61:69–90.

Johnson PJ, Qin S, Park JWR, et al. Brivenib versus sorafenib as first- line therapy in in patirnts with unresectable, advanced hepatocellular carcinoma: results from the randomized phase III brisk-Fl study. J Clin Oncol. 2013;31(28):3517–24.

Katz PO, Gerson LB, Vela MF. Guidelines for the diagnosis and management of gastroesophageal reflux disease. Off J Am College Gastroenterol. 2013;108(3):308–28.

Kim BH, Yu SJ, Kang W, Cho SB, Park SY, Kim SU, Kim DY. Expert consensus on the management of adverse events in patients receiving lenvatinib for hepatocellular carcinoma. J Gastroenterol Hepatol. 2022;37(3):428–39. https://doi.org/10.1111/jgh.15727. Epub 2021 Nov 17. PMID: 34725855; PMCID: PMC9299126

Kudo M. Immuno-oncology therapy for hepatocellular carcinoma: current status and ongoing trials. Liver Cancer. 2019;8(4):221–38.

Kudo M, Finn RS, Qin S, et al. Lenvatinib versus sorafenib in first-line treatment of patients wit unresectable hepatocellular carcinoma a randomized phase III non-inferiority trial. Lancet. 2018;391(10126):1163–73.

Kumar V, Shinagare AB, Rennke HG, et al. The safety and efficacy of checkpoint inhibitors in transplant recipients: a case series and systematic review of literature. Oncologist. 2020;25(6):505–14. https://doi.org/10.1634/theoncologist.2019-0659.

Lacouture ME, Reilly LM, Gerami P, Guitart J. Hand foot skin reaction in cancer patients treated with the multikinase inhibitors sorafenib and sunitinib. Ann Oncol. 2008;19(11):1955–61. https://doi.org/10.1093/annonc/mdn389.

Lai CL, Wu PC, Chan GC, et al. Doxorubicin versus no antitumor therapy in inoperable hepatocellular carcinoma. A prospective randomized trial. Cancer. 1988;62:479–83.

Lau GK. Hepatitis B reactivation after chemotherapy: two decades of clinical research. Hepatol Int. 2008;2(2):152–62. https://doi.org/10.1007/s12072-008-9056-3. Epub 2008 Mar 5. PMID: 19669300; PMCID: PMC2716860

Leowattana W, Leowattana T, Leowattana P. Systemic treatment for unresectable hepatocellular carcinoma. World J Gastroenterol. 2023;29(10):1551–68. https://doi.org/10.3748/wjg.v29.i10.1551. PMID: 36970588
Llovet JM, Di Bisceglie AM, Bruix J, et al. Design and endpoint of clinical trials in hepatocellular carcinoma. J Natl Cancer Inst. 2008a;100:698–711.
Llovet JM, Ricci S, Mazzaferro V, et al. Sorafenib in advanced hepatocellular carcinoma. N Engl J Med. 2008b;359(4):378–90.
Lenvima US. Prescribing information (2020). Available from: http://www.lenvima.com/pdfs/prescribing-information.pdf
Liu L, Cao Y, Chen C, et al. Sorafenib blocks the RAF/MEK/ERK pathway, inhibits tumor angiogenesisand induces tumor cell apoptosis in hepatocellular carcinoma PLC//5. Cancer Res. 2006;24:4293–300.
Lopez PM, Villanueva A, Llovet JM. Systematic review: evidence based management of hepatocellular carcinoma—an updated analysis of randomized controlled trials. Aliment Pharmacol Ther. 2006;23:1535–47.
Louafi S, Boige V, Ducreux M, et al. Gemcitabine plus oxaliplatin (GEMOX) in patients with advanced hepatocellular carcinoma (HCC): results of a phase II study. Cancer. 2007;109(7):1384–90. https://doi.org/10.1002/cncr.22532.
Mandlik DS, Mandlik SK, Choudhary HB. Immunotherapy for hepatocellular carcinoma: current status and future perspectives. World J Gastroenterol. 2023;29(6):1054–75. https://doi.org/10.3748/wjg.v29.i6.1054. PMID: 36844141; PMCID: PMC9950866
Marrero JA, Kudo M, Venock AP, et al. Observational registry of sorafenib use in clinical practice across Child-Pugh subgroups: the GIDEON study. J Hepatol. 2016 Dec;65:1140.
Mathurin P, Rixe O, Carbonell N, et al. Review article: overview of medical treatments in unresectable hepatocellular carcinoma—an impossible meta- analysis? Aliment Pharmacol Ther. 1988;12:111–26.
Maton PN. Profile and assessment of GERD pharmacotherapy. Cleve Clin J Med. 2003 Nov;1(70):S51–70.
Matsumoto K, Nagahara T, Okano J, et al. The growth inhibition of hepatocellular and cholangiocellular carcinoma cells by gemcitabine and roles of extracellular signal-regulated and checkpoints kinases. Oncol Rep. 2008;20:863–72.
Mattila P, Ahmad R, Hasan SS, Babar ZU. Availability, affordability, access, and pricing of anticancer medicines in low- and middle-income countries: a systematic review of literature. Front Public Health. 2021 Apr;30(9):628744. https://doi.org/10.3389/fpubh.2021.628744.
Miller AA, Murry DJ, Owzar K, et al. Phase I and pharmacokinetic study of Sorafenib in patients with hepatic or renal dysfunction: CALGB 60301. J Clin Oncol. 2009;27(11):1800–5.
Moye-Holz D, Saucedo RS, Dijk JPV, Reijneveld SA, Hogerzeil HV. Access to innovative cancer medicines in a middle-income country—the case of Mexico. J Pharm Policy Pract. 2018;11:25. https://doi.org/10.1186/s40545-018-0153-y.
Olweny CT, Toya T, Katongole-Mbidde E, et al. Treatment of hepatocellular carcinoma with Adriamycin, preliminary communication. Cancer. 1957;36:1250–7.
Osorio JC, Ni A, Chaft JE, et al. Antibody-mediated thyroid dysfunction during T-cell checkpoint blockade in patients with non-small-cell lung cancer. Ann Oncol. 2017;28(3):583–9. https://doi.org/10.1093/annonc/mdw640.
Parikh PM, Fuloria J, Babu G, et al. A phase II study of gemcitabine and cisplatin in patients with advanced hepatocellular carcinoma. Trop Gastroenterol. 2005;26(3):115–8.
Passat T, Touchefeu Y, Gervois N, et al. Physio pathological mechanisms of immune-related adverse events induced by anti-CTLA-4, anti-PD-1 and anti-PD-L1 antibodies in cancer treatment. Bull Cancer (Paris). 2018;105:1033–41. https://doi.org/10.1016/j.bulcan.2018.07.005.
Patel S, Dushenkov A, Jungsuwadee P, Krishnaswami A, Barac A. Team-based approach to management of hypertension associated with angiogenesis inhibitors. J Cardiovasc Transl Res. 2020;13:463–477.
Patt YZ, Hassan MM, Aguayo A, et al. Oral capecitabine for the treatment of hepatocellular carcinoma, cholangiocarcinoma and gall bladder carcinoma. Cancer. 2004;101:578–86.

Pennock GK, Chow LQ. The evolving role of immune checkpoint inhibitors in cancer treatment. Oncologist. 2015;20(7):812–22. https://doi.org/10.1634/theoncologist.2014-0422.

Peeraphatdit TB, Nkomo VT, Naksuk N, et al. Long-term outcomes after Transcatheter and surgical aortic valve replacement in patients with cirrhosis: a guide for the Hepatologist. Hepatology. 2020;72(5):1735–46. https://doi.org/10.1002/hep.31193.

Perrone F, Gallo C, Daniele B, et al. Tamoxifen in the treatment of hepatocellular carcinoma 5 year results of CLIP-1 multicenter randomized controlled trial. Curr Pharm Des. 2002;8:1013–9.

Qin S, Chen M, Cheng AL, et al. Atezolizumab plus bevacizumab versus active surveillance in patients with resected or ablated high-risk hepatocellular carcinoma (IMbrave050): a randomised, open-label, multicentre, phase 3 trial. Lancet. 2023;402(10415):1835–47. https://doi.org/10.1016/S0140-6736(23)01796-8.

Qin S, Bari Y, Lim HY, et al. Randomized, multicenter, open-label study of oxaliplatin plus fluorouracil/leucovorin versus doxorubicin as palliative chemotherapy in patients with advanced hepatocellular carcinoma from Asia. J Clin Oncol. 2013;31:3501–8.

Rimassa L, Danesi R, Pressiani T, Merle P. Management of adverse events associated with tyrosine kinase inhibitors: improving outcomes for patients with hepatocellular carcinoma. Cancer Treat Rev. 2019;77:20–8. https://doi.org/10.1016/j.ctrv.2019.05.004.

Ringelhan M, Pfister D, O'Connor T, Pikarsky E, Heikenwalder M. The immunology of hepatocellular carcinoma. Nat Immunol. 2018;19(3):222–32. https://doi.org/10.1038/s41590-018-0044-z. Epub 2018 Jan 29

Sangro B, Melero I, Wadhawan S, et al. Association of inflammatory biomarkers with clinical outcomes in nivolumab-treated patients with advanced hepatocellular carcinoma. J Hepatol. 2020;73(6):1460–9. https://doi.org/10.1016/j.jhep.2020.07.026.

Schutz FA, Je Y, Choueiri TK. Hematologic toxicities in cancer patients treated with the multi-tyrosine kinase sorafenib: a meta-analysis of clinical trials. Crit Rev Oncol Hematol. 2011;80(2):291–300. https://doi.org/10.1016/j.critrevonc.2010.11.007.

Sciarrino E, Cottone M, Dardanoni G, et al. Ultrasound in monitoring patients with hepatocellular carcinoma treated with Adriamycin. Ann Radiol (Paris). 1985;28:21–4.

Shin D, Lee S, Park J. Systemic chemotherapy with capecitabine, doxorubicin and cisplatin for metastatic hepatocellular carcinoma. (Abstract 4177); 2005 May 13–17, Orlando, FL, USA. Paper presented at the Annual Meeting of American Society of Clinical Oncology.

Sruamsiri R, Ross-DegnanD LCY, Chaiyakunapruk N, Wagner AK. Policies and programs to facilitate access to targeted cancer therapies in Thailand. PLoS One. 2015;10:e0119945. https://doi.org/10.1371/journal.pone.0119945.

Teaima MH, Al Nuseirat A, Abouhussein D, et al. Pharmaceutical policies and regulations of oral antiviral drugs for treatment of hepatitis C in Egypt case study. J Pharm Policy Pract. 2021;14:106.

Tatef M, Dorshow J, Akman S, et al. 5-Flurouracil and high dose calcium leucovorin for hepatocellular carcinoma a phase II trial. Cancer Investig. 1995;13:460–3.

Thomas MB. Systemic therapy for hepatocellular carcinoma. Cancer J. 2008;14:123–7.

Venook AP, Papandreou G, Furuse J, et al. The incidence and epidemiology of hepatocellular carcinoma: a global and regional prospective. Oncologist. 2010;Suppl 4:5–13.

Wang DY, Salem J-E, Cohen JV, et al. Fatal toxic effects associated with immune checkpoint inhibitors: a systematic review and meta-analysis. JAMA Oncol. 2018;4:1721. https://doi.org/10.1001/jamaoncol.2018.3923).

Wang K, Xia Y, Zhu Y, et al. Virological breakthrough after immune checkpoint inhibitor and nucleos(t)ide analog treatment in patients with hepatitis B surface antigen positive hepatocellular carcinoma: a real-world study. J Immuno Therap Cancer. 2021;9:e003195. https://doi.org/10.1136/jitc-2021-003195.

World Health Organization. Cancer: key facts Sheet; 2018a. Available online at: https://www.who.int/news-room/fact-sheets/detail/cancer (accessed in March 2024).

World Health Organization. Technical report: pricing of cancer medicines and its impacts: a comprehensive technical report for the world health assembly resolution 70.12: Operative

paragraph 2.9 on pricing approaches and their impacts on availability and affordability of medicines. Geneva: World Health Organization; 2018b.
Yamashita T, Kudo M, Ikeda K, et al. REFLECT—a phase 3 trial comparing efficacy and safety of lenvatinib to sorafenib for the treatment of unresectable hepatocellular carcinoma: an analysis of Japanese subset. J Gastroenterol. 2020;55:113–22. https://doi.org/10.1007/s00535-019-01642-1.
Zhu AX, Rosmordue O, Evans TR, et al. SEARRCH: a phase III, randomized, double-blind, placebo-controlled trial of Sorafenib plus Erlotinib in patients with advanced hepatocellular carcinoma. J Clin Oncol. 2015a;33(6):559–66.
Zhu AX, Park JO, Bayoo BY, et al. Ramucirumab versus placebo as a second line treatment in patients with advanced hepatocellular carcinoma following first line therapy with sorafenib (REACH): a randomized, double-blind, multicenter, Phase III trial. Lancet Oncol. 2015b;16(7):859–70.

Palliative Therapy and Supportive Care for HCC

9

Hesham Elwakiel and Khaled Abouelezz

Abstract

Hepatocellular carcinoma (HCC) is a disease associated with a heavy burden of symptoms, and a minority of patients are eligible for curative treatment. Many patients will need high-level palliative care. As most HCC patients are from LMICs, the need for palliative care is higher in these countries. Unfortunately, most of the LMICs do not have well-established palliative care programs. Pain control is one of the significant problems in these countries, with a lack of access to opioids. To improve that situation, there should be changes on different levels (governmental, political, educational, cultural, and social levels). Palliative care can be provided under different models, the choice of model based on each country's situation and needs. Palliative care has multiple domains, and providers should know them all. Effective communication is crucial to conduct such care. Caring for the caregiver is an essential part of that care. Providers dealing with patients with serious illnesses should be familiar with hospice and end-of-life care, and efficient community-based teams should be developed.

Keywords

Hepatocellular Carcinoma · Palliative care · Hospice · Low-income countries

H. Elwakiel (✉)
Medical Oncology Department, Faculty of Medicine, Ain Shams University, Cairo, Egypt

K. Abouelezz
Medical Oncology & Palliative Medicine, City of Hope Cancer Center, Phoenix, AZ, USA
e-mail: khaled.abouelezz@coh.org

R. Elwakil et al. (eds.), *Approach to Hepatocellular Carcinoma (HCC) Management in Low/Middle-Income Countries*,
https://doi.org/10.1007/978-981-96-3894-9_9

Abbreviations

APCUs	Acute palliative care units
ANH	Artificial nutrition and hydration
BCLC	Barcelona clinic liver cancer
CHWs	Community Health Workers
CPR	cardiopulmonary resuscitation
HCC	Hepatocellular carcinoma
HFSR	Hand and foot skin reaction
IASP	International Association for the Study of Pain
LMICs	Low and middle-income countries
MV	Mechanical ventilation
NCI	National Cancer Institute
NCP	National Consensus Project
USA	United State of America
WHO	World Health Organization
WHPCA	Worldwide Hospice Palliative Care Alliance

9.1 Palliative Care for HCC in LMICs

9.1.1 Definition of Palliative Care

There is no single accepted definition of palliative care among experts around the globe (Radbruch et al. 2020). World Health Organization (WHO) defined palliative care as an approach to prevent and alleviate the hardship of patients and their families who have problems related to life-threatening illnesses. To do that, there should be early identification and management of patients' physical, psychosocial, and spiritual problems. There are multiple debates about that definition; first one, who is the population that needs that care? Is it for any patient with health-related suffering or for patients with severe illness that negatively impacts the quality of life? (Lamers 2007). The other point about the timing, and if this care is provided at the end of life only or throughout the patient's illness if there is a need to alleviate suffering (Radbruch et al. 2020). For this chapter, we will use the concept of palliative care to indicate the care that the patient can get to alleviate the suffering during the course of the disease, and we will use the concept of hospice care for the care that focuses on care near the end of life.

Palliative care, according to WHO, provides control of the pain and other symptoms, supports the patients to live as actively as possible till death, improves the quality of life of the patients, supports family, utilizes a team, and can be utilized early in the disease side by side to other life-prolonging measures. The intent of this type of care is neither to speed nor delay death.

The National Consensus Project (NCP) for quality palliative care created a framework to deliver effective palliative care. Their guidelines are organized into eight domains: structure and processes, physical aspects, psychological and psychiatric aspects, social aspects, spiritual and religious aspects, cultural aspects, care near the end of life, and ethical and legal aspects (Ferrell et al. 2007).

An interdisciplinary team is required to deliver effective palliative care. That team usually includes a physician or advanced practitioner, nurse, chaplain, and social worker (Meier and Beresford 2008). A dietitian, psychiatrist, physical therapist, speech pathologist, bereavement counselor, or other specialties can be utilized according to the need (Laube et al. 2020). These team members should have special training and expertise.

9.1.2 Models of Palliative Care Delivery

There is no specific site to deliver palliative care; it can be provided anywhere. Some experts classified delivery methods of that care under five major service models: outpatient palliative care clinics, inpatient palliative care consultation teams, acute palliative care units (APCUs), community-based palliative care, and hospice care. These models complete each other to provide supportive care from diagnosis to the end of life. Each service differs in structure, care processes, patients, location of care, and reimbursement models (Hui and Bruera 2016).

Outpatient Palliative Care Clinics This model requires fewer resources. Patients can be seen early during their disease in this setting, and it can serve many patients (Finaly et al. 2018). Outpatient palliative care can be stand-alone clinics, embedded clinics, telehealth-based, or enhanced primary palliative care (Rabow et al. 2015; Hui et al. 2019).

Telehealthcare delivery can be used mainly for patients in rural areas. Clinicians can provide education and counseling and cost-effectively monitor symptoms with the potential to increase hospice referrals, minimize visits to acute care, and improve compliance (Riggs et al. 2017).

Inpatient Consultation Services Inpatient palliative care consultation teams are the core of palliative care. Approximately, 90% of National Cancer Institute (NCI)-designated cancer centers in the USA reported having inpatient consultation teams (Calton et al. 2016; Hui et al. 2010). In a randomized trial, inpatient palliative care consultation on admission was compared to routine care for patients with advanced cancer. The palliative care group showed a significant improvement regards quality of life at 12 weeks. There was no statistically significant difference in secondary outcomes (as depression incidence, intensive care unit admissions, hospice discharge, or survival), but there was a trend favoring the palliative care group (Kistler et al. 2015). Referral to inpatient palliative care can improve patient outcomes and cost of care. Multiple studies showed a lower cost of hospitalization when the palliative care team involved in the care (May et al. 2015; Morrison et al. 2011).

APCUs These are specialized units where patients with severe distress get care under the supervision of highly specialized palliative care teams. Patients in these units can get special kinds of management, like palliative sedation for patients with severe agitation. Patients with severe pain can get rapid titration of their pain medication. The palliative teams in these units can manage discussions regarding goals of care and facilitate discharge planning more efficiently (Zhang et al. 2017; Eti et al. 2013; Elsayem et al. 2011).

These units can be a site for unanswered research questions like the management of agitated delirium and detecting the signs of impending death (Hui et al. 2015).

Community-Based Palliative Care This service is done at home or in community facilities, like nursing homes. That can be done by in-person visits by the palliative care team, providing supplies, or by telephone calls. The team providing this palliative care service has special training in palliative care related topics, especially in end-of-life care, and that is different from the usual home care programs (Gomes et al. 2013).

Palliative care at home can increase the rate of terminally ill patients dying at home. That care can improve satisfaction, and controlling symptoms. The impact of that service on the cost and caregiver well-being is not clear (Gomes et al. 2013; Shepperd et al. 2016).

In certain countries in Europe, there are programs that provide daycare for patients. These day care centers can offer different kinds of support, such as physical, social, spiritual, and physical support. It provides support for caregivers as well through bereavement and respite care (Davies and Higginson 2005).

Hospice Care Although some experts consider it a palliative care model, hospice care has separate philosophy and goals. Many clinicians and patients still have the misconception that the two are the same (Hui et al. 2015).

We will discuss that type of care in detail later in this chapter.

9.1.3 Hepatocellular Carcinoma (HCC) Prognosis and Utilization of Palliative Care

Palliative care is fundamental for patients with HCC, but there are no HCC-specific guidelines for palliative care delivery. A minority of patients with HCC are candidates for curative treatment, and this may be attributed to tumor factors such as multifocality, size, and presence of metastases, patient factors such as performance status and comorbidities, or external factors such as unavailability of liver transplant (Cooper and Aloia 2013). HCC mortality-to-incidence ratio is the highest among all cancers; for example, the mortality-to-incidence ratio is 0.89 for HCC, 0.83 for pancreatic cancer. 0.72 for lung cancer, and 0.27 for colorectal cancer (Laube et al. 2020).

Patients with HCC usually have a poor prognosis. An Italian study showed that median overall survival was about 9 months. Based on the Barcelona Clinic Liver

Cancer (BCLC) classification, the median survival depends on the stage, where the survival was 38, 25, 10, 7, and 6 months for BCLC stage 0, A, B, C, and D, respectively (Giannini et al. 2014).

Palliative care can add significant support during active treatment of HCC patients or when the focus is on supportive care only, but unfortunately, HCC patients are less frequently referred to palliative care in comparison to other common cancers (Woodrell et al. 2023). Some of the aims of palliative therapies are to control symptoms, improve quality of life, and extend survival for such patients (Cunningham et al. 2013).

HCC is often asymptomatic in the early stages, but later, it can be symptomatic. Many providers are unprepared to manage symptoms related to end-stage liver disease. The most common symptoms for HCC patients who are admitted to a palliative care unit are abdominal pain (75.5%), fatigue (72.7%), anorexia or vomiting (68.2%), and ascites (64.5%) (Lin et al. 2004).

Psychological symptoms are common as well as depression and sleep disturbance; but they are often under-assessed and undertreated (Miaskowski et al. 2004).

Symptoms of decompensated liver disease as ascites, peripheral edema, encephalopathy, and gastrointestinal hemorrhage are common in HCC patients as most of these patients have underlying cirrhosis (Laube et al. 2020).

Therapy-associated symptoms are common as well. Transarterial chemoembolization (TACE) can be complicated by post-TACE syndrome, liver failure, ascites, hepatic abscess, fatigue, and gastrointestinal hemorrhage (Laube et al. 2020). Systemic therapy with tyrosine kinase inhibitors or immunotherapy can result in multiple complications including hand-foot skin reaction, hypertension, diarrhea, anorexia, weight loss, fatigue, and alopecia (Laube et al. 2020).

Symptom control can be done with both pharmacological and non-pharmacological therapy like opioid analgesics, ammonia detoxicants, and ascites drainage (Lin et al. 2004). Later, we will discuss the most common symptoms associated with HCC and their management.

Palliative care addresses the caregiver's needs as well. A few studies are addressing the needs of caregivers of HCC patients. In one study of the caregivers of HCC patients, the primary concern of caregivers was the quality of the relationship between the patient and caregiver, identification of the symptoms of the patient, the burden of managing negative assumptions of friends and other family members about the prognosis of the patient, the changing of lifestyle, lack of information about the prognosis and management, and being unprepared for end-of-life care (Hansen et al. 2017b).

Also, caregivers can give a better idea about the patients' quality of life than their healthcare providers, which can be a valuable source for evaluating patient conditions.

There are significant disparities in managing HCC, even in the USA, based on race (Wagle and Spencer 2021). The mortality rate of HCC is higher in lower-income patients (Kim et al. 2021).

9.1.4 Palliative Care in Low-Middle-Income Countries (LMICs)

Although palliative care is recognized as an integral part of primary health care (Sallnow et al. 2022), a high level of palliative care is only available to 14% of the world's population, and the availability is mainly in European countries (Clark et al. 2020).

Unfortunately, mortality from cancer is higher in LMICs due to late detection of disease and limited access to different treatment options. There is also significant inequity in the availability of palliative care services between high-income countries and LMICs (Clemens et al. 2007). For example, the number of hospices or palliative care services in the top three largest population countries in Africa, namely Nigeria, Ethiopia, and Egypt were only 17, 7, and 10 services, respectively. There are nine African countries have no hospice or palliative care services at all (Rhee et al. 2018).

In contrast, in the USA, for example, more than 60% of the hospitals in most states have palliative care programs (Hughes and Smith 2014).

Most of the patients who need palliative care in LMICs are residents in rural areas, which adds more limitations to utilizing palliative care in these countries.

9.1.5 Barriers to Develop High-Quality Palliative Care Programs in LMICs and Solutions

There are many barriers at different levels: governmental, political, health care, cultural, and communication.

Governmental and Political Barriers Without governmental and political support, it is hard to build robust palliative care programs (WHPCA 2020). Many governments and policies have low prioritization of symptom control, including pain, and focus on curative treatment (Morriss and Roques 2018).

There are also significant disparities between countries in accessing medication, especially pain medication. About 84% of the world's population has inadequate access to opioids for pain control. LMICs consume only 10% of global opioid consumption (WHPCA 2020).

Healthcare-Related Barriers HCC management is complex as many specialties can be involved in managing the disease, including oncologists, surgeons, hepatologists, and intervention radiologists. Integrating palliative care between all these providers is challenging (Gofton et al. 2022). Poor education and knowledge about palliative care referral policies and practices is a crucial factor in limiting palliative care referrals (Le et al. 2014) Providers do not refer patients to palliative care sometimes for concern of feasibility reasons as inconsistent availability of specialized palliative care team and concern of adding more appointments to the patient's schedule (Woodrell et al. 2023). Some providers do not prioritize symptoms, including pain as a priority, or they would like to manage these symptoms by themselves (Woodrell et al. 2023). HCC is considered a particular situation, as even patients with severe disease and a heavy burden of symptoms can be eligible for a liver transplant, and that can affect the decision of referral (Gofton et al. 2022).

There is a shortage of palliative care providers, which may be related to poor conditions of reimbursement, many financial constraints, and or institutional resources (Donkor et al. 2018).

Also, there is a significant lack of research on crucial palliative care issues like pain (Morriss and Roques 2018). That may delay the progress and dissemination of that field. Only a quarter of LMICs have participated in palliative care research, although four-fifths of the need for palliative care in these countries (Sallnow et al. 2022).

Communication Barriers Communication barriers include physicians' difficulties in informing patients about poor prognoses or discussing terminal illness because of various factors (Hancock et al. 2007), including the providers having too little time during their consultations, being afraid of disclosing the prognosis which might be harmful to the patients by causing distress and loss of hope (Van Vliet et al. 2013; Broom et al. 2014), and the emotional challenges in discussing death, especially in the case of young patients (Granek et al. 2013; Laryionava et al. 2018).

Lack of communication between healthcare teams can affect the patient's quality of life, especially since the care of these patients requires a multi-disciplinary team (Den Herder-Van Der Eerden et al. 2017).

Cultural and Social Barriers The cultural background of the providers, patients, and family can affect the likelihood of getting high-quality palliative care. Many healthcare providers consider palliative care inconsistent with curative therapy (Woodrell et al. 2023). Patients and families may be reluctant to accept referrals due to their idea that palliative care means terminal care (Collins et al. 2017). Even after referral and providing appropriate management, some patients may not be compliant with their medications due to cultural and social issues, as patients may suffer from pain and avoid taking appropriate pain medication for fear of addiction (Chavez et al. 2022). In many cultures, family and healthcare providers do not inform patients of their prognosis when they have a life-threatening disease (WHPCA 2020). Patients' background can affect their chances of getting palliative care; for example, patients with lower education have less chance of receiving palliative care. Also, patients with low income usually exhaust their resources in seeking curative treatment and neglect symptomatic and palliative treatment.

Disease-Related Barrier HCC can have unpredictable courses, which can delay the palliative care referral decision. Active and invasive treatment can cause more harm if used for unfit patients for such treatment (Torimura and Iwamoto 2021).

Solutions
There is no single solution to getting high-quality palliative care, but it is a complex process that needs the integration of all parties on different levels. Solutions should be tailored to LMICs, and what works for high-income countries may not work for LMICs' particular expensive strategies (Salikhanov et al. 2023). Figure 9.3 shows the public health model for the development of palliative care.

Solutions can be categorized under different levels as well:

Political and Governmental Level There should be laws to define palliative care and a national strategy to conduct that care. Palliative care should be recognized as a specialty with clinical guidelines for practicing that field (WHPCA 2020).

Only 55 countries, based on a survey in 2020, have a national strategy for palliative care. Most of these countries are in high or upper-middle-income levels (Clelland et al. 2020).

Also, there should be more funds to build strong palliative care programs (Fig. 9.1).

Conducting local studies showing the benefits of implementing palliative care programs may convince policymakers to provide more funds for these programs (Laube et al. 2020). It is known that early integration of palliative care in the treatment of lung cancer and other cancers, as well, can prolong survival and improve

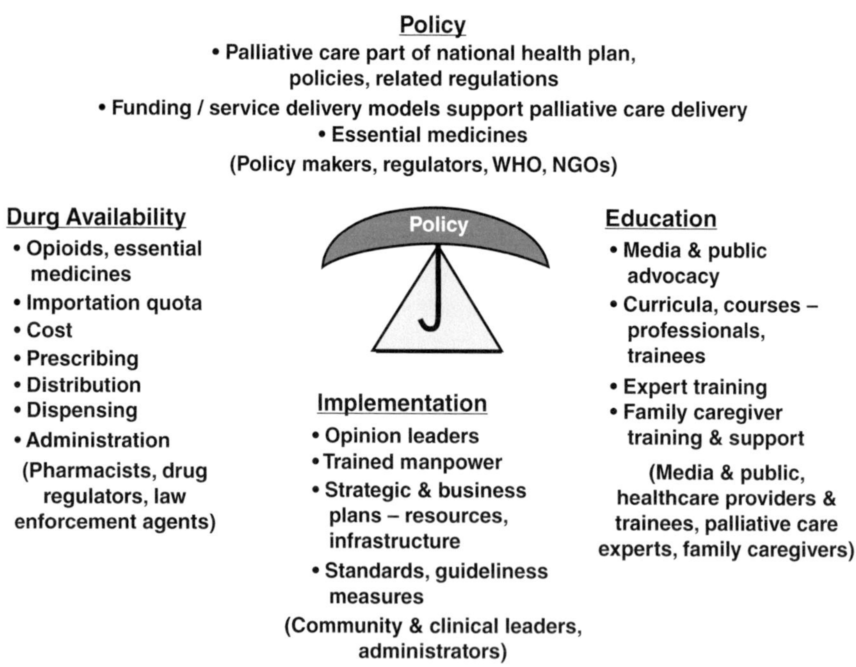

Fig. 9.1 Public Health Model for development of palliative care. Source: Worldwide Hospice Palliative Care Alliance (WHPCA) (2020) Global Atlas of Palliative Care 2nd Edition

quality of life (Bakitas et al. 2015). For conducting clinical trial, the gold standard method of clinical trial which is randomized controlled trials may not be ethical as it is not fair for some patients to hold palliative care for them. Cluster-based trials (facility-level randomization) can be an acceptable trial method. (Gofton et al. 2022).

Governments can form policies and campaigns to involve more parties to support palliative care (charities, non-governmental organizations, and volunteers) (Salikhanov et al. 2023).

For the opioid crisis, we will discuss more in the pain section.

Healthcare Level Educating providers who work in healthcare and even students about the importance of palliative care is crucial. That can be done by training workshops and conferences, educating providers as outreach areas, and providing educational materials (Laube et al. 2020). Education can be on three different levels: basic training for all health professionals, intermediate training for providers who work with patients with life-threatening illnesses, and special training for palliative care providers (Clelland et al. 2020).

There should be guidelines for the referral of patients to palliative care. For example, palliative care should be involved in the case of transitions, like patients being removed from a liver transplant list or initiation/termination of systemic therapy (Woodrell et al. 2023). Also, there should be integration of different specialties for palliative care into oncological care at the beginning of the diagnosis of advanced cancer. To decrease the burden of visits, the palliative care clinic can be located close to the oncology clinic or utilize telehealth (Woodrell et al. 2023). We also know that it is impossible to refer every HCC patient to palliative care, as there are currently not enough providers, and we are not expected to have enough providers in the near future. So, careful assessment of symptoms to identify the patients with a higher need for palliative care and conducting clinical trials to identify HCC patients or patients with end-stage liver disease with higher needs for palliative care, as in the PAL-Liver trial (Gofton et al. 2022).

Utilization of lay or community health workers (CHWs) (community members who get some training in health-related tasks but do not have professional degrees in healthcare) showed promising benefits in some areas, like infectious diseases in LMICs (Lewin et al. 2005). These workers can be utilized to support palliative or hospice services. In one review of the utilization of CHWs in LMICs, CHW's role was mainly to identify patients who need palliative care in their community, promote awareness of that service, provide psychological and spiritual support, deliver home-based care and pain management (MacRae et al. 2020). In another review, CHWs spent significant time caring for dying people, providing respite care for the families, and providing support at home (Herber and Johnston 2013). However, there were many challenges to the utilization of CHWs, including recruitment, sustainability, inadequate training in areas like managing emotional distress at the end of life, communication skills, unclear roles, burnout, financial burden, and emotional attachment (MacRae et al. 2020; Herber and Johnston 2013). There should be a good working environment and adequate training to utilize CHWs efficiently (Kang'ethe 2010).

Cultural and Social Levels
Educational programs for the population to promote and correct any misunderstanding about palliative care, patients' education classes, and individualized resources (Laube et al. 2020). There should be awareness of cultural differences even in the same country, and the palliative care team can utilize members of the patients' local communities to help understand the culture (Laube et al. 2020). Also, healthcare providers should promote the idea that patients should know their diagnosis and prognosis if they want (WHPCA 2020). However, providers should still know that some patients do not want to know that they have life-threatening conditions, or sometimes they delegate a family member or a friend to get these details. Providers must respect that and not push to tell the patient details that the patient does not want to know.

9.2 Common Symptoms in HCC and Management

9.2.1 Pain

Pain is the most common symptom patients suffer during their disease (WHPCA 2020). The definition of pain is not clear as it is highly subjective. The International Association for the Study of Pain (IASP) identified pain as "An unpleasant sensory and emotional experience associated with or resembling that associated with actual or potential tissue damage" (Raja et al. 2020). Figure 9.2 shows common symptoms of serious illness, with pain as the most common.

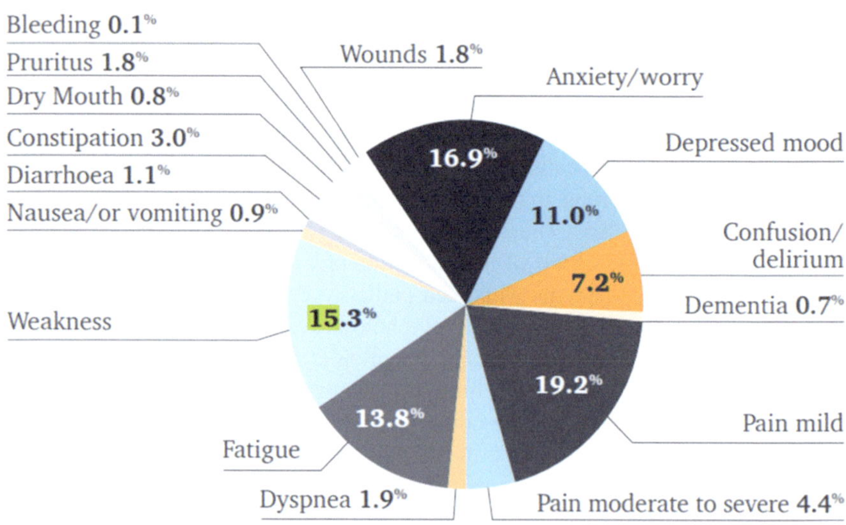

Fig. 9.2 Percentage of days that adult worldwide experiences serious health-related suffering due to 20 illness condition for common symptoms. Source Worldwide Hospice Palliative Care Alliance (WHPCA) (2020) Global Atlas of Palliative Care 2nd Edition

Patients with HCC who presented with pain may have a worse prognosis (Carr and Pujol 2010). Pain management is a challenge in hepatocellular carcinoma for many reasons, including the underlying cirrhosis that most patients have and that limits pain medication dosage due to liver dysfunction (Soleimanpour et al. 2016) Pain management is a more severe problem in LMICs due to many reasons, including that 80% of patients have little or no access to pain medication, socio-political barriers, and lack of proper training (Abu-Odah et al. 2020; Abu-Odah et al. 2020).

9.2.1.1 Common Causes of Pain in HCC and Specific Management

Pain in hepatocellular carcinoma can happen, especially at late stages, due to several reasons, including local tumor effect, metastasis, or therapy issues (Christian-Miller and Frenette 2018).

Local tumor effect: The pain from the tumor can be parietal or visceral (Christian-Miller and Frenette 2018) mainly in the right upper quadrant. Pain management depends on the patient's factor, liver condition, the severity of the pain, and availability, as mentioned above. Single 8Gy palliative radiation therapy is an option for patients with significant pain from the tumor burden (Yeung et al. 2020).

Spontaneous rupture of HCC is a rare complication in less than 4% of patients presented with acute pain and can have hypotension hemorrhagic shock as well. Management depends on the severity of the condition, but it may need intervention like TACE or liver resection (Obeidat and Wong 2022).

Pain due to cirrhosis is common, as about 80% of patients with cirrhosis are found to have pain. The most common locations are the abdomen, lower back, and large joints (Rogal et al. 2015). Abdominal pain may be related to ascites, splenomegaly, infection as spontaneous bacterial peritonitis, and hepatic capsular distension (Klinge et al. 2018). Treatment of pain is based on etiology. For ascites, the patient may need frequent paracentesis. Patients with significant splenomegaly may require partial splenic artery embolization to control their symptoms.

Metastatic disease: extrahepatic metastasis is about 15%, with the most common sites of metastases being lung 47%, lymph nodes 45%, bone 37%, and adrenal gland 12% (Uka et al. 2007). Metastases can be painful, especially in bone. 87% of bone metastasis in HCC occurs in the axial skeleton (Harding et al. 2018). The bony metastatic lesions can be presented as soft tissue masses. The pain can be from the bone or neuropathic pain due to pressure over the spinal cord and nerves (Hayashi et al. 2014). Metastatic bone disease is associated with skeletal-related events (SREs), which are events related to bone metastases, including skeletal complications such as fractures, spinal cord compression, and the need for radiation or surgery to bone. Recurrent SREs are considered an unfavorable prognosis in HCC and affect quality of life (Longo et al. 2014). Bony pain from metastasis usually has a gradual onset and progressive course and is felt mainly at night (Buga and Sarria 2012). The bone pain is most likely to get worse with movement. Bone metastasis in HCC usually consists of osteolytic lesions, so traditional bone scans may not detect these lesions (Longo et al. 2014). So, suppose there is suspicion of bone metastases, it is better to do CT or MRI, especially if radiation therapy is planned to be able to detect osteolytic lesions and soft tissue that is formed due to metastases (Kim et al. 2007).

The pain is managed based on several factors, including the patient's performance status, prognosis, comorbidities, previous treatment, and anatomy related to the metastases, including location, number of bone metastases, and bone stability. Options for treatment include analgesics, including opioids, according to the severity of pain. Corticosteroids can help with pain control as they help decrease the incidence of pain flare induced by radiation therapy if it is given before palliative radiation therapy (Hird et al. 2009). Bone modifying agents such as bisphosphonates (as zoledronic acid) and receptor activators of nuclear factor-Kappa-B ligand (RANKL) inhibitors (such as denosumab) can have some analgesic effects in patients with bone metastases. Still, these agents are usually insufficient for pain control (Poznak et al. 2017). There is not enough evidence to prefer one agent over the other. Denosumab may have a better effect on pain control than zoledronic acid, but it is not cost-effective (Xie et al. 2012). So, using zoledronic acid in low-income countries may be more reasonable.

Radiation therapy is a significant tool in treating bone metastases. Hypofractionation or single fraction may be more appropriate in countries with limited resources than for most African countries (Rick et al. 2020). The pain relief is equal using a single 8 Gy fraction versus other fractionations, but it may have more retreatment incidence (Lutz et al. 2017). The side effects of a single fraction versus the other fractionation are unclear (Lutz et al. 2017). So, a single fraction may be a convenient tool for pain management, especially near the end of life.

Paraneoplastic syndrome: prevalence around 25% in HCC patients (Chang et al. 2013; Ülger and Delik 2022). The most common manifestations are hypoglycemia, hypercholesterolemia, hypercalcemia, and erythrocytosis. Other manifestations like thrombocytosis, demyelinating disease, polyarthritis, pemphigus, and encephalomyelitis can also happen (Ülger and Delik 2022). Pain can develop secondary to hypercalcemia, polyarthritis, or pemphigus. The treatment is based on the standard treatment for each condition.

Therapy related: (pain from systemic treatment is mentioned in therapy-related side effects section.)

Locoregional therapy: Transarterial chemoembolization (TACE).

Pain is a common symptom after TACE; the incidence is 60–80% (Guan et al. 2023). It can be part of post-embolization syndrome, which manifests as abdominal pain, mainly in the right upper quadrant, ileus, and fever (Chang et al. 2020). It can be associated with nausea, fatigue, and elevation of liver enzymes as well. It is usually self-limited and happens between 24 hours and 2 weeks after the procedure (Blackburn and West 2016). Patients with older age, a higher number of embolized tumors, preoperative pain, higher preoperative prothrombin activity, higher dosage of iodized oil, and closer the lesion to the liver capsule (≤2 cm) have a higher chance of having post-procedural pain (Guan et al. 2023). Early recognition and management of pain are essential to improve outcomes.

Different therapies were examined in the management of pain around the TACE procedure. Administration of intra-arterial lidocaine pre-procedurally decreases the need for analgesics peri-procedural and may decrease admission time (Blackburn and West 2016).

IV and oral analgesics can be used to manage the pain around the procedure, including oral and IV morphine, oral oxycodone, and IV hydromorphone.

Steroids have a questionable role in the management of post-TACE pain. Still, the use of dexamethasone as a prophylactic measure before TACE may decrease the pain and post-embolization syndrome (Yang et al. 2017).

Other non-pharmacological methods like wrist-ankle acupuncture may relieve post-TACE pain as well, but that was an old study, and it was done on a small number of patients. To get standardization, that method needs to be studied in a larger group of patients (Blackburn and West 2016).

Unexplained pain: One of the unrecognized causes of pain is spiritual pain with a result of existential suffering; it is usually manifested with physical symptoms, including pain that is not explained enough with the underlying physical disease or not well controlled with the usual pain management tools. The definition of spiritual pain is not unified among experts. It can be identified as a self-identified symptom or condition in relation to the disintegration of the meaning and value that people used to understand and live (Hui et al. 2011; Illueca et al. 2023). There are many spiritual domains; the most relevant domains to supportive cancer care may include despair (versus hope), brokenness (versus wholeness), panic (versus tranquility), isolation (versus connected), meaningless (versus meaningful), guilt (versus self-forgiveness), and helpless (versus empowered) (Hui et al. 2011). There are some tools to identify spiritual suffering (TAMURA et al. 2006; Hui et al. 2011). Medical staff should be educated about spiritual pain to be able to identify it early. In one study, more than half of nurses in one Nigerian hospital had poor spiritual caring practice, so spiritual issues should be included in the training of medical staff (Bolarinwa et al. 2023).

9.2.1.2 Assessment of Pain and Choice of Therapy

In pain management, providers should consider multiple factors to manage that pain successfully; these factors include the etiology of pain, thorough assessment of pain characteristics, associated symptoms, available pain medications, and patient's condition, prognosis, and comorbidities,

Assessment for pain: A detailed analysis of pain can dramatically affect the treatment of the pain even if the etiology is the same (evaluation of intensity, location, duration, aggravating/alleviating factors, associated symptoms, and patient's beliefs about their pain). Pain intensity can be evaluated using a 0–10 scale. The location of the pain should be investigated carefully, as, for example, a patient may have a new pain related to metastasis or the patient has a localized pain that can be treated with radiation therapy. Duration and course of pain are essential; it should be apparent if the pain is acute or chronic, continuous, or comes in episodes. Aggravating/alleviating and associated symptoms will help understate that pain (Fink 2000). So, for example, for a patient with chronic abdominal pain under reasonable control, whose pain has been worse only recently, with a good analysis of pain, the clinician may find that the patient has constipation, and by treating constipation, the pain may go to its baseline.

Patient factors: general condition, prognosis, comorbidities.

Patient's condition affects the choice of pain management, as patients with short life usually have special needs (Groninger and Vijayan 2014).

Most of the patients with HCC have cirrhosis. Prescribing pain medication in patients with cirrhosis can be a challenge as sometimes drug metabolism is unpredictable (Klinge et al. 2018). There is no clear link between the degree of liver dysfunction and dose modification as in kidney failure (Soleimanpour et al. 2016).

Opioids should be used cautiously in patients with cirrhosis due to potentially serious side effects, as all opioids can precipitate hepatic encephalopathy, especially in older patients. Generally, the initial dose should be decreased, and the dose intervals should be prolonged with close assessment (Soleimanpour et al. 2016).

Choose the type and duration of pain therapy.

World Health Organization in 1986 suggested a stepwise approach for cancer pain management mainly based on the intensity of pain. The first step for mild pain is non-opioid analgesics such as non-steroidal anti-inflammatory drugs (NSAIDs) and paracetamol (acetaminophen), with the addition of adjuvant analgesics if needed. Adjuvant analgesics include antidepressants such as amitriptyline, anticonvulsants such as gabapentin, corticosteroids such as dexamethasone, and anxiolytics like benzodiazepines. The second step for moderate pain or, if progress, will be using weak opioids alone or in addition to the other non-opioid pain medications. A weak opioid is a concept that may apply to partial agonist opioids like tramadol or opioids such as codeine or hydrocodone that are produced in combination with other compounds such as acetaminophen and that limits the maximum dose that can be given (Marinangeli et al. 2004; Wickham 2017a). Step three for management of severe pain or failure of previous steps includes usually using what are called potent opioids, which include morphine, hydromorphone, methadone, buprenorphine, and fentanyl (Wickham 2017a; Marinangeli et al. 2004). Modifying this approach is reasonable based on the etiology of pain, patient condition, and availability.

9.2.1.3 Non-pharmacological, Non-opioid, and Adjuvant Modalities for Pain Management

Non-pharmacological interventions may give some relief for some types of pain. These techniques include acupuncture, hypnotherapy, massage, aromatherapy, music therapy, transcutaneous electric nerve stimulation (TENS), and cognitive behavioral therapy (CBT) (Singh and Chaturvedi 2015; Mao et al. 2022). CBT proved to improve pain in some patients. It is a reasonable option for patients with cirrhosis as that can help with other problems in these patients, like alcohol abuse, anxiety, or depression (Klinge et al. 2018).

The most common non-opioid pain medications are acetaminophen (paracetamol) and NSAIDs. For acetaminophen, limiting the dose to 2 g/day total doses in cirrhotic patients is recommended, and it can be used for a short duration for more safety (Lewis and Stine 2013).

NSAIDs are better avoided in cirrhotic patients or used very cautiously, as they can increase the risk of bleeding, including esophageal varices, and increase the possibility of renal failure. Also, some NSAIDs like diclofenac have direct hepatotoxicity effects (Lewis and Stine 2013).

Adjuvant Analgesics

Adjuvant analgesic is a term used collectively for medications whose primary indication is not pain but can be used in pain management. This category includes antidepressants, anticonvulsants, local anesthetics, steroids, bisphosphonates, calcitonin, and topical agents (Mitra and Jones 2012). WHO included some of these medications in the model lists of essential medicines, including carbamazepine and sodium valproate as anticonvulsants, ketamine and nitrous oxide as general anesthetics, bupivacaine, and lidocaine as local anesthetics (Morriss and Roques 2018).

Antidepressants such as tricyclic antidepressants (amitriptyline and nortriptyline) can be used in cancer pain and neuropathic pain, but this family has multiple side effects, especially cholinergic side effects. Nortriptyline may have fewer anticholinergic side effects (Lussier et al. 2004). This family can induce or exacerbate hepatic encephalopathy in cirrhotic patients, so this family may not be the best option for patients with liver disease (Klinge et al. 2018). If it is essential to use these drugs, the dose should be low with careful follow-up (Chandok and Watt 2010).

Other antidepressants, such as selective serotonin reuptake inhibitors (paroxetine, citalopram) and noradrenaline/serotonin reuptake inhibitors (venlafaxine), can have analgesic effects in different types of pain as well (Lussier et al. 2004). In the case of using serotonergic antidepressants, tramadol should be avoided because of the risk of serotonin syndrome (Christian-Miller and Frenette 2018).

Anticonvulsants such as gabapentin and pregabalin can be used to treat neuropathic pain related to cancer. There are few reports that pregabalin can cause liver injury, so usually, it is not the first choice (Klinge et al. 2018). Although the liver does not metabolize these two drugs, use is limited due to side effects such as sedation, dizziness, and sedation (Chandok and Watt 2010). The prescribers should slowly titrate these medications and follow-up closely.

Duloxetine, which is a serotonin and norepinephrine reuptake inhibitor, has the best evidence in the treatment of chemotherapy-induced peripheral neuropathy (Smith et al. 2013). Current drug label recommends avoiding duloxetine use in patients with chronic liver disease (Lewis and Stine 2013).

Corticosteroids have been used for cancer pain, but there is no high-level evidence that corticosteroids control that kind of pain, but they may provide some control of pain in cancer patients (Paulsen et al. 2013). They have been mainly used for bone and neuropathic pain. The effect of that family may be due to the anti-inflammatory and anti-swelling effects of corticosteroids (Leppert and Buss 2012). Corticosteroids may effectively control pain that may flare up with radiotherapy (Beuken-van Everdingen et al. 2017). The most used corticosteroid is dexamethasone, possibly due to its prolonged activity, high potency, and less mineralocorticoid activity (Leppert and Buss 2012). Side effects include increasing incidence of infection, edema, dyspepsia, weight gain, hyperglycemia, myopathy, and osteoporosis (Ettinger and Portenoy 1988). The adverse effects of corticosteroids increase with prolonged use. They may be used more liberally near the end of life as long-term side effects are unlikely due to short life expectancy. Corticosteroids should be used carefully with immune checkpoint inhibitors due to the potential impact on the immune system (Aldea et al. 2020).

Cannabis is another group that can be used to treat cancer pain. Still, there is not enough research about the safety of that group in patients with liver disease, and there is no substantial evidence that cannabis can cause harm (Klinge et al. 2018). There are multiple studies have shown that cannabis can help in cancer pain control and prolong its effectiveness by decreasing the number of opioids needed for pain control, especially THC/CBD extract (Johnson et al. 2010; Pawasarat et al. 2020).

9.2.1.4 Opioids for Pain Management

WHO listed certain opioids as essential for health care; these include morphine, fentanyl, and codeine, with methadone on the complementary list (WHO Report 2023).

Pethidine, hydrocodone, and oxycodone are sometimes used in countries with lower consumption of opioids (INCB Report 2022). Morphine is mainly metabolized by the liver and excreted by the kidney. It should be used cautiously, especially in old patients, as it can precipitate hepatic encephalopathy, and it is better to avoid long-acting forms, specifically at the beginning of therapy (Soleimanpour et al. 2016). It is recommended in cirrhotic patients to reduce the dose and the frequency by half of the usual morphine dose (Lewis and Stine 2013).

Fentanyl can be used as transdermal, IV, or oral. The hydrolysis clears it of ester, so liver dysfunction does not affect the pharmacokinetics of fentanyl, but it can affect the amount of delivered fentanyl through the transdermal route. Some experts empirically recommend fentanyl as a proper opioid, but there is no robust data to support that (Soleimanpour et al. 2016).

Tramadol should undergo biotransformation through the liver to become active metabolites so that tramadol can have less effect (Christian-Miller and Frenette 2018). Tramadol should not be given with selective serotonin reuptake inhibitors (SSRIs), serotonin-norepinephrine reuptake inhibitors (SNRIs), or TCA; it can lower seizure threshold as well (Lewis and Stine 2013). A maximum dose of 400 mg per day for non-cirrhotic patients is appropriate. For cirrhotic patients, if there are no other alternatives, starting a dose of 50 mg every 12 hours can be safe and effective (Soleimanpour et al. 2016). Meperidine (pethidine) is less addictive than morphine. It can cause seizures and hallucinations in patients with liver insufficiency (Soleimanpour et al. 2016). Bioavailability is increased in patients with cirrhosis by up to 80% due to the decreased first-pass effect, so it is better to avoid meperidine in cirrhotic patients (Christian-Miller and Frenette 2018). Figure 9.3 shows relative consumption of opioids in regions with the lowest consumption.

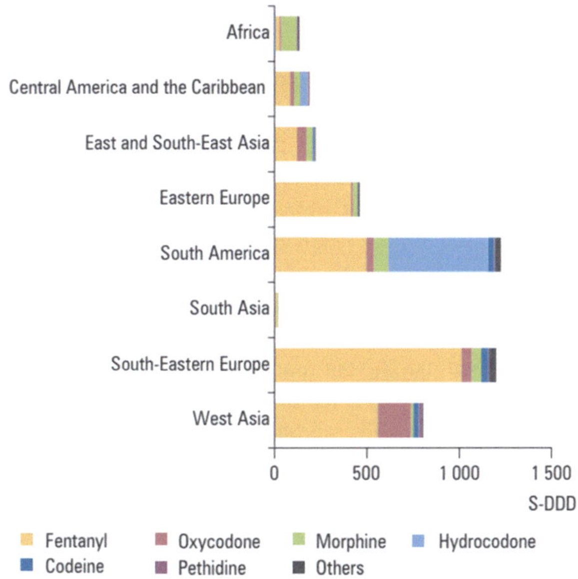

Fig. 9.3 Relative consumption of opioids in regions with the lowest consumption (defined daily doses for statistical purposes per million inhabitants per day, 2020). Source: International Narcotics Control Board INCB Report (2022) Supplement to the annual report of the Board for 2022 on the availability of internationally controlled substances. (United Nations International Narcotics Control Board report)

9.2.1.5 Challenges of Pain Management in LMICs

Patients in LMICs are more likely to get moderate to severe pain, and unfortunately, that pain is usually managed poorly in many cases (Morriss and Roques 2018). There are many challenges for pain management in LMICs. Major barriers to good pain management include lack of education of medical staff, government policies, low prioritization of pain relief, patients' attitudes, compliance, and beliefs, including fear of addiction, high cost of drugs, and lack of research in LMICs (Bond 2011; Morriss and Roques 2018).

Lack of appropriate education is a significant problem in pain management; in one survey, about 90% of doctors in LMICs do not think they had adequate undergraduate pain management education (Morriss and Roques 2018). The International Association for the Study of Pain (IASP) developed assessment criteria to fund the development of educational programs in pain management; these criteria include good organization with basic knowledge of pain management, clearly identified local needs, curriculum identified students and local needs, clear plan, and realistic budget with low social costs (Bond 2011). Medical staff should be trained on the different types of opioids and their potential side effects, including addiction (Roa et al. 2019).

Fear of addiction by cancer patients sometimes prevents them from utilizing appropriate pain medications. This fear may be due to patients' view of opioids as illicit drugs, media effects, negative experiences of friends or family members, and poor understanding of the nature of opioids and their effects (Chavez et al. 2022).

Low prioritization of pain control at governmental and global levels is a significant issue, as usually, the focus is on curative treatment and communicable diseases (Morriss and Roques 2018). Also, patients in LMICs may utilize their resources seeking curative treatment, have not enough resources to use in controlling their pain, and have less expectation of getting their pain under reasonable control as well due to poor resources for pain management (Morriss and Roques 2018).

There is a considerable disparity in accessing controlled opioid medicines all over the world (Richards et al. 2022). In comparison, the average opioid consumption in the Americas is 144 mg/person, while in Africa, only 1.4 mg/person. WHO listed minimum pain medications that are needed for the basic health care system, that include for non-opioids: acetylsalicylic acid (suppository and tablet forms), ibuprofen (liquid and tablet forms), and paracetamol/acetaminophen (liquid, suppository, and tablet forms), for opioids analgesics: codeine (tablet form), fentanyl (transdermal patch), and morphine (granules, injection, liquid, slow-release tablet, and immediate release tablet form), with hydromorphone and oxycodone as therapeutic alternatives for morphine, and methadone in the complementary list (WHO Report 2023). Only 14% of low-income countries have access to oral morphine (Coghlan et al. 2021). Approval and utilization of opioids in LMICs can be a complicated process. Many of these countries do not have the capacity to manufacture or even evaluate the safety and effectiveness of a drug (Ruff et al. 2016).

So, establishing educational programs for medical staff with pain-related courses, building robust infrastructure to help with promoting the education of pain management, changing media view of pain management for cancer patients, establishing national plan and guidelines for pain management, updating the opioid policy for cancer pain management, manufacturing and distributing pain medications, and education of stakeholder about the situation of pain management may be tools to improve the pain control in LMICs (Abu-Odah et al. 2020; Goh and Lee 2018; Morriss and Roques 2018). Hospice Africa Uganda is an example of an efficient strategy to make opioids available to patients who need them (Merriman and Harding 2010).

9.2.2 Hepatic Encephalopathy

Hepatic encephalopathy most likely occurs due to changes in ammonia metabolism and is associated with neurologic disturbance. These symptoms can be mild, such as subclinical impairment, or severe, such as coma. Cancer can affect ammonia metabolism in multiple ways, such as infiltration of hepatic tissue, treatment toxicities, viral hepatitis activation, shunting, and TACE (Willson et al. 2013). Patients with hepatic tumors can develop portosystemic shunt and develop encephalopathy (Hashimoto et al. 2011).

Sorafenib can cause encephalopathy that can be reversible by stopping the drug (Marks et al. 2009).

The excess ammonia is converted to glutamine in the brain through glutamine synthetase. The accumulation of osmotically active glutamine causes intra-astrocytic edema and Alzheimer's type II change in the brain (Shah et al. 2008; Häussinger and Schliess 2008). Cytokine release and hyponatremia can increase the change of astrocytic swelling and increase the effects of hyperammonemia (Häussinger et al. 2000).

Hepatic encephalopathy can range from minimal symptoms like cognitive impairment to coma (Xu et al. 2019b). Encephalopathy can significantly impact the quality of life of patients and caregivers with substantial financial burdens (Bajaj et al. 2011). Hepatic encephalopathy can be prevented by avoiding dehydration, electrolyte imbalance, and constipation. Early recognition of infection and bleeding can also prevent the progression of encephalopathy (Xu et al. 2019b).

Management of encephalopathy depends on the prognosis of the patient. If a patient is close to end of life, it is more appropriate to focus on distressing symptoms than addressing encephalopathy. Treatment with nonabsorbable disaccharides such as lactulose or rifaximin (nonabsorbable antibiotic) can be used for other patients. Rifaximin costs much more than lactulose, which is not superior to it, but some patients can better tolerate it (Jiang et al. 2008).

9.2.3 Gastrointestinal (GI) Symptoms

GI symptoms are common in patients with advanced HCC, especially at the terminal stage. Anorexia and vomiting are the most common GI symptoms, as about 75% of hospice patients with HCC develop these symptoms (Lin et al. 2004). Anorexia can be related to cancer itself or the treatment, but sometimes reversible factors can contribute to anorexia, like chronic nausea, constipation, and depression. Treatment of these factors can improve anorexia (Sun and Sarna 2008). Some pharmacological agents can help patients with anorexia. Low-dose olanzapine (5 mg) can improve cancer patients' appetite and weight gain (Roeland et al.,(Roeland et al. 2023). If olanzapine does not work, megestrol acetate can be used. However the weight gain from megestrol acetate is primarily from increasing adipose tissue and body fluid with little effect on muscle mass (Evans 2007).

Constipation is a common symptom in cancer patients, as up to 60% of patients can develop constipation (Wickham 2017b). Frequency of constipation in HCC patients is about 20% (Hansen et al. 2017a). Non-pharmacological management includes lifestyle modifications like taking fibers with plenty of fluid and adjusting the timing of defecation (Wickham 2017b). Patients who use opioids should use pharmacological agents prophylactically to reduce the incidence of constipation. Fentanyl may cause less constipation than morphine (Christian-Miller and Frenette 2018). Pharmacological agents include bulking agents like fibers, stool softeners like docusate sodium and mineral oil, osmotic agents like magnesium citrate, lactulose, and polyethylene glycol, and stimulants like senna and bisacodyl (Wickham 2017b). Patients more likely to get hepatic encephalopathy may benefit more from lactulose.

Diarrhea is a common symptom in HCC patients as well, with an incidence of about 30% (Hansen et al. 2017a). It can be iatrogenic from the medications that are commonly used in association with HCC, like lactulose and sorafenib. About 40% of patients who use sorafenib develop diarrhea. Dose modification or interruption is indicated if the patient has grade 3 or 4 diarrhea. Mild and moderate diarrhea can be treated with hydration, electrolyte correction, dietary changes, or pharmacological agents like loperamide and diphenoxylate if indicated (Kornblau et al. 2000; Li et al. 2015).

9.2.4 Depression

Depression and anxiety are common in patients with HCC (Lee et al. 2017). These conditions are associated with poorer survival outcomes and reduced QOL for patients and family members (Rice et al. 2021; Smith 2015). The prevalence of depression in patients with cancer is higher in LMICs than in other countries (Walker et al. 2021).

The prevalence of depression and anxiety in patients with HCC is about 24%. There is a difference in the prevalence of depression in the different WHO regions, where the lowest in the Americas (16.44%) and the highest in South-East Asia (66.67%) (Tan et al. 2022).

Many factors can cause or increase the risk of depression in HCC cancer patients. The risk of depression in HCC patients can increase with the psychological effect of cancer diagnosis, the stress of repeated hospital visits, and the complications of different treatments (Lee et al. 2017).

The risk of anxiety can increase as well due to the fear of being terminally and progression of the disease (Ghand et al. 2014).

Alcohol consumption and cirrhosis were associated with higher chance of getting depression (Lynskey and Agrawal 2008). Cirrhosis is associated with a poor QOL due to both physical and psychological health change (Bianchi et al. 2005).

There are contradictory data about the relationship between education and depression, while a study in the USA suggested that people with higher education have a higher chance of developing depression (Strine et al. 2008), other studies suggesting higher rates of depression in cancer patients with lower education level in LMICs (Walker et al. 2021).

In two studies in LMICs, agriculture workers were found to have more depressive symptoms in comparison to office workers (Walker et al. 2021).

Due to the high prevalence of psychological conditions in HCC patients, healthcare providers should have a low threshold to screen patients with HCC for depression and anxiety. The diagnosis of depression may be self-reported, self-assessment, or clinician-rated diagnoses. Self-reported diagnosis included identification of depression from medical history. Self assessment diagnosis of depression using different scales, including the Hospital Anxiety and Depression Scale (HADS). Clinician-rated diagnosis depends on depression diagnosed by the psychiatrist (Ismail et al. 2017). The downside of self-rated tools for diagnosis of depression is that they cannot diagnose major depression (Mohamed et al. 2014), while physician-rated diagnosis is the key method of diagnosing psychological disorders (Li and He 2018). Prospective studies are needed to identify the best screening tools for depression and anxiety in HCC patients (Tan et al. 2022).

Providers should pay attention to conditions that can mimic depression to manage correctly, like hypothyroidism, anemia, grief, medication side effects, and CNS involvement.

Management of depression is essential in cancer patients, as it not only affects the social and well-being of the patient, but also makes it harder to manage physical symptoms (Wilson et al. 2007).

Healthcare providers should consider early referral of potential patients with depression to psychological services for cognitive behavioral therapy and pharmacological treatment.

Treatment of physical symptoms of cancer patients, including pain, should be done before or with the treatment of depression (Rodin et al. 2007). Different non-pharmacological and pharmacological methods can be used to treat depression. Among patients with mood disorders, preemptive non-pharmacological strategies such as more comprehensive education and supportive services may be instituted (Wang et al. 2019). Psychological therapies and yoga showed improvement in depressive symptoms in some of LMICs as well (Walker et al. 2021).

There is no robust data examining pharmacological therapy for the treatment of depression in cancer patients who are living in LMICs (Walker et al. 2021). The prevalence of use of antidepressant medication in high-income countries is 2–4 times higher than LMICs (Kazdin et al. 2023).

There is no strong evidence of the superiority of an antidepressant agent over another. The choice mainly depends on tolerability and the side effects of the medicine (Rodin et al. 2007).

The choice and dosing of antidepressants should be in consideration of liver function since most HCC patients have liver dysfunction. Selective serotonin reuptake inhibitors (SSRIs) can be used in liver dysfunction. This class of drugs may be the safest class to use in patients with chronic liver disease (Mullish et al. 2014). However, the usual recommended dose is 50% of that used for patients without liver dysfunction, especially in the maintenance setting (Menon et al. 2022). Tricyclic antidepressants (TCAs) can be used as well, with particular consideration of their side effect profile, especially sedation (Mullish et al. 2014).

9.2.5 Common Side Effects from HCC Therapy

As palliative care should be an integral part in the management of patients with HCC at all stages (Agarwal and Epstein 2017), palliative care providers should be aware of symptoms related to common therapies in HCC. Both localized and systemic therapies can have multiple complications. For local therapy, TACE can cause mild side effects in up to 83% of patients, such as nausea, vomiting, fever, and abdominal (can call it post-embolization syndrome). Severe complications can happen, but that is uncommon, such as hepatic artery complications (7.2%), new ascites (6.1%), hepatic failure (1.0%), hepatic abscess (0.9%), and acute renal impairment (0.6%) (Lencioni et al. 2016; Yang and Si 2018). TACE may also provoke psychological symptoms including fatigue and depression, which can result in early discontinuation of therapy (Lan et al. 2015).

There are no clear guidelines to manage these symptoms, steroids have questionable rule in management of this condition, but one study found 3 days of intravenous dexamethasone and granisetron, significantly reduced post-embolization symptoms with no significant adverse effects (Ogasawara et al. 2018).

Systemic therapies are utilized now more in HCC, the two main groups that are utilized are multikinase inhibitors (MKI) and immune checkpoint inhibitors. MKIs come at the expense of frequent side effects. Sorafenib and Lenvatinib used to be the first line therapies before ICIs. In the trial that showed non-inferiority of Lenvatinib to soraenib, 75% and 67% of patients had grade 3 or higher side effects to Lenvatinib and sorafenib, respectively. The most common side effects were palmar-planter erythrodysesthesia, diarrhea, hypertension, poor appetite, weight loss, and fatigue (Kudo et al. 2018). So skin manifestations are one of the most common side effect of MKIs, these skin manifestation include nail, and hair changes, rash, dry skin, stomatitis, and hand and foot skin reaction (HFSR). HFSR that happens with MKIs is different histologically and clinically from classic hand and foot syndrome that happen with some cytotoxic chemotherapies. HFSR is usually presented as plaques in friction or high-pressure areas like heels, fingers, and over joints. These plaques are usually painful, yellowish, and hyperkeratotic (Kwakman et al. 2020). HFSR usually appears early in the treatment, usually between 2 and 4 weeks of treatment. Prevention of HFSR from MKIs can include removal of hyperkeratotic skin, avoiding pressure points, avoiding rubbing, and using moistures and keratolytic creams like urea-based or salicylic-based creams (McLellan et al. 2015). Treatment is usually based on the grade; for grade one and two keratolytics, topical analgesics like lidocaine patch or gel and topical corticosteroids like clobetasol 0.05% can be used. MKI dose can be placed on hold or decreased as well. For higher grades, MKI should be placed on hold or discontinued permanently (McLellan et al. 2015).

ICIs is another family that has best outcome so far in treatment of HCC. This family may be associated with the development of immune-related adverse effects (irAEs) such as hepatitis, diarrhea, and endocrine dysfunction (Xu et al. 2019a). These symptoms are common anyway in patient with HCC, so providers should do clear evaluation before blaming ICIs as a cause of these symptoms (Song et al. 2023). The treatment of ICIs side effects depends on the grade of toxicity as well, ICI can be continued or placed on hold for early grades, but usually for higher grade especially grade four, ICI is discontinued permanently except in endocrine irAEs. Immunosuppression with corticosteroids and/or immunomodulators such as mycophenolate and tumor necrosis factor inhibitors may be required for higher grades of toxicity as well.

Unfortunately, multikinase inhibitors and immune checkpoint inhibitors are not always available in LMICs. Cytotoxic chemotherapy option is included in some guidelines in case of unavailability of targeted therapies (Torimura and Iwamoto 2022). Oxaliplatin based regimen specifically showed some benefits in certain populations (Abouelezz et al. 2020). One of the most common side effects of oxaliplatin is peripheral neuropathy. Duloxetine has the best evidence in treatment of chemotherapy-induced peripheral neuropathy (Smith et al. 2013), but the use is limited by current drug label recommendations to avoid in chronic liver disease (Lewis and Stine 2013).

9.3 Geriatric Patients with HCC in LMICs

More than half of newly diagnosed cancers occur in patients aged >65 years, and this older population accounts for nearly three-fourths of cancer deaths (Yancik 2005). There is an estimation that most of the world population who are above 60 years old will live in LMICs by 2030 (Goodman-Palmer et al. 2023). For elderly HCC patients, there are more incidences of women and non-viral etiology (Honda et al. 2011). Elderly patients are less often treated with surgery or locoregional treatment in comparison to younger patients (Guo et al. 2017). Compared with younger patients, older patients with cancer are more likely to be undertreated and experience earlier discontinuation of treatment for their stage of cancer. In a Korean study of 3492 elderly HCC patients, 1-year survival rates were 92%, 65%, 37%, 20%, and 7% for BCLC stages 0, A, B, C, D, respectively (Yoo et al. 2023).

Poor symptoms management and inadequate social support may be the reason of suboptimal treatment of these patients, but research is needed to address this complicated population (Neugut et al. 2006; Sargent et al. 2001). Older patients usually have unique situation related to their physical function, comorbid conditions, medication management, prognosis, and coping (Nipp et al. 2017; Cheung et al. 2011). There is significant mismatch between the research projects related to elderly between high income and LMICs (Goodman-Palmer et al. 2023).

Interventions targeting geriatric-specific palliative care concerns are lacking (Mohile et al. 2018).

Integration of palliative care in management of elderly HCC patients specifically can help in many aspects, including understanding the nature of their disease, symptoms control, psychological support, and decision making (Woodrell et al. 2018).

9.4 Communication Issues in Low- and Middle-Income Countries

Effective communication between members of the health care team and between the care team and patients plays a crucial role in the delivery of high-quality care. Most medical errors happen due to ineffective communication between healthcare teams (Burgener 2020). Effective communication between healthcare providers and patients improves the outcome as well (King and Hoppe 2013). Good communications improve the patient satisfaction and the adherence to the treatment plan; poor communication results in insufficient information and feeling of lack of empathy (King and Hoppe 2013). Unfortunately, there is poor communication between healthcare providers and patients in some of developing countries (Unger et al.

2003). Also, research in areas related to communication in low-income countries is limited due to many reasons, including the instability of the political situation in many of these countries, limitation of academic freedom, and poverty (Mheidly and Fares 2020). There are many barriers that can affect the quality of communication with patients, including general differences between the provider and the patient like age, sex, race, and education; culture differences like roots, religion, and ethnicity; language barriers like using scientific terms and using a translator (Quill 1989). There are several maneuvers to overcome these barriers, but basically, providers should recognize, acknowledge, and explore the barrier, then the provider should show empathy and legitimize the patient's situation (Quill 1989). There are many ways to teach healthcare providers effective communication; these methods include didactic lectures, reflective discussions, and role-playing (Anderson et al. 2016).

9.5 Ethics

The ethical principles recognized universally are autonomy, beneficence, nonmaleficence, and justice. These "four principles" are common in Eastern and Western cultures. These principles application and importance may be different from an area to another (Cavalieri 2001).

For HCC patients, to make an ethical decision there are some basics that must be clear before any intervention. The information about diagnosis and prognosis should be clear and discussed with the patient; providers should know what the patient wants; The impact of the intervention on the quality of life should be communicated with the patient; providers should pay attention to any other special considerations like the cost of the intervention and its availability (van Leeuwen and van Delden 2015).

Autonomy is the right to self-determination. An essential principle of medical ethics is to respect patient autonomy (Crane et al. 2005). For patients who have lost the ability to make decisions, their autonomy can be protected by using methods like advance directives (ADs).

ADs examples are living wills, health care proxies, and "do not resuscitate" (DNR) orders (Kessler and McClellan 2004; Crane et al. 2005).

If a patient has not previously documented his or her wishes and becomes terminally ill, the end-of-life decision is made by the patient's physician with consultations with next of kin or the patient's health care proxy (Crane et al. 2005).

Beneficence requires physicians to support the most helpful intervention for the patient.

Nonmaleficence is the principle of avoiding unnecessary harm. Harm may be justified if the benefit of the medical intervention outweighs the harm to the patient and the intervention is not intended to cause harm (Kessler and McClellan 2004).

Providers do not have to do futile medical procedures for their patient. Medical futility is defined as a clinical action serving no useful purpose in attaining a specified goal for a given patient (Clark 2007).

Justice is about ensuring a fair distribution of health resources and delivery of health services (Kessler and McClellan 2004).

Healthcare providers have an ethical obligation to advocate for fair and appropriate treatment of patients at the end of life. Providers should be honest, but sensitive in providing critical information near the end of life.

Patient-centered communication skills help physicians learn and meet the demands of their patients (Ngo-Metzger et al. 2008). In some cultures, families try not to inform the patient about the cancer diagnosis, factors that may contribute to that include lower education, rural area residence, and the belief that the patient is unaware of the diagnosis (Alsirafy et al. 2016). Providers when they encounter that situation should explore more to be able to solve that issue as we mentioned in the communication section.

Life-prolonging measures close to the end of life have been always a critical issue. These procedures include CPR, artificial nutrition and hydration (ANH), mechanical ventilation (MV), and circulatory support.

The use of CPR may not be appropriate for dying patients and may lead to complications and worsen the patients' quality of life. There are multiple factors, such as patient preferences, the estimated success rate, the risks of the procedure, and the perceived benefit, that can affect the decision for CPR (Cook et al. 2017). Some patients refuse to undergo CPR and this is called do-not-resuscitate (DNR). There are many LMICs have no legal regulation on DNR orders (Hüseyin et al. 2023).

ANH involves giving food and water to patients who are comatosed or unable to swallow (Slomka 2003). Artificial nutrition can be given through enteral feeding by tube or parenteral feeding. The bros and cons of ANH should be explained to the patient or the family in details (Slomka 2003).

There are other multiple ethical situations that can be debatable like euthanasia and physician-assisted suicide (Nunes and Rego 2016). Terminal sedation is a medical intervention used in terminally ill patients, usually as a last effort to alleviate suffering when death is inevitable. The purpose of terminal sedation is not to cause or accelerate death but to relieve pain that does not respond to other measures.

9.6 Hospice and End-of-Life Care

There is no agreement on one definition for hospice care (Hui et al. 2013). It can be defined as a type of care that provides comprehensive care for patients near the end of life utilizing an interdisciplinary approach (Batchelor 2010). Hospice care can be described in multiple terms, such as a system, a program, a philosophy, or a facility. That service can be community based, or inpatient; there is high emphasis of the role of volunteers, bereavement care, and community care in that type of care (Hui et al. 2013). So this service can be provided at home, care facilities like nursing home, or in hospitals in certain cases. Caring of caregivers is a part of this care as well.

The term "end of life" definition is not clear; for a patient to be eligible for hospice care in the USA, two physicians should certify that the patient with life-limiting illness has a life expectancy of 6 months or less (Batchelor 2010). According to American Medicare regulations, most patients are enrollment only at final weeks or days of life, about16% died within 3 days of hospice enrollment in 2012 (O'Connor et al. 2014). There is high need for this type of care. According to Global Atlas of Palliative Care at the End of life that was released by WHO in 2014, there is about 20.4 million people needs palliative care at the end of life. Figure 9.4 shows world map with global distribution rates for people who need palliative care at end of life. The majority of deaths are in LMICs without adequate access to a palliative care. There is inequality in palliative and hospice care services between high-income countries and other countries (Clemens et al. 2007). End-of-life care is limited in LMICs as that care is not integrated into the national health system in many of these countries (Cruz-Oliver et al. 2017). Treatment in the last period of life is expensive, and in countries without unified health care coverage, families may fall in poverty due to these expenses (Sallnow et al. 2022). Figure 9.4 shows the world map with global distribution of rates of people who need palliative care at end of life.

For HCC patients, in one small prospective trial, the most common distressing symptoms near the end of life were lack of energy and pain. The other symptoms include drowsiness, sexual-related problems, insomnia, and itching (Hansen et al. 2017a). In another study, nausea/vomiting cachexia, peripheral edema, and ascites are common symptoms as well (Lin et al. 2004). As many patients with HCC have liver cirrhosis, patients can manifest with ascites, jaundice, hepatic encephalopathy, and variceal bleeding as well (Hashmi et al. 2023).

Utilization of palliative and hospice care was found to reduce healthcare resource utilization, which includes the cost of hospitalization, visits to the emergency room,

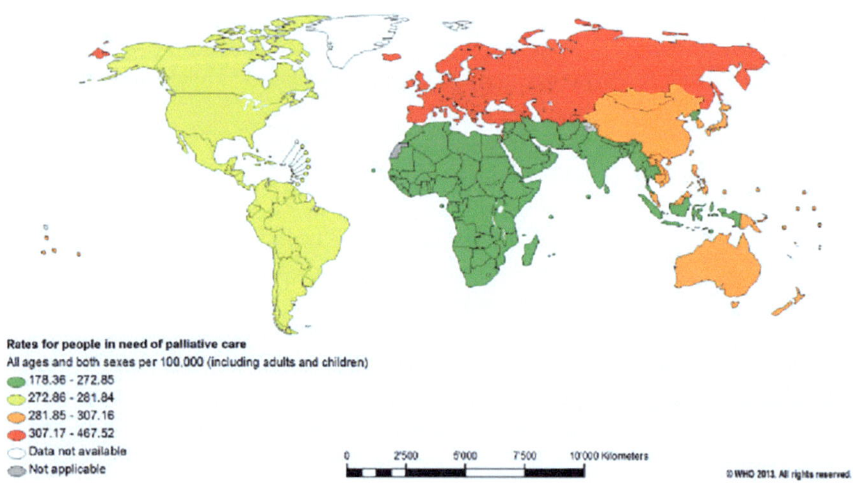

Fig. 9.4 World map with global distribution of rates of people who need palliative care at end of life. Source: Worldwide Hospice Palliative Care Alliance Global Atlas of Palliative Care at the End of Life

and admission to the critical care unit. HCC patients who utilize this service are less likely to die in the hospital and get resuscitation. There is no difference in survival most likely between patients who get hospice care and the patients who get usual care (Mudumbi et al. 2018).

HCC patients near the end of life do not react the same; some have a fighting view and want to do whatever aggressive intervention is available, like TKIs or TACE; other patients want quality of life and prefer not to go with interventions with side effects without clear benefits (Hansen et al. 2015). Providers should be aware of this difference and discuss with their patients' pros and cons of any interventions in details.

Management of these patients depends on the type of symptoms with consideration of the prognosis. Management of pain usually with opioids, non-opioid, and adjuvant medications as we mentioned before. Treatment of encephalopathy with lactulose, or polyethylene glycol with adding rifaximin sometimes, but the usage of the latter is limited due to the cost. Ascites can be treated with diuretics, sodium restriction, and repeated paracentesis (Miller et al. 2023). Long-term catheter for refractory ascites can be used, but it increases the risk of infection if they stay for a long time, usually more than 3 months (Reinglas et al. 2016). So, there should be careful choice of patients who are eligible for that procedure. However, there are no robust studies to show the clear benefit of interventions like enema, blood transfusion antibiotics, or abdominal paracentesis near the end of life in HCC patients (Lin et al. 2004). There should be studies to clarify the benefits of these interventions.

Other than physical symptoms, psychological symptoms should be evaluated. Advanced care planning, like a preferred place of death, and resuscitation preference, should be discussed earlier as cirrhosis that usually accompanies HCC usually has an unpredictable course (Miller et al. 2023). Patients near the end of life depend heavily on informal caregivers (family members or friends), especially in low-income countries, due to limited resources to get professional caregivers. These caregivers can suffer from physical, psychological, social, and spiritual challenges and need support (Wan et al. 2022). Online social support groups can be a modern method to support caregivers (Benson et al. 2020).

The location of care is a crucial matter in hospice care. The preferred place of death for patients with incurable cancer is usually home, which is applicable to LMICs as well (Alsirafy et al. 2019).

9.7 Conclusion

There are no well stablished guidelines for palliative care for HCC patients, especially in LMICs. Providers should be aware of common symptoms accompanied by HCC and treat or refer patients to palliative care as needed. There are many challenges facing implementation of palliative care in LMICs in general as we discussed. There should be active roadmap on different levels to improve that situation with efficient utilization of the limited resources. The strategies used in high-income countries may not be applicable to LMICs, so there should be robust research projects and careful planning to achieve suitable strategies. Some effective ideas like local production of generic pain medication, training primary care providers on palliative care, utilization of CHWs, and conducting home-based services, can be adopted.

References

Abouelezz K, Khanapara D, Batiha GE, et al. Cytotoxic chemotherapy as an alternative for systemic treatment of advanced hepatocellular carcinoma in developing countries. Cancer Manag Res. 2020;12:12239–48. https://doi.org/10.2147/CMAR.S280631.

Abu-Odah H, Molassiotis A, Liu J. Challenges on the provision of palliative care for patients with cancer in low- and middle-income countries: a systematic review of reviews. BMC Palliat Care. 2020;19(1):55. https://doi.org/10.1186/s12904-020-00558-5.

Agarwal R, Epstein AS. The role of palliative Care in Oncology. Semin Interv Radiol. 2017;34(4):307–12. https://doi.org/10.1055/s-0037-1608702.

Aldea M, Orillard E, Mansi L, et al. How to manage patients with corticosteroids in oncology in the era of immunotherapy? Eur J Cancer. 2020;141:239–51. https://doi.org/10.1016/j.ejca.2020.09.032.

Alsirafy SA, Abdel-Kareem SS, Ibrahim NY, et al. Cancer diagnosis disclosure preferences of family caregivers of cancer patients in Egypt: cancer diagnosis disclosure preference. Psycho Oncol Chichester, UK. 2016;26:1758–62. https://doi.org/10.1002/pon.4206.

Alsirafy SA, Hammad AM, Ibrahim NY, et al. Preferred place of death for patients with incurable cancer and their family caregivers in Egypt. Am J Hosp Palliat Med. 2019;36(5):423–8. https://doi.org/10.1177/1049909118813990.

Anderson PF, Wescom E, Carlos RC. Difficult doctors, difficult patients: building empathy. J Am Coll Radiol. 2016;13(12):1590–8. https://doi.org/10.1016/j.jacr.2016.09.015.

Bajaj JS, Wade JB, Gibson DP, et al. The multi-dimensional burden of cirrhosis and hepatic encephalopathy on patients and caregivers. Am J Gastroenterol. 2011;106(9):1646–53. https://doi.org/10.1038/ajg.2011.157.

Bakitas MA, Tosteson TD, Li Z, et al. Early versus delayed initiation of concurrent palliative oncology care: patient outcomes in the ENABLE III randomized controlled trial. JCO. 2015;33(13):1438.

Batchelor NH. Palliative or hospice care? Understanding the similarities and differences. Rehabil Nurs. 2010;35(2):60–4. https://doi.org/10.1002/j.2048-7940.2010.tb00032.x.

Benson JJ, Oliver DP, Washington KT, et al. Online social support groups for informal caregivers of hospice patients with cancer. Eur J Oncol Nurs Off J Eur Oncol Nurs Soc. 2020;44:101698. https://doi.org/10.1016/j.ejon.2019.101698.

Beuken-van Everdingen MHJ, Graeff A, Jongen JLM, et al. Pharmacological treatment of pain in cancer patients: the role of adjuvant analgesics, a systematic review. Pain Pract. 2017;17(3):409–19. https://doi.org/10.1111/papr.12459.

Bianchi G, Marchesini G, Nicolino F, et al. Psychological status and depression in patients with liver cirrhosis. Dig Liver Dis. 2005;37(8):593–600. https://doi.org/10.1016/j.dld.2005.01.020.

Blackburn H, West S. Management of postembolization syndrome following hepatic transarterial chemoembolization for primary or metastatic liver cancer. Cancer Nurs. 2016;39(5):E1–E18. https://doi.org/10.1097/NCC.0000000000000302.

Bolarinwa FI, Esan DT, Bolarinwa OA. Assessment of spiritual care practices among nurses caring for cancer patients in a tertiary Hospital in Nigeria. SAGE Open Nurs. 2023;9:23779608221150600. https://doi.org/10.1177/23779608221150600.

Bond M. Pain education issues in developing countries and responses to them by the International Association for the Study of Pain. Pain Res Manag. 2011;16(6):404–6. https://doi.org/10.1155/2011/654746.

Broom A, Kirby E, Good P, et al. The troubles of telling: managing communication about the end of life. Qual Health Res. 2014;24(2):151–62. https://doi.org/10.1177/1049732313519709.
Buga S, Sarria JE. The management of pain in metastatic bone disease. Cancer Contr J Moffitt Cancer Center. 2012;19:2. https://doi.org/10.1177/107327481201900210.
Burgener AM. Enhancing communication to improve patient safety and to increase patient satisfaction. Health Care Manag. 2020;39(3):128–32. https://doi.org/10.1097/HCM.0000000000000298.
Calton BA, Alvarez-Perez A, Portman DG, et al. The current state of palliative care for patients cared for at leading US cancer centers: the 2015 NCCN palliative care survey. J Natl Compr Cancer Netw. 2016;14(7):859.
Carr BI, Pujol L. Pain at presentation and survival in hepatocellular carcinoma. J Pain. 2010;11(10):988–93. https://doi.org/10.1016/j.jpain.2010.01.265.
Cavalieri TA. Ethical issues at the end of life. J Am Osteopath Assoc. 2001;101(10):616–22.
Chandok N, Watt KDS. Pain management in the cirrhotic patient: the clinical challenge. Mayo Clin Proc. 2010;85(5):451–8. https://doi.org/10.4065/mcp.2009.0534.
Chang PE, Ong WC, Lui HF, et al. Epidemiology and prognosis of paraneoplastic syndromes in hepatocellular carcinoma. ISRN Oncol. 2013;2013:684026–8. https://doi.org/10.1155/2013/684026.
Chang Y, Jeong SW, Young Jang J, et al. Recent updates of Transarterial Chemoembolilzation in hepatocellular carcinoma. Int J Mol Sci. 2020;21(21):8165. https://doi.org/10.3390/ijms21218165.
Chavez MN, Tyson DM, Lake PW, et al. 'They say you can get addicted': exploring factors that fuel the fear of addiction to prescription opioids among cancer survivors. Eur J Cancer Care. 2022;31(3):e13582. https://doi.org/10.1111/ecc.13582.
Cheung WY, Le LW, Gagliese L, et al. Age and gender differences in symptom intensity and symptom clusters among patients with metastatic cancer. Support Care Cancer. 2011;19(3):417–23. https://doi.org/10.1007/s00520-010-0865-2.
Christian-Miller N, Frenette C. Hepatocellular cancer pain: impact and management challenges. J Hepatocell Carcinoma. 2018;5:75–80. https://doi.org/10.2147/JHC.S145450.
Clark PA. Medical futility: legal and ethical analysis. Virtual Ment. 2007;9(5):375–83. https://doi.org/10.1001/virtualmentor.2007.9.5.msoc1-0705.
Clark D, Baur N, Clelland D, et al. Mapping levels of palliative care development in 198 countries: the situation in 2017. J Pain Symptom Manag. 2020;59(4):794.
Clelland D, Van Steijn D, Whitelaw S, et al. Palliative care in public policy: results from a global survey. Palliat Med Rep. 2020;1(1):183.
Clemens KE, Kumar S, Bruera E, et al. Palliative care in developing countries: what are the important issues? Palliat Med. 2007;21(3):173.
Coghlan R, Shamieh O, Bloomer MJ. Inequities of palliative care availability and access to opioids in low- and middle-income countries. Palliat Med. 2021;36:NP1. https://doi.org/10.1177/02692163211034083.
Collins A, McLachlan S, Philip J. Initial perceptions of palliative care: an exploratory qualitative study of patients with advanced cancer and their family caregivers. Palliat Med. 2017;31(9):825–32. https://doi.org/10.1177/0269216317696420.
Cook I, Kirkup AL, Langham LJ, et al. End of life care and do not resuscitate orders: how much does age influence decision making? A systematic review and meta-analysis. Gerontol Geriatr Med. 2017;3:2333721417713422.
Cooper A, Aloia TA. Surgical resection for hepatocellular carcinoma. Transl Cancer Res. 2013; https://doi.org/10.3978/j.issn.2218-676X.2013.09.03.
Crane MK, Wittink M, Doukas DJ. Respecting end-of-life treatment preferences. Am Fam Physician. 2005;72(7):1263–8.
Cruz-Oliver DM, Little MO, Woob J, et al. End-of-life care in low-and middle-income countries. Bull World Health Organ. 2017;95(11):731. https://doi.org/10.2471/BLT.16.185199.
Cunningham SC, Choti MA, Bellavance EC et al. Palliation of hepatic tumors (2013).

Davies E, Higginson IJ. Systematic review of specialist palliative day-care for adults with cancer. Support Care Cancer. 2005;13(8):607.

Den Herder-Van Der Eerden M, Ewert B, Hodiamont F, et al. Towards accessible integrated palliative care: perspectives of leaders from seven European countries on facilitators, barriers and recommendations for improvement. J Integ Care Brighton, UK. 2017;25(3):222–32. https://doi.org/10.1108/JICA-03-2017-0006.

Donkor A, Luckett T, Aranda S, et al. Barriers and facilitators to implementation of cancer treatment and palliative care strategies in low- and middle-income countries: systematic review. Int J Public Health. 2018;63(9):1047–57. https://doi.org/10.1007/s00038-018-1142-2.

Elsayem A, Calderon BB, Camarines EM, et al. A month in an acute palliative care unit. Am J Hosp Palliat Care. 2011;28(8):550.

Eti S, O'Mahony S, Mchugh M, et al. Outcomes of the acute palliative care unit in an Academic Medical Center. Am J Hosp Palliat Care. 2013;31(4):380.

Ettinger AB, Portenoy RK. The use of corticosteroids in the treatment of symptoms associated with cancer. J Pain Symptom Manag. 1988;3(2):99–103. https://doi.org/10.1016/0885-3924(88)90167-4.

Evans WJ. Megestrol acetate use for weight gain should be carefully considered. J Clin Endocrinol Metab. 2007;92(2):420–1. https://doi.org/10.1210/jc.2006-2734.

Ferrell B, Connor SR, Cordes A, et al. The National Agenda for quality palliative care: the National Consensus Project and the National Quality Forum. J Pain Symptom Manag. 2007;33(6):737–44. https://doi.org/10.1016/j.jpainsymman.2007.02.024.

Finaly E, Rabow M, Buss MK. Finalay OP palliaitve care. Am Soc Clin Oncol Educ Book. 2018; https://doi.org/10.1200/EDBK_200775.

Fink R. Pain assessment: the cornerstone to optimal pain management. Proc (Bayl Univ Med Cent). 2000;13:236. https://doi.org/10.1080/08998280.2000.11927681.

Ghand S, Khubchandani S, Lyer R. Quality of life and hepatocellular carcinoma. J Gastrointest Oncol. 2014;5:296. https://doi.org/10.3978/j.issn.2078-6891.2014.046.

Giannini EG, Farinati F, Ciccarese F, et al. Prognosis of untreated hepatocellular carcinoma. Hepatology. 2014;61(1):184.

Gofton C, Agar M, George J. Early implementation of palliative and supportive care in hepatocellular carcinoma. Semin Liver Dis. 2022;42(04):514.

Goh CR, Lee S. Education in pain and palliative care in the low- and middle-income countries of the Asia Pacific region. Pain. 2018;159(1):S74.

Gomes B, Calanzani N, Curiale V, et al. Effectiveness and cost-effectiveness of home palliative care services for adults with advanced illness and their caregivers. Cochrane Database Syst Rev. 2013;2013(6):CD007760.

Goodman-Palmer D, Ferriolli E, Gordon AL, et al. Health and wellbeing of older people in LMICs: a call for research-informed decision making. Lancet Glob Health. 2023;11(2):e191–2. https://doi.org/10.1016/S2214-109X(22)00546-0.

Granek L, Krzyzanowska MK, Tozer R, et al. Oncologists' strategies and barriers to effective communication about the end of life. J Oncol Pract. 2013;9(4):e129–35. https://doi.org/10.1200/JOP.2012.000800.

Groninger H, Vijayan J. Pharmacologic Management of Pain at the end of life. Am Fam Physician. 2014;90(1):26–32.

Guan Y, Tian Y, Fan Y. Pain management in patients with hepatocellular carcinoma after transcatheter arterial chemoembolisation: a retrospective study. World J Gastrointest Surg. 2023;15(3):374–86. https://doi.org/10.4240/wjgs.v15.i3.374.

Guo H, Wu T, Lu Q, et al. Hepatocellular carcinoma in elderly: clinical characteristics, treatments and outcomes compared with younger adults. PLoS One. 2017;12(9):e0184160. https://doi.org/10.1371/journal.pone.0184160.

Hancock K, Clayton JM, Parker SM, et al. Truth-telling in discussing prognosis in advanced life-limiting illnesses: a systematic review. Palliat Med. 2007;21(6):507–17.

Hansen L, Dieckmann NF, Kolbeck KJ, et al. Symptom distress in patients with hepatocellular carcinoma toward the end of life. Oncol Nurs Forum. 2017a;44(6):665–73. https://doi.org/10.1188/17.ONF.665-673.
Hansen L, Rosenkranz S, Wherity K, et al. Living with hepatocellular carcinoma near the end of life: family caregivers' perspectives. ONF. 2017b;44(5):562.
Hansen L, Rosenkranz SJ, Vaccaro GM, et al. Patients with hepatocellular carcinoma near the end of life: a longitudinal qualitative study of their illness experiences. Cancer Nurs. 2015;38(4):E19–27. https://doi.org/10.1097/NCC.0000000000000188.
Harding JJ, Abu-Zeinah G, Chou JF, et al. Frequency, morbidity, and mortality of bone metastases in advanced hepatocellular carcinoma. J Natl Compr Cancer Netw. 2018;16(1):50.
Hashimoto N, Akahoshi T, Shoji T, et al. Successful treatment for hepatic encephalopathy aggravated by portal vein thrombosis with balloon-occluded retrograde Transvenous obliteration. Case Rep Gastroenterol. 2011;5(2):366–71. https://doi.org/10.1159/000330287.
Hashmi IN, Lee HM, Wedd JP, et al. A narrative review of supportive and end of life care considerations in advanced hepatocellular carcinoma. Ann Palliat Med. 2023;12(6):1260.
Häussinger D, Schliess F. Pathogenetic mechanisms of hepatic encephalopathy. Gut. 2008;57(8):1156–65. https://doi.org/10.1136/gut.2007.122176.
Häussinger D, Kircheis G, Fischer R, et al. Hepatic encephalopathy in chronic liver disease: a clinical manifestation of astrocyte swelling and low-grade cerebral edema? J Hepatol. 2000;32(6):1035–8.
Hayashi S, Tanaka H, Hoshi H. Palliative external-beam radiotherapy for bone metastases from hepatocellular carcinoma. World J Hepatol. 2014;6(12):923–9. https://doi.org/10.4254/wjh.v6.i12.923.
Herber OR, Johnston BM. The role of healthcare support workers in providing palliative and end-of-life care in the community: a systematic literature review. Health Soc Care Community. 2013;21(3):225–35. https://doi.org/10.1111/j.1365-2524.2012.01092.x.
Hird A, Zhang L, Holt T, et al. Dexamethasone for the Prophylaxis of Radiation-induced Pain Flare after Palliative Radiotherapy for Symptomatic Bone Metastases: a Phase II Study. Clin Oncol Royal College Radiol Gr Brit. 2009;21(4):329–35. https://doi.org/10.1016/j.clon.2008.12.010.
Honda T, Miyaaki H, Ichikawa T, et al. Clinical characteristics of hepatocellular carcinoma in elderly patients. Oncol Lett. 2011;2(5):851–4. https://doi.org/10.3892/ol.2011.359.
Hughes MT, Smith TJ. The growth of palliative care in the United States. Annu Rev Public Health. 2014;35(1):459.
Hui D, Bruera E. Integrating palliative care into the trajectory of cancer care. Nat Rev Clin Oncol. 2016;13(3):159.
Hui D, De La Cruz M, Mori M, et al. Concepts and definitions for "supportive care," "best supportive care," "palliative care," and "hospice care" in the published literature, dictionaries, and textbooks. Support Care Cancer. 2013;21(3):659–85. https://doi.org/10.1007/s00520-012-1564-y.
Hui D, de la Cruz M, Thorney S, et al. The frequency and correlates of spiritual distress among patients with advanced cancer admitted to an acute palliative care unit. Am J Hospice Palliat Med. 2011;28(4):264–70. https://doi.org/10.1177/1049909110385917.
Hui D, Dos Santos R, Chisholm G, et al. Bedside clinical signs associated with impending death in patients with advanced cancer: preliminary findings of a prospective, longitudinal cohort study. Cancer. 2015;121(6):960.
Hui D, Elsayem A, Palla S, et al. Discharge outcomes and survival of patients with advanced cancer admitted to an acute palliative care unit at a Comprehensive Cancer Center. J Palliat Med. 2010;13(1):49.
Hui D, Hannon BL, Zimmermann C, et al. Improving patient and caregiver outcomes in oncology: team-based, timely, and targeted palliative care. CA A Cancer J Clinicians. 2019;68(5):356.
Hüseyin GC, Pelin KA, Canan YGA. Physician perspectives on the DNR order in Turkey: a survey of physicians in internal medicine. Afr Health Sci. 2023;23(1):667–77. https://doi.org/10.4314/ahs.v23i1.71.
Illueca M, Bradshaw YS, Carr DB. Spiritual pain: a symptom in search of a clinical definition. J Relig Health. 2023;62(3):1920–32. https://doi.org/10.1007/s10943-022-01645-y.

INCB Report. Supplement to the annual report of the Board for 2022 on the availability of internationally controlled substances. (United Nations International Narcotics Control Board report) (2022).
Ismail Z, Elbayoumi H, Fischer CE, et al. Prevalence of depression in patients with mild cognitive impairment: a systematic review and meta-analysis. JAMA Psych Chicago, IL. 2017;74(1):58–67. https://doi.org/10.1001/jamapsychiatry.2016.3162.
Jiang Q, Jiang X, Zheng M, et al. Rifaximin versus nonabsorbable disaccharides in the management of hepatic encephalopathy: a meta-analysis. Eur J Gastroenterol Hepatol. 2008;20(11):1064–70. https://doi.org/10.1097/MEG.0b013e328302f470.
Johnson JR, et al. Multicenter, double-blind, randomized, placebo-controlled, parallel-group study of the efficacy, safety, and tolerability of THC:CBD extract and THC extract in patients with intractable cancer-related pain. J Pain Symptom Manag. 2010;39(2):167–79. https://doi.org/10.1016/j.jpainsymman.2009.06.008.
Kang'ethe SM. Validating that palliative care giving is a stressful occupation: the case of the Kanye community home-based care programme, Botswana. South Afr Family Pract. 2010;52(6):548–56. https://doi.org/10.1080/20786204.2010.10874046.
Kazdin AE, Wu C, Hwang I, et al. Antidepressant use in low- middle- and high-income countries: a world mental health surveys report. Psychol Med. 2023;53(4):1583–91. https://doi.org/10.1017/S0033291721003160.
Kessler DP, McClellan MB. Advance directives and medical treatment at the end of life. J Health Econ. 2004;23(1):111–27. https://doi.org/10.1016/j.jhealeco.2003.08.006.
Kim S, Chun M, Wang H, et al. Bone metastasis from primary hepatocellular carcinoma: characteristics of soft tissue formation. Cancer Res Treat. 2007;39(3):104–8. https://doi.org/10.4143/crt.2007.39.3.104.
Kim DJ, Yoo JW, Chang JW, et al. Does low income effects 5-year mortality of hepatocellular carcinoma patients? Int J Equity Health. 2021;20(1):151.
King A, Hoppe RB. "Best practice" for patient-centered communication: a narrative review. J Grad Med Educ. 2013;5(3):385–93. https://doi.org/10.4300/jgme-d-13-00072.1.
Kistler EA, Sean Morrison R, Richardson LD, et al. Emergency department–triggered palliative Care in Advanced Cancer: proof of concept. Acad Emerg Med. 2015;22(2):237.
Klinge M, Coppler T, Liebschutz JM, et al. The assessment and Management of Pain in cirrhosis. Curr Hepatology Rep. 2018;17(1):42–51. https://doi.org/10.1007/s11901-018-0389-7.
Kornblau S, Benson AB, Catalano R, et al. Management of cancer treatment–related diarrhea: issues and therapeutic strategies. J Pain Symptom Manag. 2000;19(2):118–29. https://doi.org/10.1016/S0885-3924(99)00149-9.
Kudo M, Finn RS, Qin S, et al. Lenvatinib versus sorafenib in first-line treatment of patients with unresectable hepatocellular carcinoma: a randomised phase 3 non-inferiority trial. Lancet (British edition). 2018;391(10126):1163–73. https://doi.org/10.1016/S0140-6736(18)30207-1.
Kwakman JJM, Elshot YS, Punt CJA, et al. Management of cytotoxic chemotherapy-induced hand-foot syndrome. Oncol Rev. 2020;14(1):57–63. https://doi.org/10.4081/ONCOL.2020.442.
Lamers WM. Defining palliative care, cancer without pain, when to contact hospice, when to treat multiple myeloma, meaning of physical signs, pneumonia at end-of-life. J Pain Palliat Care Pharmacother. 2007;21(1):85–90. https://doi.org/10.1080/J354v21n01_19.
Lan S, Lin Y, Chen S, et al. Effects of acupressure on fatigue and depression in hepatocellular carcinoma patients treated with Transcatheter arterial chemoembolization: a quasi-experimental study. Evid Based Complement Alternat Med. 2015;2015:496485–10. https://doi.org/10.1155/2015/496485.
Laryionava K, Heußner P, Hiddemann W, et al. "Rather one more chemo than one less…": oncologists and oncology nurses' reasons for aggressive treatment of Young adults with advanced cancer. Oncol Dayton, OH. 2018;23(2):256–62. https://doi.org/10.1634/theoncologist.2017-0094.
Laube R, Sabih A, Strasser SI, et al. Palliative care in hepatocellular carcinoma. J Gastro Hepatol. 2020;36(3):618.

Le BHC, Mileshkin L, Doan K, et al. Acceptability of early integration of palliative care in patients with incurable lung cancer. J Palliat Med. 2014;17(5):553–8. https://doi.org/10.1089/jpm.2013.0473.

Lee K, Lin J, Shi H. Anxiety and depression are associated with long-term outcomes of hepatocellular carcinoma: a nationwide study of a cohort from Taiwan. World J Biol Psychiatry. 2017;19(6):431.

Lencioni R, de Baere T, Soulen MC, et al. Lipiodol transarterial chemoembolization for hepatocellular carcinoma: a systematic review of efficacy and safety data. Hepatology. 2016;64(1):106–16. https://doi.org/10.1002/hep.28453.

Leppert W, Buss T. The role of corticosteroids in the treatment of pain in cancer patients. Curr Pain Headache Rep. 2012;16(4):307–13. https://doi.org/10.1007/s11916-012-0273-z.

Lewin SA, Dick J, Pond P, et al. Lay health workers in primary and community health care. Cochrane Database Syst Rev. 2005;1:CD004015. https://doi.org/10.1002/14651858.CD004015.pub2.

Lewis JH, Stine JG. Review article: prescribing medications in patients with cirrhosis—a practical guide. Alim Pharmacol Therap. 2013;37(12):1132–56. https://doi.org/10.1111/apt.12324.

Li F, He H. Assessing the accuracy of diagnostic tests. Gen Psych. 2018;30(3):207–12. https://doi.org/10.11919/j.issn.1002-0829.218052.

Li Y, Gao Z, Qu X. The adverse effects of Sorafenib in patients with advanced cancers. Basic Clin Pharmacol Toxicol. 2015;116(3):216–21. https://doi.org/10.1111/bcpt.12365.

Lin M, Wu P, Tsai S, et al. Hospice palliative care for patients with hepatocellular carcinoma in Taiwan. Palliat Med. 2004;18(2):93–9. https://doi.org/10.1191/0269216304pm851oa.

Longo V, Brunetti O, D'Oronzo S, et al. Bone metastases in hepatocellular carcinoma: an emerging issue. Cancer Metastasis Rev. 2014;33(1):333–42. https://doi.org/10.1007/s10555-013-9454-4.

Lussier D, Huskey AG, Portenoy RK. Adjuvant analgesics in cancer pain management. Oncol Dayton, OH. 2004;9(5):571–91. https://doi.org/10.1634/theoncologist.9-5-571.

Lutz S, Balboni T, Jones J, et al. Palliative radiation therapy for bone metastases: update of an ASTRO evidence-based guideline. Pract Radiat Oncol. 2017;7(1):4–12. https://doi.org/10.1016/j.prro.2016.08.001.

Lynskey M, Agrawal A. Differential criterion functioning of alcohol use symptomatology in major depressive disorder? Psychol Med. 2008;38(3):441–9. https://doi.org/10.1017/S003329170700178X.

MacRae MC, Fazal O, O'Donovan J. Community health workers in palliative care provision in low-income and middle-income countries: a systematic scoping review of the literature. BMJ Glob Health. 2020;5(5):e002368. https://doi.org/10.1136/bmjgh-2020-002368.

Mao JJ, Ismaila N, Bao T, et al. Integrative medicine for pain management in oncology: society for integrative oncology-ASCO guideline. J Clin Oncol. 2022;40(34):3998–4024.

Marinangeli F, Ciccozzi A, Leonardis M, et al. Use of strong opioids in advanced cancer pain: a randomized trial. J Pain Symptom Manag. 2004;27(5):409–16. https://doi.org/10.1016/j.jpainsymman.2003.10.006.

Marks A, Gerard R, Fournier P, et al. Sorafenib-induced hepatic encephalopathy. Ann Pharmacother. 2009;43(12):2121. https://doi.org/10.1345/aph.1M457.

May P, Garrido MM, Cassel JB, et al. Prospective cohort study of hospital palliative care teams for inpatients with advanced cancer: earlier consultation is associated with larger cost-saving effect. JCO. 2015;33(25):2745.

McLellan B, Ciardiello F, Lacouture ME, et al. Regorafenib-associated hand–foot skin reaction: practical advice on diagnosis, prevention, and management. Ann Oncol. 2015;26(10):2017–26. https://doi.org/10.1093/annonc/mdv244.

Meier DE, Beresford L. The palliative care team. J Palliat Med. 2008;11(5):677–81. https://doi.org/10.1089/jpm.2008.9907.

Menon V, Ransing R, Praharaj SK. Management of psychiatric disorders in patients with hepatic and gastrointestinal diseases. Indian J Psych. 2022;64(Suppl 2):S379–93.

Merriman A, Harding R. Pain control in the African context: the Ugandan introduction of affordable morphine to relieve suffering at the end of life. PEHM. 2010;5(1):10. https://doi.org/10.1186/1747-5341-5-10.

Mheidly N, Fares J. Health communication in low-income countries: a 60-year bibliometric and thematic analysis. J Educ Heal Prom. 2020;9(1):163. https://doi.org/10.4103/jehp.jehp_384_20.
Miaskowski C, Dodd M, Lee K. Symptom clusters: the new frontier in symptom management research. J Natl Cancer Inst Monogr. 2004;2004(32):17.
Miller K, Barman P, Kappus M. Palliative care and end of life care in decompensated cirrhosis. Clin Liver Dis Malden, MA. 2023;22(1):10–3. https://doi.org/10.1097/CLD.0000000000000044.
Mitra R, Jones S. Adjuvant analgesics in cancer pain: a review. Am J Hosp Palliat Med. 2012;29(1):70–9. https://doi.org/10.1177/1049909111413256.
Mohamed S, Sabki ZA, Zainal NZ. Depression and psychosocial correlates of liver transplant candidates: a systematic review. Asia Pac Psychiatry. 2014;6(4):447–53. https://doi.org/10.1111/appy.12145.
Mohile SG, Dale W, Somerfield MR, et al. Practical assessment and management of vulnerabilities in older patients receiving chemotherapy: Asco guideline for geriatric oncology. J Clin Oncol. 2018;36(22):2326–47. https://doi.org/10.1200/JCO.2018.78.8687.
Morrison RS, Dietrich J, Ladwig S, et al. Palliative care consultation teams cut hospital costs for medicaid beneficiaries. Health Aff. 2011;30(3):454.
Morriss WW, Roques CJ. Pain management in low- and middle-income countries. BJA Educ. 2018;18(9):265–70. https://doi.org/10.1016/j.bjae.2018.05.006.
Mudumbi SK, Bourgeois CE, Hoppman NA, et al. Palliative care and hospice interventions in decompensated cirrhosis and hepatocellular carcinoma: a rapid review of literature. J Palliat Med. 2018;21(8):1177–84. https://doi.org/10.1089/jpm.2017.0656.
Mullish BH, Kabir MS, Thursz MR, et al. Review article: depression and the use of antidepressants in patients with chronic liver disease or liver transplantation. Alimen Pharmacol Therap. 2014;40(8):880–92. https://doi.org/10.1111/apt.12925.
Neugut AI, Matasar M, Wang X, et al. Duration of adjuvant chemotherapy for colon cancer and survival among the elderly. J Clin Oncol. 2006;24(15):2368–75. https://doi.org/10.1200/JCO.2005.04.5005.
Ngo-Metzger Q, August KJ, Srinivasan M, et al. End-of-life care: guidelines for patient-centered communication. Am Fam Physician. 2008;77(2):167–74.
Nipp RD, Greer JA, El-Jawahri A, et al. Coping and prognostic awareness in patients with advanced cancer. J Clin Oncol. 2017;35(22):2551–7. https://doi.org/10.1200/JCO.2016.71.3404.
Nunes R, Rego G. Euthanasia: a challenge to medical ethics. J Clin Res Bioethic. 2016;7(4) https://doi.org/10.4172/2155-9627.1000282.
Obeidat AE, Wong LL. Spontaneous rupture of hepatocellular carcinoma: new insights. J Clin Exp Hepatol. 2022;12(2):483–91. https://doi.org/10.1016/j.jceh.2021.05.010.
O'Connor NR, Hu R, Harris PS, et al. Hospice admissions for cancer in the final days of life: independent predictors and implications for quality measures. JCO. 2014;32(28):3184.
Ogasawara S, Chiba T, Ooka Y, et al. A randomized placebo-controlled trial of prophylactic dexamethasone for transcatheter arterial chemoembolization. Hepatology. 2018;67(2):575–85. https://doi.org/10.1002/hep.29403.
Paulsen Ø, Aass N, Kaasa S, et al. Do corticosteroids provide analgesic effects in cancer patients? A systematic literature review. J Pain Symptom Manag. 2013;46(1):96–105. https://doi.org/10.1016/j.jpainsymman.2012.06.019.
Pawasarat IM, Schultz EM, Frisby JC, et al. The efficacy of medical marijuana in the treatment of cancer-related pain. J Palliat Med. 2020;23(6):809–16. https://doi.org/10.1089/jpm.2019.0374.
Poznak CV, Somerfield MR, Barlow WE, et al. Role of bone-modifying agents in metastatic breast cancer: an American society of Clinical Oncology-cancer care Ontario focused guideline update. J Clin Oncol. 2017;35:3978.
Quill TE. Recognizing and adjusting to barriers in doctor-patient communication. Ann Intern Med. 1989;111(1):51–7. https://doi.org/10.7326/0003-4819-111-1-51.
Rabow MW, Dahlin C, Ritchie C. New frontiers in outpatient palliative care for patients with cancer. Cancer Contr. 2015;22:465.

Radbruch L, De Lima L, Knaul F, et al. Redefining palliative care—a new consensus-based definition. J Pain Symptom Manag. 2020;60(4):754–64. https://doi.org/10.1016/j.jpainsymman.2020.04.027.
Raja SN, Carr DB, Cohen M, et al. The revised International Association for the Study of Pain definition of pain: concepts, challenges, and compromises. Pain. 2020;161(9):1976.
Reinglas J, Amjadi K, Petrcich B, et al. The palliative Management of Refractory Cirrhotic Ascites Using the PleurX © catheter. Can J Gastroenterol Hepatol. 2016;2016:4680543–7. https://doi.org/10.1155/2016/4680543.
Rhee JY, Luyirika E, Namisango E et al. The African Palliative Care Association (APCA) atlas of palliative care development in Africa: a comparative analysis; 2018.
Rice DR, Dalmacy D, Hyer JM, et al. Impact of psychiatric illness on survival among patients with hepatocellular carcinoma. J Gastrointest Surg. 2021;25(12):3242–3. https://doi.org/10.1007/s11605-021-05029-7.
Richards GC, Aronson JK, Mahtani KR, et al. Global, regional, and national consumption of controlled opioids: a cross-sectional study of 214 countries and non-metropolitan territories. Br J Pain. 2022;16(1):34–40. https://doi.org/10.1177/20494637211013052.
Rick TJ, Habtamu B, Tigeneh W, et al. RADIATION ONCOLOGY original reports Radiotherapy practice for treatment of bone metastasis in Ethiopia. JCO Glob Oncol. 2020;6:1422.
Riggs A, Breuer B, Dhingra L, et al. Hospice enrollment after referral to community-based, specialist palliative care: impact of telephonic outreach. J Pain Symptom Manag. 2017;54(2):219.
Roa J, Guevara A, Guevara C, et al. Physician's role in prescribing opioids in developing countries Global health. BMJ Case Rep. 2019;12(6):e227072.
Rodin G, Katz M, Lloyd N, et al. Treatment of depression in cancer patients. Curr Oncol. 2007;14(5):180–8. https://doi.org/10.3747/co.2007.146.
Roeland EJ, Bohlke K, Baracos VE, et al. Cancer cachexia: ASCO guideline rapid recommendation update. J Clin Oncol. 2023;41(25):4178–9. https://doi.org/10.1200/JCO.23.01280.
Rogal SS, Bielefeldt K, Wasan AD, et al. Inflammation, psychiatric symptoms, and opioid use are associated with pain and disability in patients with cirrhosis. Clin Gastroenterol Hepatol. 2015;13(5):1009–16. https://doi.org/10.1016/j.cgh.2014.10.029.
Ruff P, Al-Sukhun S, Blanchard C, et al. Access to cancer therapeutics in low- and middle-income countries. Am Soc Clin Oncol Educ Book. 2016;35(36):58–65. https://doi.org/10.1200/EDBK_155975.
Salikhanov I, Katapodi MC, Kunirova G, et al. Improving palliative care outcomes in remote and rural areas of LMICs through family caregivers: lessons from Kazakhstan. Front Public Health. 2023;11:1186107. https://doi.org/10.3389/fpubh.2023.1186107.
Sallnow L, Smith R, Ahmedzai SH, et al. Report of the lancet commission on the value of death: bringing death back into life. Lancet (British edition). 2022;399(10327):837–84. https://doi.org/10.1016/S0140-6736(21)02314-X.
Sargent DJ, Goldberg RM, Jacobson SD, et al. A pooled analysis of adjuvant chemotherapy for resected colon cancer in elderly patients. N Engl J Med. 2001;345(15):1091–7. https://doi.org/10.1056/NEJMoa010957.
Shah NJ, Neeb H, Kircheis G, et al. Quantitative cerebral water content mapping in hepatic encephalopathy. Neuro Image Orlando, FL. 2008;41(3):706–17. https://doi.org/10.1016/j.neuroimage.2008.02.057.
Shepperd S, Gonçalves-Bradley DC, Straus SE, et al. Hospital at home: home-based endof-life care. Cochrane Database Syst Rev. 2016;2:CD009231. https://doi.org/10.1002/14651858.CD009231.pub2.
Singh P, Chaturvedi A. Complementary and alternative medicine in cancer pain management: a systematic review. Indian J Palliat Care. 2015;21(1):105–15. https://doi.org/10.4103/0973-1075.150202.
Slomka J. Withholding nutrition at the end of life: clinical and ethical issues. Cleve Clin J Med. 2003;70(6):548–52. https://doi.org/10.3949/ccjm.70.6.548.

Smith EML, Pang H, Cirrincione C, et al. Effect of duloxetine on pain, function, and quality of life among patients with chemotherapy-induced painful peripheral neuropathy: a randomized clinical trial. JAMA. 2013;309(13):1359–67. https://doi.org/10.1001/jama.2013.2813.

Smith HR. Depression in cancer patients: pathogenesis, implications and treatment (review). Oncol Lett. 2015;9(4):1509–14. https://doi.org/10.3892/ol.2015.2944.

Soleimanpour H, Safari S, Shahsavari Nia K, et al. Opioid drugs in patients with liver disease: a systematic review. Hepat Mon. 2016;16(4):e32636. https://doi.org/10.5812/hepatmon.32636.

Song Y, Yoo J, Kim SG, et al. Complications of immunotherapy in advanced hepatocellular carcinoma. J Liver Cancer. 2023; https://doi.org/10.17998/jlc.2023.11.21.

Strine TW, Mokdad AH, Dube SR, et al. The association of depression and anxiety with obesity and unhealthy behaviors among community-dwelling US adults. Gen Hosp Psychiatry. 2008;30(2):127–37. https://doi.org/10.1016/j.genhosppsych.2007.12.008.

Sun VCY, Sarna L. Symptom management in hepatocellular carcinoma. Clin J Oncol Nurs. 2008;12(5):759–66. https://doi.org/10.1188/08.CJON.759-766.

Tamura K, Ichihara K, Maetaki E, et al. Development of a spiritual pain assessment sheet for terminal cancer patients: targeting terminal cancer patients admitted to palliative care units in Japan. Palliat Support Care. 2006;4(2):179–88. https://doi.org/10.1017/S147895150606024X.

Tan DJH, Quek SXZ, Yong JN, et al. Global prevalence of depression and anxiety in patients with hepatocellular carcinoma: systematic review and meta-analysis. Clin Mol Hepatol. 2022;28(4):864.

Torimura T, Iwamoto H. Optimizing the management of intermediate-stage hepatocellular carcinoma: current trends and prospects. Clin Mol Hepatol. 2021;27(2):236.

Torimura T, Iwamoto H. Treatment and the prognosis of hepatocellular carcinoma in Asia. Liver Int. 2022;42(9):2042–54. https://doi.org/10.1111/liv.15130.

Ülger Y, Delik A. Paraneoplastic syndrome frequency and prognostic effect in hepatocellular carcinoma patients. Eur J Gastroenterol Hepatol. 2022;34(7):769–73. https://doi.org/10.1097/MEG.0000000000002341.

Uka K, Aikata H, Takaki S, et al. Clinical features and prognosis of patients with extrahepatic metastases from hepatocellular carcinoma. World J Gastroenterol. 2007;13(3):414–20.

Unger J, Ghilbert P, Fisher JP. Doctor-patient communication in developing countries. BMJ. 2003;327(7412):450. https://doi.org/10.1136/bmj.327.7412.450-a.

van Leeuwen DJ, van Delden OM. Ethics and informed consent in patients with hepatocellular carcinoma: changing roles for hepatologist and radiologist: hepatocellular carcinoma. Clin Liver Dis (Malden, MA). 2015;6(5):122–5. https://doi.org/10.1002/cld.513.

Van Vliet LM, Van Der Wall E, Plum NM, et al. Explicit prognostic information and reassurance about nonabandonment when entering palliative breast cancer care: findings from a scripted video-vignette study. J Clin Oncol. 2013;31(26):3242–9. https://doi.org/10.1200/JCO.2012.45.5865.

Wagle NS, Spencer JC. Challenges for measuring cost-effectiveness of immunotherapy in unresectable hepatocellular carcinoma. JAMA Netw Open. 2021;4(4):e215476.

Walker ZJ, Xue S, Jones MP, et al. Depression, anxiety, and other mental disorders in patients with cancer in low- and lower-middle–income countries: a systematic review and meta-analysis. JCO Glob Oncol. 2021;7(7):1233–50. https://doi.org/10.1200/GO.21.00056.

Wan A, Lung E, Ankita A, et al. Support for informal caregivers in Canada: a scoping review from a hospice and palliative/end-of-life care lens. J Palliat Care. 2022;37(3):410–8. https://doi.org/10.1177/08258597221078370.

Wang J, Yan C, Fu A. A randomized clinical trial of comprehensive education and care program compared to basic care for reducing anxiety and depression and improving quality of life and survival in patients with hepatocellular carcinoma who underwent surgery. Medicine. 2019;98(44):e17552. https://doi.org/10.1097/MD.0000000000017552.

WHO Report. The selection and use of essential medicines 2023: Executive summary of the report of the 24th WHO Expert Committee on the Selection and Use of Essential Medicines; 2023.

WHPCA. Global atlas of palliative care at the end of life. 2nd ed. WHPCA; 2020.

Wickham RJ. Cancer pain management: opioid analgesics, part 2. J Adv Pract Oncol. 2017a;8(6):588–607. https://doi.org/10.6004/jadpro.2017.8.6.3.
Wickham RJ. Managing constipation in adults with cancer. J Adv Pract Oncol. 2017b;8(2):149–61. https://doi.org/10.6004/jadpro.2017.8.2.3.
Willson KJ, Nott LM, Broadbridge VT, et al. Hepatic encephalopathy associated with cancer or anticancer therapy. Gastrointest Cancer Res. 2013;6(1):11–6.
Wilson KG, Chochinov HM, Skirko MG, et al. Depression and anxiety disorders in palliative cancer care. J Pain Symptom Manag. 2007;33(2):118–29. https://doi.org/10.1016/j.jpainsymman.2006.07.016.
Woodrell CD, Hansen L, Schiano TD, et al. Palliative care for people with hepatocellular carcinoma, and specific benefits for older adults. Clin Ther. 2018;40(4):512–25. https://doi.org/10.1016/j.clinthera.2018.02.017.
Woodrell CD, Mulholland CN, Goldstein NE, et al. Clinician perspectives on palliative care for people with hepatocellular carcinoma: facilitators of and barriers to referral. Cancers. 2023;15(14)
Xie J, Diener M, Sorg R, et al. Cost-effectiveness of Denosumab compared with Zoledronic acid in patients with breast cancer and bone metastases. Clin Breast Cancer. 2012;12(4):247–58. https://doi.org/10.1016/j.clbc.2012.04.001.
Xu W, Liu K, Chen M, et al. Immunotherapy for hepatocellular carcinoma: recent advances and future perspectives. Ther Adv Med Oncol. 2019a;11:1758835919862692.
Xu XY, Ding HG, Li WG, et al. Chinese guidelines on management of hepatic encephalopathy in cirrhosis. World J Gastroenterol. 2019b;25(36):5403–22. https://doi.org/10.3748/wjg.v25.i36.5403.
Yancik R. Population aging and cancer: a cross-national concern. Cancer J Sudbury, MA. 2005;11(6):437–41. https://doi.org/10.1097/00130404-200511000-00002.
Yang Y, Si T. Yttrium-90 transarterial radioembolization versus conventional transarterial chemoembolization for patients with hepatocellular carcinoma: a systematic review and meta-analysis. Cancer Biol Med. 2018;15(3):299–310. https://doi.org/10.20892/j.issn.2095-3941.2017.0177.
Yang H, Seon J, Sung PS, et al. Dexamethasone prophylaxis to alleviate Postembolization syndrome after Transarterial chemoembolization for hepatocellular carcinoma: a randomized, double-blinded, placebo-controlled study. J Vasc Interv Radiol. 2017;28(11):1503–1511.e2. https://doi.org/10.1016/j.jvir.2017.07.021.
Yeung CSY, Chiang CL, Wong NSM, et al. Palliative liver radiotherapy (RT) for symptomatic hepatocellular carcinoma (HCC). Sci Rep. 2020;10(1):1254.
Yoo J, Lee J, Choi GH, et al. A nationwide study on the current treatment status and natural prognosis of hepatocellular carcinoma in elderly. Sci Rep. 2023;13(1):14584. https://doi.org/10.1038/s41598-023-41771-5.
Zhang H, Barysauskas C, Rickerson E, et al. The intensive palliative care unit: changing outcomes for hospitalized cancer patients in an Academic Medical Center. J Palliat Med. 2017;20(3):285.

Prevention of HCC

10

Ashraf Albreedy, Mohamed Kamal Shaker,
and Medhat Elsahhar

Abstract

Understanding the risk factors for hepatocellular carcinoma (HCC) offers a critical opportunity to develop and implement effective prevention strategies aimed at reducing the global burden of the disease. Prevention efforts can be categorized into three levels: primary prevention, which targets risk factors and their early management; secondary prevention, which focuses on treating underlying liver diseases to prevent HCC development; and tertiary prevention, which aims to reduce the risk of recurrence following curative treatment. This chapter discusses the available methods for HCC prevention—primary, secondary, and tertiary—in the context of low- and middle-income countries (LMICs).

Keywords

Aflatoxin · Hepatitis B virus · Hepatitis C virus · Hepatocellular carcinoma
Nonalcoholic fatty liver disease · Nonalcoholic steatohepatitis · Prevention

Abbreviations

AASLD	American Association for The Study of Liver Disease
AFB1	Aflatoxin B1
AFP	Alpha-fetoprotein
ALT	Alanine transaminase
APASL	The Asian Pacific Association for the Study of the Liver

A. Albreedy (✉) · M. K. Shaker · M. Elsahhar
Tropical Medicine Department, Ain Shams University, Cairo, Egypt

R. Elwakil et al. (eds.), *Approach to Hepatocellular Carcinoma (HCC) Management in Low/Middle-Income Countries*,
https://doi.org/10.1007/978-981-96-3894-9_10

cccDNA	Covalently closed circular DNA
CHB	Chronic hepatitis B
CI	Confidence interval
CRISPR	Clustered Regularly Interspaced Short Palindromic Repeats
CT	Computed tomography
DAA	Direct-acting antiviral
DCP	Desgamma-carboxy prothrombin
DNA	Deoxyribonucleic acid
EASD	European Association for the Study of Diabetes
EASL	European Association for The Study of Liver
EASO	European Association for the Study of Obesity
ELF	Enhanced liver fibrosis
ESMO	European Society of Medical Oncology
FIB-4	Fibrosis-4
GLP-1 RAs	Glucagon-like peptide-1 receptor agonists
HBV	Hepatitis B virus
HBeAg	Hepatitis B e antigen
HBsAg	Hepatitis B surface antigen
HCC	Hepatocellular carcinoma
HCV	Hepatitis C virus
HIV/AIDS	human immunodeficiency virus/acquired immunodeficiency syndrome
HR	Hazard ratio
IFN	Interferon
IFN-λ3	Interferon lambda-3
LAM	Lamivudine
LSM	Liver stiffness measurement
MRI	Magnetic resonance imaging
MRE	Magnetic resonance elastography
NA	Nucleos(t)ide analogs
NAFLD	Nonalcoholic fatty liver disease
NASH	Nonalcoholic steatohepatitis
NCCN	National comprehensive cancer network
NITs	Noninvasive tests
PUFA	Polyunsaturated fatty acids
RCTs	Randomized controlled trials
RFS	Recurrence-free survival
RNA	Ribonucleic acid
SVR	Sustained virological response
T2DM	Type 2 diabetes mellitus
TAF	Tenofovir alafenamide
TDF	Tenofovir disoproxil fumarate
TZDs	Thiazolidinediones
VCTE	Vibration-controlled elastography
WHO	World Health Organization

10.1 Introduction and Types of Prevention

When considering the urgent need to prevent tumors, two compelling factors emphasize hepatocellular carcinoma (HCC) as one of the most critical cancers globally: its high incidence and its devastating prognosis. HCC frequently grows rapidly, particularly among Black African and Chinese populations, and often remains asymptomatic in the early stages. As a result, patients typically present with an advanced tumor at the time of diagnosis. Given its high prevalence, particularly in many densely populated, low-resource countries, and its poor outcomes when symptomatic, prevention of HCC has become a critical global health priority. Encouragingly, almost all cases of HCC are theoretically preventable since the etiology is known in over 90% of patients, with the majority of these causes being potentially preventable (Kew 2010).

Although global efforts to prevent HCC are still evolving, it appears increasingly feasible that most cases of this prevalent and deadly tumor could be prevented in the near future. In regions with high HCC rates, particularly those with limited healthcare resources, pragmatic and cost-effective interventions must be prioritized. Furthermore, because the patterns of tumor causation vary geographically, tailored prevention strategies are necessary for different regions (Kew 2010).

This chapter provides an overview of current strategies in primary, secondary, and tertiary prevention of HCC.

10.2 Primary Prevention

Primary prevention, defined as halting the carcinogenic process by preventing exposure to etiological agents, remains the most effective method for cancer prevention. It is particularly effective in combating cancers caused by chemical, physical, and viral factors. Given that oncogenic hepatitis viruses are responsible for over 80% of all HCC cases worldwide, preventing chronic viral infections could substantially reduce HCC incidence globally (Kew 2010).

10.2.1 Active and Passive Immunization against HBV

From a global perspective, primary prevention is essential—and arguably the only sustainable strategy—for reducing the burden of HCC in low-resource countries where viral hepatitis is endemic and healthcare resources are limited. In endemic regions, hepatitis B virus (HBV) is mainly transmitted through contact with infected blood, often vertically from mother to infant during pregnancy or delivery, and horizontally among infants and young children (Yang and Roberts 2010).

Chronic HBV infection accounts for over 50% of HCC cases worldwide (EASL 2012). A systematic review and meta-analysis have shown that the risk of HCC varies with disease stage: incidence rates among asymptomatic carriers range from 0.07 to 0.42 per 100 person-years; among inactive carriers, 0.03 to 0.17; among patients with chronic hepatitis, 0.12 to 0.49; and among patients with decompensated cirrhosis, 2.03 to 3.37 (Raffetti et al. 2016). Other cofactors, including serum HBV DNA levels, significantly affect the risk of HCC (El-Serag 2012).

The cornerstone of HCC primary prevention is preventing HBV infection. As most chronic HBV cases are vertically transmitted, active immunization of newborns is critical. The World Health Organization (WHO) recommends that all newborns receive a "timely birth dose" of the HBV vaccine within 24 hours of delivery, followed by two or three additional doses within the first 6 months of life (WHO 2017). Taiwan, the first country to introduce routine neonatal HBV vaccination in 1984, subsequently saw a 75% reduction in HCC incidence among vaccinated cohorts (Chang et al. 1997; Chang 2011).

In some countries, passive immunization with hepatitis B immune globulin alongside the HBV vaccine is also recommended, particularly for infants born to mothers with high viral loads. Studies have shown that this combined approach is significantly more effective than either intervention alone (Lee et al. 2006a, b).

Prior to universal newborn vaccination, vertical transmission rates among HBeAg-positive mothers were 70–100% in Asia and 40% in Africa, while rates among HBeAg-negative mothers were 5–30% (Asia) and 5% (Africa). After the introduction of neonatal immunization programs, these rates fell dramatically to 20% and 0%, respectively (Lee et al. 2006a, b; Machaira et al. 2015). Nevertheless, substantial gaps remain: Africa's vaccination coverage is about 75%, mainly due to factors such as inadequate delivery services and competing healthcare priorities (Hainaut et al. 2019).

For highly viremic mothers (HBV DNA >6 $\log_{10}$ copies/mL and HBeAg positive), vaccine failure remains a risk. Major international guidelines (Brown Jr et al. 2016; Pan et al. 2016; Terrault et al. 2018; EASL 2017) recommend treating these mothers with effective antivirals (e.g., tenofovir disoproxil fumarate) during pregnancy to further reduce vertical transmission risks.

Following the global introduction of HBV vaccination in the 1980s–2000s, the prevalence of chronic HBV infection among children under five dropped from 4.7% to 1.3% by 2015. However, prevalence remains relatively high (around 3.0%) in young African children.

Multiple studies underscore the protective effect of neonatal HBV vaccination on HCC incidence. In Thailand, children over 10 years old who were vaccinated had a standardized HCC incidence of 0.07 per million compared to 0.88 per million in unvaccinated peers (Wichajarn et al. 2008). Similarly, a Taiwanese cohort study found that the relative risk of HCC among vaccinated children was 0.31 compared to nonvaccinated children, after adjusting for age and gender (Chang et al. 2009). Factors linked to vaccine failure included incomplete vaccination (OR, 29.5) and absence of hepatitis B immune globulin administration in high-risk infants (OR, 9.43).

A large cohort study from Hong Kong involving 695,925 subjects showed a reduction in chronic HBV prevalence from 14.3% in 1970 to 6.7% in 1988. Although

HCC events remained rare, vaccinated individuals consistently showed numerically lower incidences of hepatic events and HCC, even after adjusting for confounding factors (Wong et al. 2022).

10.2.2 Primary Prevention of HCV-Related HCC

Despite extensive efforts over many years, the development of a vaccine against hepatitis C virus (HCV) remains a distant goal. Several factors have complicated progress in this area, including the virus's high genetic diversity, the constant presence of numerous quasispecies in infected individuals, and the significant variability in the viral genome—especially within its hypervariable regions. Furthermore, the absence of a consistently effective neutralizing antibody response further hinders vaccine development efforts (Kew 2010).

10.2.3 Other Strategies for Primary Prevention of Hepatitis B and C Virus Infections

In the absence of an available HCV vaccine, alternative preventive measures become crucial. These interventions may, in fact, offer a greater opportunity to prevent HCV-related hepatocellular carcinoma compared to HBV-related cases. Unlike chronic HBV infections, which are usually contracted during early childhood in endemic areas, most HCV infections occur later in life, primarily in adulthood. Because of this difference, preventive strategies can target behavioral and environmental risk factors more directly and effectively (Heathcote 2004).

For the foreseeable future, prevention of this virus's infection and spread through non-vaccination methods will remain a crucial strategy. The main goals of HCV infection prevention should be to stop the virus's spread by identifying and testing those who are more susceptible to infection as well as by lowering the frequency of new infections and the likelihood that these infections will progress to chronic liver disease (Kew et al. 2004). It is recommended that the following procedures be implemented as broadly as feasible:

Safe injection practices enhancing injection and infusion safety among healthcare providers—including medical, dental, and paramedical professionals—is a key strategy to prevent hepatitis virus transmission. Educational initiatives stress the importance of using needles and syringes only once whenever possible. If reuse is unavoidable, strict sterilization protocols must be followed. Proper handling of multi-dose vials is also critical to minimize infection risks. Additionally, reducing healthcare-associated infections through the safe disposal of used needles and promoting the use of "safety-engineered" disposal-proof needles are recommended.

Preventing HBV and HCV infections among people who inject drugs remains complex and sometimes controversial. A fundamental strategy is to promote safer injection practices, including large-scale needle and syringe exchange programs that provide not only sterile needles but also clean injection paraphernalia. Such interventions aim to reduce the sharing of contaminated equipment, a major driver of infection spread (Kew et al. 2004).

Screening of Donated Blood for Hepatitis Viruses
Infection through blood transfusions has been virtually eliminated in high-income countries by screening donated blood for hepatitis B and C viruses using highly sensitive tests. Unfortunately, in many low-resource settings, particularly in sub-Saharan Africa, a significant proportion—up to 45%—of transfusions are not screened. This gap poses a major risk for the continued transmission of hepatitis viruses, highlighting the urgent need for widespread blood screening to curb HCC cases related to transfusion-transmitted infections (WHO 2000).

10.2.4 Prevention of NAFLD-Associated HCC

The link between nonalcoholic fatty liver disease (NAFLD) and hepatocellular carcinoma (HCC) is complex and not yet fully understood. Unlike other chronic liver diseases where cirrhosis often precedes HCC, NAFLD-related HCC can sometimes occur without underlying cirrhosis.

Lifestyle changes and chemoprevention strategies have the potential to reduce the risk of HCC by addressing modifiable factors such as obesity, diabetes, dyslipidemia, and hypertension—all metabolic conditions that are strongly associated with increased HCC risk (Lange et al. 2021; Kanwal et al. 2018). Positive health behaviors like healthy diet, regular physical activity, and avoiding smoking and excessive alcohol consumption have been shown to reduce cancer risk in general, including liver cancer (Lee et al. 2009).

10.2.5 Primary Prevention of Aflatoxin B1-Induced Hepatocellular Carcinoma

In wealthier countries, stringent food safety regulations prevent aflatoxin B1 (AFB1) contamination of staple foods, effectively reducing public exposure. In contrast, in many low-income regions, especially among subsistence farming communities, contaminated crops often enter local markets without regulatory oversight. This results in widespread exposure to AFB1 through diet, significantly contributing to the risk of hepatotoxicity and HCC (Hamid et al. 2013). Globally, around 45 million people are estimated to be regularly exposed to aflatoxins (Williams et al. 2004).

Prevention efforts should aim at minimizing fungal contamination throughout crop production and storage. Strategies such as selecting crops less prone to fungal infection, improving irrigation, applying fungicides, and modifying harvesting practices can lower AFB1 levels. For instance, switching to a rice-based diet was shown to substantially reduce AFB1 exposure in a study conducted in China (Wild and Gong 2010). However, large-scale dietary changes are challenging in most low-resource settings.

More feasible interventions include simple post-harvest measures like sun-drying crops on cloth instead of the ground, careful hand-sorting to remove moldy produce, and using improved storage facilities. Training farmers and providing basic resources are crucial to ensure the success of these approaches (Turner et al. 2005; Wild and Gong 2010).

10.3 Secondary Prevention

Secondary prevention of HCC involves strategies that interfere with the activity or metabolism of carcinogens before they can damage tissue DNA or initiate carcinogenesis. This may include interventions that inhibit the activation of carcinogens, prevent their binding to DNA, or enhance detoxification pathways.

10.3.1 Chemoprevention of HBV-Induced HCC

Recent advancements in HBV antiviral therapy suggest that a significant proportion of HBV-induced hepatocellular carcinoma (HCC) cases may now be preventable. The primary treatment goal for chronic HBV infection is to reduce the risk of liver-related complications, such as HCC and cirrhosis progression. Current international guidelines no longer recommend lamivudine, adefovir, or telbivudine—agents with a low genetic barrier to resistance—as first-line treatments due to high rates of drug-resistant mutations and common treatment-emergent adverse events (de Fraga et al. 2020). Instead, entecavir, tenofovir disoproxil fumarate (TDF), and tenofovir alafenamide (TAF) are now recommended first-line nucleos(t)ide analogs (NAs), given their potent antiviral effects and high genetic barrier to resistance (Lampertico et al. 2017; Sarin et al. 2016; Terrault et al. 2018).

Long-term NA treatment has been shown to reduce HCC incidence, as demonstrated in a meta-analysis (Singal et al. 2013). Key findings include: (1) in chronic hepatitis B (CHB) patients, lamivudine (LAM) treatment over a median of 43 months reduced HCC incidence by over 50%, from 9.7% annually in untreated controls to 3.3% annually in treated patients; (2) in over 10,000 patients on oral antivirals, the overall HCC incidence was 1.4%, regardless of the agent used; and (3) patients who were older, cirrhotic, or had detectable HBV-DNA at treatment end were at higher risk for HCC. These findings underscore the importance of sustained HBV suppression to improve patient outcomes.

According to the latest treatment guidelines, antiviral therapy is recommended for individuals aged 30–40 years with HBV DNA >2000 IU/mL, even without significant fibrosis or elevated ALT (Lampertico et al. 2017; Sarin et al. 2016;

Terrault et al. 2018). Nevertheless, long-term NA therapy does not entirely eliminate HCC risk. Data show a persistent annual HCC risk of 0.5–1.4% in non-cirrhotic and 0.7–5.0% in cirrhotic patients, even after prolonged viral suppression (Papatheodoridis et al. 2015). Notably, a reduction in HCC incidence typically becomes evident only after 5 years of NA therapy (Papatheodoridis et al. 2015, 2017).

Mechanistic data suggest earlier antiviral intervention may be beneficial. In young, immune-tolerant CHB patients, HBV DNA integration—an oncogenic driver of HCC—is frequently observed (Tu et al. 2017), alongside HBV-specific T cell responses and hepatic necroinflammation (Kennedy et al. 2012). These findings imply that hepatocarcinogenesis may begin during the immune-tolerant phase, supporting a "test-and-treat" strategy for early intervention.

Treating young CHB patients could offer additional benefits, including reducing HBV transmission and simplifying management. This would shift the clinical approach from complex diagnostic evaluations to a straightforward "test-and-treat" model. Given the reduced cost of generic NAs, early antiviral therapy is also cost-effective (Kim et al. 2020). However, challenges persist: ~90% of chronic HBV patients are unaware of their infection, and linkage to care remains suboptimal (Razavi-Shearer et al. 2018). Additionally, the necessity for lifelong therapy poses compliance challenges.

While entecavir and TDF are both recommended first-line treatments for treatment-naïve CHB patients, emerging evidence has questioned their comparative efficacy in HCC chemoprevention. A Korean nationwide cohort study (n = 24,156) and validation cohort (n = 2701) found that TDF was associated with a lower risk of HCC than entecavir (HR 0.68) (Choi et al. 2019). However, another multicenter study in South Korea (n = 2897) found no significant difference (HR 1.02) (Kim et al. 2019). Subsequent studies and meta-analyzes have shown mixed results—some favoring TDF, others finding no significant difference.

Biologically, TDF may offer advantages: stronger virological suppression, greater HBsAg reduction (Choi et al. 2019), higher ALT normalization rates, and possibly enhanced antitumor immunity via increased interferon lambda-3 (IFN-λ3) induction (Murata et al. 2018; Abushahba et al. 2010). However, these biological hypotheses require validation in human cohorts before practice-changing recommendations can be made. Large, randomized controlled trials with long follow-up would provide the highest quality evidence, but such trials are unlikely (Yip et al. 2020).

Additionally, TAF—a modified version of TDF with superior safety and ALT normalization profiles—may further refine strategies for HCC chemoprevention (Byun et al. 2022).

Despite these advances, NAs do not completely eliminate HCC risk, even with prolonged viral suppression, due to possible pre-existing genetic or epigenetic alterations (Takeda et al. 2017). Thus, novel antiviral therapies targeting cccDNA and HBV entry, alongside strategies to restore anti-HBV immunity, are under development (Lee et al. 2020a, b, c; Fanning et al. 2019).

10.3.2 Chemoprevention of HCV-Induced HCC

Like HBV, active HCV infection drives hepatocarcinogenesis, making viral eradication the cornerstone of HCC secondary prevention. During the interferon (IFN) era, achieving a sustained virological response (SVR) significantly reduced the annual HCC risk from 2–8% to 0.5–1% in cirrhotic patients (Brown 2000). However, IFN-based therapies had limitations: only about 50% achieved SVR, and toxicity limited their use in cirrhotic patients.

The introduction of IFN-free direct-acting antivirals (DAAs) revolutionized HCV treatment. These therapies achieve SVR rates exceeding 95%, improve liver function and fibrosis, and reduce portal hypertension (Baumert et al. 2019). They are also safe for use in decompensated cirrhosis. Achieving SVR at any fibrosis stage confers benefits, though in decompensated cirrhosis, HCC risk persists post-SVR (Terrault and Hassanein 2016). The concept of a "point of no return," where irreversible liver damage leads to ongoing HCC risk, underscores the importance of continued surveillance (Bruno et al. 2016).

HCC Occurrence after DAA Therapy

Initial studies raised concerns about high HCC incidence post-DAA SVR (Reig et al. 2016; Conti et al. 2016; Cardoso et al. 2016; Ravi et al. 2017). These studies reported HCC rates ranging from 3.6% to 9% within 6–12 months post-SVR, prompting speculation that DAAs might promote hepatocarcinogenesis.

However, larger retrospective studies, such as that by Singer et al. (2018), refuted these concerns. They found a lower HCC risk in DAA-treated patients compared to untreated controls and IFN-treated patients after adjusting for age and cirrhosis status. Similarly, Nahon et al. (2018) reported a higher unadjusted HCC incidence in DAA-treated patients compared to IFN-SVR patients, but this was likely due to differences in baseline characteristics (i.e., older, more cirrhotic DAA cohort).

Subsequent prospective studies further reinforced that DAAs reduce HCC risk. A French study of 7344 DAA-treated patients showed a significant HCC risk reduction (adjusted HR 0.66) (Carrat et al. 2019). In Latin America, a cohort of 1400 patients showed a 73% relative risk reduction for de novo HCC post-SVR (Piñero et al. 2019).

Thus, the current evidence supports that achieving SVR with DAAs substantially reduces HCC risk in chronic HCV patients. Early concerns may have reflected undiagnosed subclinical HCCs at baseline or altered immune surveillance dynamics following rapid viral clearance (Colombo and Boccaccio 2018).

10.3.3 Chemoprevention of AFB1-Induced HCC and Dietary Change

The goal of cancer chemoprevention is to develop agents that inhibit or reverse carcinogenic processes. In the case of aflatoxin B1 (AFB1)-induced malignant transformation, the aim is to lessen the impact of unavoidable dietary exposure to the toxin by adjusting the balance between metabolic activation and detoxification of reactive AFB1 metabolites, specifically AFB1–8,9-exo-epoxide and AFB1-FABY. Numerous chemopreventive drugs have shown effectiveness against AFB1-induced malignancy in experimental animals; however, few are suitable for human use (Kew 2010).

Chlorophyllin is one promising agent. Sodium copper chlorophyllin, a water-soluble derivative of natural chlorophylls, exhibits strong anti-carcinogenic properties in experimental models of AFB1-induced hepatocellular carcinoma (HCC) (Simonich et al. 2007). Chlorophyllin can bind tightly to aflatoxins, acting as an "interceptor molecule" that reduces their bioavailability. In vitro, it is also a potent inhibitor of cytochrome P450 enzymes involved in the bioactivation of various carcinogens and functions as an antioxidant (Simonich et al. 2007). Chlorophyllin is most effective when administered in molar excess at or near the time of carcinogen exposure (Morel et al. 1993).

A randomized, double-blind, placebo-controlled trial in Qidong County, China, demonstrated that chlorophyllin, given three times daily for 4 months, resulted in a 55% reduction in the median urinary excretion of the AFB1-N-gua biomarker, compared to placebo. No adverse side effects were reported, and adherence was high (Egner et al. 2001). Further trials are needed to assess the long-term safety and feasibility of chlorophyllin use. Alternatively, increasing dietary intake of chlorophyll-rich foods, such as spinach and other leafy greens, may offer a practical preventive strategy.

Another chemopreventive approach involves enhancing AFB1 detoxification. **Oltipraz**, an anti-schistosomal drug structurally similar to dithiolethiones from cruciferous vegetables, has shown promise (Itoh et al. 1999). Oltipraz induces glutathione-S-transferase (GST), a phase II detoxifying enzyme, and upregulates genes encoding other conjugating and antioxidative enzymes. It disrupts the KEAP1-NRF2 interaction, facilitating NRF2 translocation to the nucleus, where it promotes expression of detoxifying enzymes. Recent studies also suggest oltipraz inhibits phase I enzymes such as CYP1A2 and CYP3A4, thereby reducing AFB1 activation (Sofowora et al. 2001).

In a randomized, placebo-controlled trial among adults in Qidong County with detectable serum aflatoxin-albumin adducts, oltipraz administration resulted in a 2.6-fold increase in urinary excretion of AFB1-mercapturic acid, an AFB1–8,9-exo-epoxide metabolite (Jacobson et al. 1997). Another study showed that weekly oltipraz treatment for one month decreased urinary aflatoxin M1 levels and promoted AFB1 conjugation (Wang et al. 1999). However, cost and safety concerns may limit the widespread use of oltipraz for secondary prevention of HCC.

Natural products are also under investigation for their potential to counteract aflatoxicosis and AFB1-associated HCC. For instance, a mouse study demonstrated that cactus cladode extract (CCE) from *Opuntia ficus indica* exerted a protective effect against AFB1-induced liver damage (Brahmi et al. 2011).

There is ample evidence that dietary antioxidants confer protection against HCC in animal models. The anticancer properties of fruits and vegetables have been well documented. Apiaceous vegetables (e.g., carrots, parsnips, celery, and parsley) were found to inhibit human cytochrome P450 1A2 (hCYP1A2), an enzyme involved in the activation of procarcinogens including AFB1 (Peterson et al. 2006). Regular consumption of these vegetables may therefore reduce AFB1-induced hepatocarcinogenesis.

Similarly, grapefruits have been shown to reduce liver DNA damage by decreasing hepatic CYP3A activity in F344 rats exposed to AFB1 (Miyata et al. 2004). Coffee has also been reported to induce detoxifying enzymes such as glutathione synthetase transferases and aldo-keto reductase (AKR), providing potential protection against AFB1 cytotoxicity and genotoxicity (Cavin et al. 2008).

Furthermore, recent studies have demonstrated that natural compounds such as **sulforaphane (SFN)** and **phenethyl isothiocyanate (PEITC)** can exert chemoprotective effects against AFB1-DNA adduct formation in human primary hepatocytes (Gross-Steinmeyer et al. 2010).

10.3.4 Iron Storage Diseases

Phlebotomy remains the gold standard for treating hereditary hemochromatosis (HH), as it mobilizes iron for erythropoiesis and thereby reduces iron overload (Adams and Barton 2010). When initiated before the development of cirrhosis or diabetes, phlebotomy significantly reduces morbidity and mortality (Prabhu et al. 2020).

Repeated venesection in HH patients not only reverses iron accumulation but may also exert a secondary preventive effect against HCC by preventing fibrosis and cirrhosis, regardless of whether excess hepatic iron directly promotes hepatocarcinogenesis. The primary goal of therapy is to lower and maintain serum ferritin within the normal range.

Iron Storage Diseases

Phlebotomy remains the gold standard for treating hemochromatosis by mobilizing iron for erythropoiesis, thus reducing iron accumulation in the body (Adams and Barton 2010). Initiating treatment before the onset of cirrhosis and/or diabetes significantly reduces morbidity and mortality (Prabhu et al. 2020). Repeated venesection (phlebotomy) in patients with hereditary hemochromatosis (HH) is expected to have a secondary preventive effect against hepatocellular carcinoma (HCC) formation by reversing iron accumulation and preventing the development of fibrosis and cirrhosis, irrespective of whether excess hepatic iron is directly hepatocarcinogenic. The therapeutic goal is to reduce and maintain serum ferritin at a normal level.

Available evidence suggests that phlebotomy may also help alleviate symptoms like arthralgias and fatigue and improve liver function tests. In some cases, it may even promote regression of liver fibrosis and cirrhosis. Clinical and cohort studies have demonstrated that therapeutic phlebotomy improves survival (Milman et al. 2001). However, there remains a lack of conclusive data regarding its impact on quality of life, and its effectiveness in reducing the risk of liver cancer, diabetes, or cardiovascular disease (Prabhu et al. 2020). Furthermore, no large-scale initiatives have been undertaken to address secondary prevention of hepatic iron overload resulting from dietary causes.

10.3.5 Prevention of NAFLD/NASH-Associated HCC

Carcinogenic processes leading to HCC development in nonalcoholic fatty liver disease (NAFLD) and nonalcoholic steatohepatitis (NASH) are complex and not fully understood. Unlike most chronic liver diseases, where HCC typically develops after cirrhosis, NAFLD-associated HCC can occur even without cirrhosis (Stine et al. 2018). Several modifiable risk factors in the NAFLD population can be targeted through chemoprevention or lifestyle interventions, potentially offering broader health benefits.

Weight Loss

Although direct evidence that weight loss reduces HCC risk in NAFLD is lacking, clinical studies have shown that weight reduction improves NAFLD activity and may lead to fibrosis regression (Vilar-Gomez et al. 2015). A large meta-analysis examining weight loss following bariatric surgery in NAFLD patients found that 40%, 50%, and 66% of patients experienced resolution of fibrosis, inflammation, and steatosis, respectively (Lee et al. 2019). However, it remains uncertain if these histological improvements correlate with reduction of HCC risk.

Diet

Various diets, nutrients, and food groups have been studied in the context of NAFLD and HCC (George et al. 2021). Higher adherence to the Mediterranean diet has consistently been associated with a lower risk of HCC in several studies (Turati et al. 2014; Li et al. 2014; Bogumil et al. 2019). However, a large American prospective cohort study did not find a statistically significant association (HR 0.75; 95% CI 0.49–1.15). European guidelines recommend the Mediterranean diet for patients with NAFLD (EASL-EASD-EASO 2016).

Physical Activity

Independent of weight loss, physical activity appears to reduce HCC risk. Proposed mechanisms include improved mitochondrial function (e.g., autophagy and biogenesis), reduction in NAFLD/NASH activity, and modulation of carcinogenic signaling pathways (Guarino et al. 2020; Saran et al. 2018). The European Prospective Investigation into Cancer and Nutrition (EPIC) study found that individuals who engaged in at least 2 hours of vigorous physical activity per week had a lower risk of HCC, regardless of body weight and other common risk factors (Baumeister et al. 2019a, b). A meta-analysis confirmed these findings, showing a significantly lower HCC risk in physically active individuals (HR 0.75; 95% CI 0.63–0.89) (Baumeister et al. 2019a, b).

Alcohol and Smoking

Alcohol consumption shares pathophysiological pathways with NAFLD/NASH and can synergistically increase HCC risk, particularly when combined with obesity and diabetes (Ganne-Carrié and Nahon 2019). Studies have demonstrated a supra-additive interaction between alcohol use and obesity for HCC development (Loomba et al. 2010; Loomba et al. 2013). Case-control studies have shown high odds ratios for HCC among individuals with both diabetes and heavy alcohol use (Hassan et al. 2002; Yuan et al. 2004).

Smoking is generally associated with increased HCC risk, although specific data for NAFLD populations are limited. A meta-analysis of 81 studies found that current smokers (OR 1.55; 95% CI 1.46–1.65) and former smokers (OR 1.39; 95% CI 1.26–1.52) had higher HCC risks compared to never smokers (Abdel-Rahman et al. 2017). Importantly, individuals who quit smoking over 30 years ago had HCC risks comparable to never smokers (HR 1.09; 95% CI 0.74–1.61) (Petrick et al. 2018). Thus, cessation of alcohol use and smoking should be prioritized for NAFLD-HCC prevention.

Pharmacological Interventions

Several medications have been proposed to improve NAFLD/NASH and potentially lower HCC risk, though direct evidence for chemoprevention is limited. It is believed that addressing key drivers of fibrogenesis and histological features of NASH may ultimately prevent cirrhosis and HCC (Brunt et al. 2019).

Metformin has been associated with reduced HCC risk in patients with type 2 diabetes mellitus (T2DM), although it does not appear to significantly improve NASH or fibrosis (Cunha et al. 2020). A network meta-analysis reported that metformin use reduced HCC risk compared to sulfonylureas and insulin (RR 0.45 and 0.28, respectively) (Zhou et al. 2016). Moreover, metformin may hinder HCC progression in high-fat diet models by modulating innate immune responses and restoring tumor surveillance (de Oliveira et al. 2019). Nonetheless, these findings require further validation and should be interpreted cautiously.

10.3.6 Coffee for HCC Prevention

Numerous studies have consistently demonstrated that coffee consumption is associated with a reduced incidence of hepatocellular carcinoma (HCC). A significant Japanese population-based cohort study found that daily coffee drinkers had a lower risk of HCC compared to those who almost never drank coffee (hazard ratio [HR] 0.49; 95% confidence interval [CI] 0.36–0.66); this inverse association was also observed in patients with chronic hepatitis C (Inoue et al. 2005). Similarly, a hospital-based case-control study conducted in Italy reported a lower risk of HCC irrespective of its etiology (Gelatti et al. 2005), findings later confirmed by meta-analyzes of case-control and cohort studies from Southern Europe and Japan (Bravi et al. 2007; Bravi et al. 2013).

Another meta-analysis showed that increasing daily coffee consumption by two cups was associated with a 43% reduction in liver cancer risk (relative risk [RR] 0.57; 95% CI 0.49–0.67) (Larsson and Wolk 2007). Furthermore, a nested case-control study reported an inverse association between coffee consumption and HCC (risk ratio for four or more cups vs. less than two cups: 0.25; 95% CI 0.11–0.62) (Aleksandrova et al. 2015).

Beyond HCC, high coffee consumption has also been linked to lower rates of chronic liver disease mortality and a lower incidence of HCC in the U.S. Multiethnic Cohort (over 215,000 individuals) (Setiawan et al. 2015). Importantly, no studies have demonstrated harmful effects of coffee consumption on the liver. Based on the accumulating evidence, the European Association for the Study of the Liver (EASL) has recommended coffee consumption for patients with chronic liver diseases to reduce the risk of liver-related death and HCC development. However, a precise dosage recommendation cannot yet be made (EASL 2018).

10.3.7 Statins and Aspirin for HCC Prevention

Statins

Several large observational studies have investigated the association between statin use and the risk of HCC. A matched case-control study using Taiwan's National Health Insurance Research Database found a significant inverse association between statin use and HCC risk (odds ratio [OR] 0.62; 95% CI 0.42–0.91) (Chiu et al. 2011). Subsequent studies, regardless of geographic location, also reported the chemopreventive effects of statins on HCC risk (McGlynn et al. 2015; Tran et al. 2020). A meta-analysis of 11 studies found that statin users had a 46% lower risk of HCC, although there was significant heterogeneity among studies ($I^2 = 96.8\%$) (Chang et al. 2020).

Research in high-risk populations, particularly patients with HBV or HCV infections, mostly based on retrospective cohort studies also showed that statins may reduce the risk of HCC (Tsan et al. 2012; Tsan et al. 2013). The protective effect appeared consistent or even more pronounced in HBV patients receiving nucleos(t)ide analogs (Goh et al. 2020). In HCV-infected patients, adding statins to direct-acting antiviral (DAA) therapy was associated with higher sustained virologic response rates (OR 1.44; 95% CI 1.29–1.61), reduced progression to cirrhosis (HR 0.56; 95% CI 0.50–0.63), and lower risk of HCC development (HR 0.51; 95% CI 0.34–0.76) (Butt et al. 2015).

While many of these patients may also have had NAFLD-related HCC, studies specifically examining the impact of statins on NAFLD-related HCC are limited. However, available evidence suggests a significant protective effect of statin use against HCC in NAFLD patients (Zou et al. 2023; Pinyopornpanish et al. 2021). Nonetheless, more prospective randomized controlled trial (RCT) data, including from two ongoing clinical trials (NCT02968810 and NCT03024684), are needed to establish the risk-benefit profile of statins for HCC prevention (Goh and Sinn 2022).

Aspirin

Most studies evaluating the effect of aspirin on HCC risk have focused on patients with cirrhosis or viral hepatitis, who have a higher baseline risk. As with statins, these studies were largely retrospective.

In a Korean hospital-based cohort, antiplatelet therapy was associated with a 56% reduced risk of HCC in 1624 HBV patients on nucleos(t)ide analogue treatment. Specifically, aspirin use was significantly protective (HR 0.26; 95% CI 0.09–0.74), whereas clopidogrel or dual therapy showed no significant associations (Lee et al. 2017). A more recent cohort study in Hong Kong with 35,111 HBV patients reported a dose-response relationship, with longer aspirin use associated with greater HCC risk reduction (HR 0.65, 0.63, and 0.41 for 0.25–2, 2–5, and ≥5 years, respectively) (Hui et al. 2021).

Among HCV patients, a Taiwanese cohort study found that aspirin use reduced HCC risk by approximately 50% (Liao et al. 2020). Similar results were reported in a second Taiwanese study, although significance was not achieved in the cirrhotic subgroup (Lee et al. 2020a, b, c). A pooled analysis of seven matched cohort and case-control studies (n = 1799) showed a 49% reduction in HCC risk with aspirin use (HR 0.51; 95% CI 0.36–0.72) (Tan et al. 2021). A more recent meta-analysis further confirmed that aspirin use was associated with a lower risk of HCC in patients with HBV or HCV infections (Li et al. 2021), though it also highlighted a potential increase in gastrointestinal bleeding risk. These findings warrant confirmation through future clinical trials.

10.3.8 Surveillance of High-Risk Populations

HCC surveillance represents a key secondary prevention strategy, aiming to detect tumors early when curative treatment is still possible.

Although there are no high-quality RCTs, a meta-analysis of 47 studies (n = 15,158) found that HCC surveillance is associated with improved overall survival due to earlier tumor detection (Singal et al. 2014). However, the U.S. National Cancer Institute remains cautious, stating that there is only "fair evidence" that screening reduces HCC mortality (National Cancer Institute 2019). This cautious stance stems from the lack of high-quality evidence, despite observational studies consistently suggesting a survival benefit with surveillance (Singal et al. 2014).

Ethical and practical challenges likely prevent a randomized trial on HCC surveillance, as patients informed of the risks generally opt for regular monitoring (Poustchi et al. 2011).

Current guidelines recommend HCC surveillance for:

- Patients with Child A or B cirrhosis of any cause.
- Patients with Child C cirrhosis listed for liver transplantation.

- Patients with non-cirrhotic chronic HBV infection who have high-risk characteristics (e.g., Asian men >40 years, Asian women >50 years, those with a family history of HCC, and individuals of African or North American Black descent) (EASL 2018; Singal et al. 2023; Omata et al. 2017).

EASL guidelines also recommend using the PAGE-B score, based on platelet count, age, and gender, to stratify risk in chronic HBV patients treated with entecavir or tenofovir (EASL 2018).

The standard surveillance protocol endorsed by liver societies includes **liver ultrasonography with or without alpha-fetoprotein (AFP) testing every 6 months** (EASL 2018; Singal et al. 2023; Omata et al. 2017).

In Japan, biomarkers such as DCP and AFP-L3 have been routinely utilized alongside AFP for hepatocellular carcinoma (HCC) surveillance (Marrero et al. 2009; Lok et al. 2010). The GALAD score, which incorporates gender, age, AFP, AFP-L3, and DCP, has been introduced as an effective tool for early HCC detection. A multicenter phase II study in 2018 demonstrated that the GALAD model outperformed ultrasound in detecting HCC (Yang et al. 2019). A recent systematic review and meta-analysis further validated the diagnostic strength of GALAD across all stages of HCC, particularly in early-stage disease. Incorporating GALAD into ultrasound-based surveillance strategies may enhance detection rates (Guan et al. 2023). Given its simple calculation using basic demographic and serum biomarker data, the GALAD score has strong potential as a screening tool, especially in settings where imaging access is limited. Prospective studies are needed to compare its performance directly against imaging modalities and to assess its cost-effectiveness.

HCC Surveillance in NAFLD/NASH Populations

Inadequate surveillance among patients with NAFLD remains a pressing issue, particularly given the difficulty in identifying high-risk individuals prior to cirrhosis. An analysis of the U.S. Veterans Administration HCC cohort revealed that surveillance uptake three years prior to diagnosis was lower in NAFLD-related HCC compared to HCV- and alcohol-related HCC (Mittal et al. 2015).

Importantly, HCC can occur in non-cirrhotic NAFLD patients. Mittal et al. (2016) reported that approximately 13% of HCC cases arose in the absence of cirrhosis, with NAFLD patients facing a significantly higher risk than those with HCV. Another meta-analysis (Tan et al. 2022) confirmed that NAFLD-related HCC patients more often presented without cirrhosis and were less likely to have been under surveillance, often presenting with larger tumors. This rising burden of NAFLD highlights the need for refined risk stratification to guide surveillance strategies (Norero and Dufour 2023).

In primary care settings, most NAFLD patients fall into a low-risk category, characterized by a FIB-4 score below 1.3 or a liver stiffness measurement (LSM) under 8.0 kPa (Kanwal et al. 2018; Lomonaco et al. 2021; Barb et al. 2021). Systematic HCC screening for non-cirrhotic NAFLD is currently not recommended by major liver societies (EASL-EASD-EASO 2016; Rinella et al. 2023; Eslam et al.

2020). For low-risk patients, reassessment every 2–3 years is suggested, whereas patients with diabetes or multiple metabolic risk factors may warrant FIB-4 evaluation more frequently, around every 1–2 years (Rinella et al. 2023).

Approximately 30%–40% of screened patients are classified as indeterminate risk, based on a FIB-4 between 1.3 and 2.67 or an LSM between 8.0 and 12.0 kPa (Kanwal et al. 2018; Barb et al. 2021). Patients with multiple metabolic risk factors, even without cirrhosis, seem to have a higher risk of HCC (Stine et al. 2018; Kanwal et al. 2018). Additional inflammatory or fibrotic stimuli may be needed to drive carcinogenesis in this group (Plaz Torres et al. 2020).

For patients with FIB-4 ≥1.3, further risk stratification using vibration-controlled transient elastography (VCTE) or enhanced liver fibrosis (ELF) testing is recommended. Direct referral to hepatology should be considered if FIB-4 >2.67 or persistent aminotransferase elevations are observed. In cases where noninvasive testing yields inconclusive results or advanced disease is suspected, magnetic resonance elastography (MRE) is advisable (Rinella et al. 2023).

High-risk patients, defined by a FIB-4 >2.67, LSM >12.0 kPa, or biopsy-proven fibrosis stage ≥F2, comprise around 10% of screened populations (Kanwal et al. 2018). For those diagnosed with cirrhosis, HCC surveillance and esophageal varices screening should be initiated. Patients with "at-risk" NASH (activity score ≥ 4, fibrosis stage ≥2) may be candidates for emerging therapies. While liver biopsy remains the gold standard, it can be avoided if noninvasive tools strongly indicate cirrhosis.

Patients with advanced fibrosis (≥F2) should be prioritized for pharmacologic interventions as they become available, while all patients should receive counseling on lifestyle modifications. Noninvasive test (NIT) cut-offs are approximations meant to guide clinical management rather than serve as absolute diagnostic thresholds (Rinella et al. 2023).

Routine 6-month surveillance with ultrasound ± AFP is recommended for NASH-cirrhosis patients by all major societies (EASL-EASD-EASO 2016; Rinella et al. 2023; Eslam et al. 2020).

Tertiary Prevention Strategies

Tertiary prevention in HCC aims to lower recurrence rates, reduce mortality, and improve survival following curative treatments (Nan et al. 2023). Strategies include vigilant monitoring of etiological factors and recurrence risk stratification to facilitate early intervention and prolong survival.

Surveillance Post-Curative Treatment

Dynamic imaging (contrast-enhanced CT, MRI, or contrast-enhanced ultrasound) should be performed 1–2 months post-treatment to assess response. Ongoing surveillance with AFP and imaging every 3–6 months during the first 2 years, and every 6–12 months thereafter, is recommended (Benson III et al. 2017; Vogel et al. 2018; Singal et al. 2023).

Adjuvant and Neoadjuvant Therapy

Currently, neoadjuvant therapies are not recommended outside clinical trials for patients undergoing resection, ablation, or transplantation (EASL 2018; Singal et al. 2023). However, the IMbrave050 trial demonstrated that atezolizumab plus bevacizumab as adjuvant therapy improved recurrence-free survival in high-risk patients after resection or ablation (Hack et al. 2020; Roche 2023; Qin et al. 2023). This combination is now considered for high-risk patients.

Surveillance Following Liver Transplantation

Post-transplant recurrence most commonly involves the lung and liver. Thus, abdominal and chest imaging (CT or MRI) is preferred over ultrasound. Additional imaging modalities may be considered in cases of elevated AFP without detectable recurrence (Lee et al. 2020a, b, c). Risk stratification models may help refine surveillance intervals.

Calcineurin inhibitors are associated with increased HCC recurrence risk, while mTOR inhibitors may confer anti-tumor benefits (Rodriguez-Peralvarez et al. 2013). The SiLVER trial did not show a benefit of sirolimus across all patients but did report improved outcomes in select subgroups (Geissler et al. 2016; Schnitzbauer et al. 2020).

Antiviral Therapy

In HBV-related HCC, nucleos(t)ide analogs (NAs) and/or interferon therapy post-curative treatment have been shown to prolong recurrence-free survival (Qi et al. 2020; Huang et al. 2018). Patients with positive HBsAg and/or HBV DNA should receive first-line NAs, while PEG-IFNα may be considered in eligible patients (Kao et al. 2020).

Earlier concerns that DAA therapy might increase HCC recurrence in HCV-infected patients have been refuted by subsequent studies. DAAs were shown to lower both de novo and recurrent HCC incidence and to improve survival after curative HCC therapy (Lin et al. 2020; Singal et al. 2019; Lui et al. 2020; Frazzoni et al. 2021). Thus, DAA therapy is recommended after curative HCC treatment in patients with positive HCV RNA (Nan et al. 2023).

10.4 Conclusion

The landscape of hepatocellular carcinoma (HCC) epidemiology has shifted significantly over the past decade, driven largely by advancements in the prevention and treatment of viral hepatitis. This trend is expected to continue as viral-related liver diseases become better controlled. Conversely, the incidence of HCC associated with alcohol-related liver disease (ALD) and nonalcoholic fatty liver disease (NAFLD) continues to rise steadily. Moving forward, a major challenge will be the development of effective surveillance and intervention strategies aimed at preventing HCC, particularly among individuals who remain at risk even without progression to cirrhosis. Increasing awareness and early identification of these high-risk populations will be crucial in mitigating the future burden of HCC.

References

Abdel-Rahman O, Helbling D, Schöb O, Eltobgy M, Mohamed H, Schmidt J, et al. Cigarette smoking as a risk factor for the development of and mortality from hepatocellular carcinoma: an updated systematic review of 81 epidemiological studies. J Evid Based Med. 2017;10(4):245–54.

Abushahba W, Balan M, Castaneda I, et al. Antitumor activity of type I and type III interferons in BNL hepatoma model. Cancer Immunol Immunother. 2010;59:1059–71.

Adams PC, Barton JC. How I treat hemochromatosis. Blood. 2010;116:317–25.

Aleksandrova K, Bamia C, Drogan D, Lagiou P, Trichopoulou A, Jenab M, et al. The association of coffee intake with liver cancer risk is mediated by biomarkers of inflammation and hepatocellular injury: data from the European prospective investigation into cancer and nutrition. Am J Clin Nutr. 2015;102:1498–508.

Barb D, Repetto EM, Stokes ME, Shankar SS, Cusi K. Type 2 diabetes mellitus increases the risk of hepatic fibrosis in individuals with obesity and nonalcoholic fatty liver disease. Obesity (Silver Spring). 2021;29:1950–60.

Baumeister SE, Schlesinger S, Aleksandrova K, Jochem C, Jenab M, Gunter MJ, et al. Association between physical activity and risk of hepatobiliary cancers: a multinational cohort study. J Hepatol. 2019a;70(5):885–92.

Baumeister SE, Leitzmann MF, Linseisen J, Schlesinger S. Physical activity and the risk of liver cancer: a systematic review and meta-analysis of prospective studies and a bias analysis. J Natl Canc Inst. 2019b;111(11):1142–51.

Baumert TF, Berg T, Lim JK, Nelson DR. Status of direct-acting antiviral therapy for hepatitis C virus infection and remaining challenges. Gastroenterology. 2019;156:431–45.

Benson AB III, D'Angelica MI, Abbott DE, et al. NCCN guidelines insights: hepatobiliary cancers, Version 1.2017. J Natl Compr Cancer Netw. 2017;15(5):563–73.

Bogumil D, Park S-Y, Le Marchand L, Haiman CA, Wilkens LR, Boushey CJ, et al. High-quality diets are associated with reduced risk of hepatocellular carcinoma and chronic liver disease: the multiethnic cohort. Hepatol Commun. 2019;3(3):437–47.

Brahmi D, Bouaziz C, Ayed Y, Ben Mansour H, Zourgui L, Bacha H. Chemopreventive effect of cactus Opuntia ficus indica on oxidative stress and genotoxicity of aflatoxin B1. Nutr Metab (Lond). 2011;8:73.

Bravi F, Bosetti C, Tavani A, Bagnardi V, Gallus S, Negri E, et al. Coffee drinking and hepatocellular carcinoma risk: a meta-analysis. Hepatology. 2007;46:430–5.

Bravi F, Bosetti C, Tavani A, Gallus S, La Vecchia C. Coffee reduces risk for hepatocellular carcinoma: an updated meta-analysis. Clin Gastroenterol Hepatol. 2013;11:1413–21.

Brown JL. Interferon therapy reduces the risk for hepatocellular carcinoma. Gut. 2000;47:610–1.

Brown RS Jr, McMahon BJ, Lok AS, et al. Anti viral therapy in chronic hepatitis B viral infection during pregnancy: a systematic review and meta-analysis. Hepatology. 2016;63:319–33.

Bruno S, Boccaccio V, Russo ML, Maisonneuve P. Is the benefit of treating patients with cirrhosis proven? Liver Int. 2016;36:21–7.

Brunt EM, Kleiner DE, Wilson LA, Sanyal AJ. Neuschwander-Tetri BA; nonalcoholic steatohepatitis clinical research network. Improvements in histologic features and diagnosis associated with improvement in fibrosis in nonalcoholic steatohepatitis: results from the nonalcoholic steatohepatitis clinical research network treatment trials. Hepatology. 2019;70(2):522–31.

Butt AA, Yan P, Bonilla H, Abou-Samra AB, Shaikh OS, Simon TG, et al. Effect of addition of statins to antiviral therapy in hepatitis C virus-infected persons: results from ERCHIVES. Hepatology. 2015;62:365–74.

Byun KS, Choi J, Kim JH, Lee YS, Lee HC, Kim YJ, Yoo BC, Kwon SY, Gwak GY, Lim YS. Tenofovir Alafenamide for drug-resistant hepatitis B: a randomized trial for switching from Tenofovir Disoproxil fumarate. Clin Gastroenterol Hepatol. 2022;20(2):427–37.

Cardoso H, Vale AM, Rodrigues S, Gonçalves R, Albuquerque A, Pereira P, Lopes S, Silva M, Andrade P, Morais R, et al. High incidence of hepatocellular carcinoma following successful interferon-free antiviral therapy for hepatitis C associated cirrhosis. J Hepatol. 2016;65:1070–1.

Carrat F, Fontaine H, Dorival C, Simony M, Diallo A, Hezode C, De Ledinghen V, Larrey D, Haour G, Bronowicki J-P, et al. Clinical outcomes in patients with chronic hepatitis C after direct-acting antiviral treatment: a prospective cohort study. Lancet. 2019;393:1453–64.

Cavin C, Marin-Kuan M, Langouët S, et al. Induction of Nrf2-mediated cellular defenses and alteration of phase I activities as mechanisms of chemoprotective effects of coffee in the liver. Food Chem Toxicol. 2008;46:1239–48.

Chang MH. Hepatitis B virus and cancer prevention. Recent Results Cancer Res. 2011;188:75–84.

Chang MH, Chen CJ, Lai MS, Hsu HM, Wu TC, Kong MS, Liang DC, Shau WY, Chen DS. Universal hepatitis B vaccination in Taiwan and the incidence of hepatocellular carcinoma in children. Taiwan Childhood Hepatoma Study Group. N Eng J Med. 1997;336:1855–9.

Chang MH, You SL, Chen CJ, et al. Taiwan Hepatoma Study Group. Decreased incidence of hepatocellular carcinoma in hepatitis B vaccinees: a 20-year follow-up study. J Natl Cancer Inst. 2009;101:1348–55.

Chang Y, Liu Q, Zhou Z, Ding Y, Yang M, Xu W, et al. Can statin treatment reduce the risk of hepatocellular carcinoma? A systematic review and meta-analysis. Technol Cancer Res Treat. 2020;19:1533033820934881.

Chiu HF, Ho SC, Chen CC, Yang CY. Statin use and the risk of liver cancer: a population-based case–control study. Am J Gastroenterol. 2011;106:894–8.

Choi J, Kim HJ, Lee J, et al. Risk of hepatocellular carcinoma in patients treated with entecavir vs tenofovir for chronic hepatitis B: a Korean nationwide cohort study. JAMA Oncol. 2019;5:30–6.

Colombo M, Boccaccio V. HCV therapy and risk of liver cancer recurrence: who to treat? Nat Rev Gastroenterol Hepatol. 2018;15:392–3.

Conti F, Buonfiglioli F, Scuteri A, Crespi C, Bolondi L, Caraceni P, Foschi FG, Lenzi M, Mazzella G, Verucchi G, et al. Early occurrence and recurrence of hepatocellular carcinoma in HCV-related cirrhosis treated with direct-acting antivirals. J Hepatol. 2016;65:727–33.

Cunha V, Cotrim HP, Rocha R, Carvalho K, Lins-Kusterer L. Metformin in the prevention of hepatocellular carcinoma in diabetic patients: a systematic review. Ann Hepatol. 2020;19(3):232–7.

de Fraga RS, Van Vaisberg V, Mendes LCA, et al. Adverse events of nucleos(t)ide analogues for chronic hepatitis B: a systematic review. J Gastroenterol. 2020;55:496–514.

de Oliveira S, Houseright RA, Graves AL, Golenberg N, Korte BG, Miskolci V, Huttenlocher A. Metformin modulates innate immune-mediated inflammation and early progression of NAFLD-associated hepatocellular carcinoma in zebrafish. J Hepatol. 2019;70:710–21.

Egner PA, Wang J-B, Zu YR, Yhang BC, Wu Y, Zhang QY, Qian GS, et al. Chlorophyllin intervention reduces aflatoxin-DNA adducts in individuals at high risk of liver can¬cer. Proc Natl Acad Sci USA. 2001;98:14601–6.

El-Serag HB. Epidemiology of viral hepatitis and hepatocellular carcinoma. Gastroenterology. 2012;142(1264):1273.e1.

Eslam M, Sarin SK, Wong VW, Fan JG, Kawaguchi T, Ahn SH, Zheng MH, Shiha G, Yilmaz Y, Gani R, Alam S, Dan YY, Kao JH, Hamid S, Cua IH, Chan WK, Payawal D, Tan SS, Tanwandee T, Adams LA, Kumar M, Omata M, George J. The Asian Pacific Association for the Study of the liver clinical practice guidelines for the diagnosis and management of metabolic associated fatty liver disease. Hepatol Int. 2020;14:889–919.

European Association for the Study of the Liver. European Organisation for Research and Treatment of Cancer: EASL-EORTC clinical practice guidelines: management of hepatocellular carcinoma. J Hepatol. 2012;56:908–43.
EASL. EASL 2017 Clinical Pratice Guidelines on the management of hepatitis B virus infection. J Hepatol. 2017;67:370–98.
EASL. EASL clinical practice guidelines: management of hepatocellular carcinoma. J Hepatol. 2018;69:182–236.
EASL-EASD-EASO. Clinical Practice Guidelines for the management of non-alcoholic fatty liver disease. J Hepatol. 2016;64(6):1388–402.
Fanning GC, Zoulim F, Hou J, Bertoletti A. Therapeutic strategies for hepatitis B virus infection: towards a cure. Nat Rev Drug Discov. 2019;18:827–44.
Frazzoni L, Sikandar U, Metelli F, Sadalla S, Mazzella G, Bazzoli F, Fuccio L, Azzaroli F. Hepatocellular carcinoma recurrence after hepatitis C virus therapy with direct-acting antivirals. A systematic review and meta-analysis. J Clin Med. 2021;10:1694.
Ganne-Carrié N, Nahon P. Hepatocellular carcinoma in the setting of alcohol-related liver disease. J Hepatol. 2019;70(2):284–93.
Gelatti U, Covolo L, Franceschini M, Pirali F, Tagger A, Ribero ML, et al. Coffee consumption reduces the risk of hepatocellular carcinoma independently of its aetiology: a case-control study. J Hepatol. 2005;42:528–34.
Geissler EK, Schnitzbauer AA, Zulke C, Lamby PE, Proneth A, Duvoux C, et al. Sirolimus use in liver transplant recipients with hepatocellular carcinoma: a randomized, multicenter, open-label phase 3 trial. Transplantation. 2016;100:116–25.
George ES, Sood S, Broughton A, Cogan G, Hickey M, Chan WS, et al. The association between diet and hepatocellular carcinoma: a systematic review. Nutrients. 2021;13(1):172.
Goh MJ, Sinn DH. Statin and aspirin for chemoprevention of hepatocellular carcinoma: time to use or wait further? Clin Mol Hepatol. 2022;28(3):380–95.
Goh MJ, Sinn DH, Kim S, Woo SY, Cho H, Kang W, et al. Statin use and the risk of hepatocellular carcinoma in patients with chronic hepatitis B. Hepatology. 2020;71:2023–32.
Gross-Steinmeyer K, Stapleton PL, Tracy JH, Bammler TK, Strom SC, Eaton DL. Sulforaphane- and phenethyl isothiocyanate-induced inhibition of aflatoxin B1-mediated genotoxicity in human hepatocytes: role of GSTM1 genotype and CYP3A4 gene expression. Toxicol Sci. 2010;116:422–32.
Guan MC, Zhang SY, Ding Q, Li N, Fu TT, Zhang GX, He QQ, Shen F, Yang T, Zhu H. The performance of GALAD score for diagnosing hepatocellular carcinoma in patients with chronic liver diseases: a systematic review and meta-analysis. J Clin Med. 2023;12(3):949.
Guarino M, Kumar P, Felser A, Terracciano LM, Guixé-Muntet S, Humar B, et al. Exercise attenuates the transition from fatty liver to steatohepatitis and reduces tumor formation in mice. Cancers (Basel). 2020;12(6)
Hack SP, Spahn J, Chen M, Cheng AL, Kaseb A, Kudo M, Lee HC, Yopp A, Chow P, Qin S. IMbrave 050: a Phase III trial of atezolizumab plus bevacizumab in high-risk hepatocellular carcinoma after curative resection or ablation. Future Oncol. 2020;16(15):975–89.
Hainaut P, Amadou A, Gormally E. Cancer prevention and control: hepatocellular carcinoma. E Cancer Med Sci. 2019;13:949.
Hamid AS, Tesfamariam IG, Zhang Y, Zhang ZG. Aflatoxin B1-induced hepatocellular carcinoma in developing countries: geographical distribution, mechanism of action and prevention. Oncol Lett. 2013;5(4):1087–92.
Hassan MM, Hwang L-Y, Hatten CJ, Swaim M, Li D, Abbruzzese JL, et al. Risk factors for hepatocellular carcinoma: synergism of alcohol with viral hepatitis and diabetes mellitus. Hepatology. 2002;36(5):1206–13.
Heathcote EJ. Prevention of hepatitis C virus-related hepatocellular carcinoma. Gastroenterology. 2004;127:S294–302.
Huang G, Li PP, Wan YL, et al. Antiviral therapy reduces hepatocellular carcinoma recurrence in patients with low HBV-DNA levels: a randomized controlled trial. Ann Surg. 2018;268(6):943–54.

Hui VW, Yip TC, Wong VW, Tse YK, Chan HL, Lui GC, et al. Aspirin reduces the incidence of hepatocellular carcinoma in patients with chronic hepatitis b receiving oral nucleos(t)ide analog. Clin Transl Gastroenterol. 2021;12:e00324.

Inoue M, Yoshimi I, Sobue T, Tsugane S. Influence of coffee drinking on subsequent risk of hepatocellular carcinoma: a prospective study in Japan. J Natl Cancer Inst. 2005;97:293–300.

Itoh K, Wakabayashi N, Kotoh H, Ishii T, Iganashi K, Enge JP, Yamamoto M, et al. Keap1 represses nuclear activa¬tion of antioxidant responsive elements by Nrf2 through binding to the amino-terminal Nrf2 domain. Genes Dev. 1999;13:76–86.

Jacobson LP, Zhang BC, Zhu YR, Wang JB, Wu Y, Zhang QN, Yu LY, Qian GS, Kuang SY, Li YF, Fang X, Zarba A, Chen B, Enger C, Davidson NE, Gorman MB, Gordon GB, Prochaska HJ, Egner PA, Groopman JD, Muñoz A, Helzlsouer KJ, Kensler TW. Oltipraz chemoprevention trial in Qidong, People's Republic of China: study design and clinical outcomes. Cancer Epidemiol Biomarkers Prev. 1997;6(4):257–65.

Kanwal F, Kramer JR, Mapakshi S, Natarajan Y, Chayanupatkul M, Richardson PA, et al. Risk of hepatocellular cancer in patients with nonalcoholic fatty liver disease. Gastroenterology. 2018;155(6):1828–1837.e2.

Kao JH, Hu TH, Jia J, et al. East Asia expert opinion on treatment initiation for chronic hepatitis B. Aliment Pharmacol Ther. 2020;52(10):1540–50.

Kennedy PT, Sandalova E, Jo J, Gill U, Ushiro-Lumb I, Tan AT, Naik S, Foster GR, Bertoletti A. Preserved TCell function in children and young adults with immune-tolerant chronic hepatitis B. Gastroenterology. 2012;143:637–45.

Kew MC. Prevention of hepatocellular carcinoma. Ann Hepatol. 2010;9(2):120–32.

Kew MC, Francois G, Lavanchy D, Margolis H, van Damme P, Grob P, Hallauer J, et al. Prevention of hepatitis C virus infection. J Med Virol. 2004;11:198–205.

Kim SU, Seo YS, Lee HA, et al. A multicenter study of entecavir vs tenofovir on prognosis of treatment-naive chronic hepatitis B in South Korea. J Hepatol. 2019;71:456–64.

Kim H-L, Kim G-A, Park J-A, Kang H-R, Lee E-K, Lim Y-S. Cost-effectiveness of antiviral treatment in adult patients with immune-tolerant phase chronic hepatitis B. Gut. 2020;70:2172–82.

Lampertico P, Agarwal K, Berg T, Buti M, Janssen HL, Papatheodoridis G, Zoulim F, Tacke F. EASL 2017 Clinical Practice Guidelines on the management of hepatitis B virus infection. J Hepatol. 2017;67:370–98.

Lange NF, Radu P, Dufour J. Prevention of NAFLD-associated HCC: role of lifestyle and chemoprevention. J Hepatol. 2021;75:1217–27.

Larsson SC, Wolk A. Coffee consumption and risk of liver cancer: a meta-analysis. Gastroenterology. 2007;132(5):1740–5.

Lee C, Gong Y, Brok J, et al. Effect of hepatitis B immunisation in newborn infants of mothers positive for hepatitis B surface antigen: systematic review and meta-analysis. BMJ. 2006a;332:328–36.

Lee C, Gong Y, Brok J, et al. Hepatitis B immunisation for newborn infants of hepatitis B surface antigen-positive mothers. Cochrane Database Syst Rev. 2006b;2:CD004790.

Lee DD, Sapisochin G, Mehta N, Gorgen A, Musto KR, Hajda H, et al. Surveillance for HCC after liver transplantation: increased monitoring May yield aggressive treatment options and improved postrecurrence survival. Transplantation. 2020a;104:2105–12.

Lee HW, Lee JS, Ahn SH. Hepatitis B virus cure: targets and future therapies. Int J Mol Sci. 2020b;22(1):213.

Lee M, Chung GE, Lee JH, Oh S, Nam JY, Chang Y, et al. Antiplatelet therapy and the risk of hepatocellular carcinoma in chronic hepatitis B patients on antiviral treatment. Hepatology. 2017;66:1556–69.

Lee TY, Hsu YC, Tseng HC, Lin JT, Wu MS, Wu CY. Association of daily aspirin therapy with hepatocellular carcinoma risk in patients with chronic hepatitis C virus infection. Clin Gastroenterol Hepatol. 2020c;18:2784–2792.e7.

Lee Y-CA, Cohet C, Yang Y-C, Stayner L, Hashibe M, Straif K. Meta-analysis of epidemiologic studies on cigarette smoking and liver cancer. Int J Epidemiol. 2009;38(6):1497–511.

Lee Y, Doumouras AG, Yu J, Brar K, Banfield L, Gmora S, et al. Complete resolution of nonalcoholic fatty liver disease after bariatric surgery: a systematic review and meta-analysis. Clin Gastroenterol Hepatol. 2019;17(6):1040–1060.e11.

Li W-Q, Park Y, McGlynn KA, Hollenbeck AR, Taylor PR, Goldstein AM, et al. Index-based dietary patterns and risk of incident hepatocellular carcinoma and mortality from chronic liver disease in a prospective study. Hepatology. 2014;60(2):588–97.

Li X, Wu S, Yu Y. Aspirin use and the incidence of hepatocellular carcinoma in patients with hepatitis B virus or hepatitis C virus infection: a meta-analysis of cohort studies. Front Med (Lausanne). 2021;7:569759.

Liao YH, Hsu RJ, Wang TH, Wu CT, Huang SY, Hsu CY, et al. Aspirin decreases hepatocellular carcinoma risk in hepatitis C virus carriers: a nationwide cohort study. BMC Gastroenterol. 2020;20:6.

Lin W-C, Lin Y-S, Chang C-W, Chang C-W, Wang T-E, Wang H-Y, Chen M-J. Impact of direct-acting antiviral therapy for hepatitis C–related hepatocellular carcinoma. PLoS One. 2020;15:e0233212.

Lok AS, Sterling RK, Everhart JE, Wright EC, Hoefs JC, Di Bisceglie AM, Morgan TR, Kim HY, Lee WM, Bonkovsky HL, Dienstag JL, HALT-C Trial Group. Des-gamma-carboxy prothrombin and alpha-fetoprotein as biomarkers for the early detection of hepatocellular carcinoma. Gastroenterology. 2010;138(2):493–502.

Lomonaco R, Godinez Leiva E, Bril F, Shrestha S, Mansour L, Budd J, Portillo Romero J, Schmidt S, Chang KL, Samraj G, Malaty J, Huber K, Bedossa P, Kalavalapalli S, Marte J, Barb D, Poulton D, Fanous N, Cusi K. Advanced liver fibrosis is common in patients with type 2 diabetes followed in the outpatient setting: the need for systematic screening. Diabetes Care. 2021;44:399–406.

Loomba R, Yang H-I, Su J, Brenner D, Iloeje U, Chen C-J. Obesity and alcohol synergize to increase the risk of incident hepatocellular carcinoma in men. Clin Gastroenterol Hepatol. 2010;8(10):891–8.

Loomba R, Yang H-I, Su J, Brenner D, Barrett-Connor E, Iloeje U, et al. Synergism between obesity and alcohol in increasing the risk of hepatocellular carcinoma: a prospective cohort study. Am J Epidemiol. 2013;177(4):333–42.

Lui FH, Moosvi Z, Patel A, Hussain S, Duong A, Duong J, Nguyen DL. Decreased risk of hepatocellular carcinoma recurrence with directacting antivirals compared with no treatment for hepatitis C: a meta-analysis, vol. 33. Gastroenterol: Ann; 2020. p. 293.

Machaira M, Papaevangelou V, Vouloumanou EK, et al. Hepatitis B vaccine alone or with hepatitis B immunoglobulin in neonates of HBsAg+/HBeAg- mothers: a systematic review and meta-analysis. J Antimicrob Chemother. 2015;70:396–404.

Marrero JA, Feng Z, Wang Y, Nguyen MH, Befeler AS, Roberts LR, Reddy KR, Harnois D, Llovet JM, Normolle D, Dalhgren J, Chia D, Lok AS, Wagner PD, Srivastava S, Schwartz M. Alpha-fetoprotein, des-gamma carboxyprothrombin, and lectin-bound alpha-fetoprotein in early hepatocellular carcinoma. Gastroenterology. 2009;137(1):110–8.

McGlynn KA, Hagberg K, Chen J, Graubard BI, London WT, Jick S, et al. Statin use and risk of primary liver cancer in the clinical practice research datalink. J Natl Cancer Inst. 2015;107:djv009.

Milman N, Pedersen P, Steig T, Byg KE, Graudal N, Fenger K. Clinically overt hereditary hemochromatosis in Denmark 1948–1985: epidemiology, factors of significance for long-term survival, and causes of death in 179 patients. Ann Hematol. 2001;80:737–44.

Mittal S, Sada YH, El-Serag HB, Kanwal F, Duan Z, Temple S, May SB, Kramer JR, Richardson PA, Davila JA. Temporal trends of nonalcoholic fatty liver disease-related hepatocellular carcinoma in the veteran affairs population. Clin Gastroenterol Hepatol. 2015;13:594–601.e1.

Mittal S, El-Serag HB, Sada YH, Kanwal F, Duan Z, Temple S, May SB, Kramer JR, Richardson PA, Davila JA. Hepatocellular carcinoma in the absence of cirrhosis in United States veterans is associated with nonalcoholic fatty liver disease. Clin Gastroenterol Hepatol. 2016;14:124–31.e1.

Miyata M, Takano H, Guo LQ, Nagata K, Yamazoe Y. Grapefruit juice intake does not enhance but rather protects against aflatoxin B1-induced liver DNA damage through a reduction in hepatic CYP3A activity. Carcinogenesis. 2004;25:203–9.

Morel F, Fardel O, Meyer DJ, Langouet S, Gilmore KS, Meunier B, Tu CP, et al. Preferential increase of glutathione-S-transferase class alpha transcripts in cultured human hepatocytes by phenobarbital, 3-methylcholanthrene and dithiolethiones. Cancer Res. 1993;53:231–4.

Murata K, Asano M, Matsumoto A, et al. Induction of IFNlambda3 as an additional effect of nucleotide, not nucleoside, analogues: a new potential target for HBV infection. Gut. 2018;67:362–71.

Nahon P, Layese R, Bourcier V, Cagnot C, Marcellin P, Guyader D, Pol S, Larrey D, De Lédinghen V, Ouzan D, et al. Incidence of hepatocellular carcinoma after direct antiviral therapy for HCV in patients with cirrhosis included in surveillance programs. Gastroenterology. 2018;155:1436–50.

Nan Y, Xu X, Dong S, Yang M, Li L, Zhao S, Duan Z, Jia J, Wei L, Zhuang H, Chinese Society of Hepatology, Chinese Medical Association. Consensus on the tertiary prevention of primary liver cancer. Hepatol Int. 2023;17(5):1057–71.

National Cancer Institute (ed.). PDQ cancer information summaries, 2019. https://www.ncbi.nlm.nih.gov/books/NBK65785/ (NCBI 2019).

Norero B, Dufour JF. Should we undertake surveillance for HCC in patients with MAFLD? Ther Adv Endocrinol Metab. 2023;28(14):20420188231160389.

Omata M, Cheng AL, Kokudo N, Kudo M, Lee JM, Jia J, Tateishi R, Han KH, Chawla YK, Shiina S, Jafri W, Payawal DA, Ohki T, Ogasawara S, Chen PJ, Lesmana CRA, Lesmana LA, Gani RA, Obi S, Dokmeci AK, Sarin SK. Asia-Pacific clinical practice guidelines on the management of hepatocellular carcinoma: a 2017 update. Hepatol Int. 2017;11(4):317–70.

Pan CQ, Duan Z, Dai E, et al. China Study Group for the Mother-to- Child Transmission of hepatitis B. Tenofovir to prevent hepatitis B transmission in mothers with high viral load. N Engl J Med. 2016;374:2324–34.

Papatheodoridis GV, Chan HL-Y, Hansen BE, Janssen HL, Lampertico P. Risk of hepatocellular carcinoma in chronic hepatitis B: assessment and modification with current antiviral therapy. J Hepatol. 2015;62:956–67.

Papatheodoridis GV, Idilman R, Dalekos GN, Buti M, Chi H, Van Boemmel F, Calleja-Panero JL, Sypsa V, Goulis J, Manolakopoulos S, et al. The risk of hepatocellular carcinoma decreases after the first 5 years of entecavir or tenofovir in Caucasians with chronic hepatitis B. Hepatology. 2017;66:1444–53.

Peterson S, Lampe JW, Bammler TK, Gross-Steinmeyer K, Eaton DL. Apiaceous vegetable constituents inhibit human cytochrome P-450 1A2 (hCYP1A2) activity and hCYP1A2-mediated mutagenicity of aflatoxin B1. Food Chem Toxicol. 2006;44:1474–84.

Petrick JL, Campbell PT, Koshiol J, Thistle JE, Andreotti G, Beane- Freeman LE, et al. Tobacco, alcohol use and risk of hepatocellular carcinoma and intrahepatic cholangiocarcinoma: the Liver Cancer Pooling Project. Br J Canc. 2018;118(7):1005–12.

Piñero F, Mendizabal M, Ridruejo E, Wolff FH, Ameigeiras B, Anders M, Schinoni MI, Reggiardo V, Palazzo A, Videla M, et al. Treatment with direct-acting antivirals for HCV decreases but does not eliminate the risk of hepatocellular carcinoma. Liver Int. 2019;39:1033–43.

Pinyopornpanish K, Al-Yaman W, Butler RS, Carey W, McCullough A, Romero-Marrero C. Chemopreventive effect of statin on hepatocellular carcinoma in patients with nonalcoholic steatohepatitis cirrhosis. Am J Gastroenterol. 2021;116:2258–69.

Plaz Torres MC, Bodini G, Furnari M, Marabotto E, Zentilin P, Strazzabosco M, Giannini EG. Surveillance for hepatocellular carcinoma in patients with non-alcoholic fatty liver disease: universal or selective? Cancers (Basel). 2020;12

Poustchi H, Farrell GC, Strasser SI, Lee AU, McCaughan GW, George J. Feasibility of conducting a randomized control trial for liver cancer screening: is a randomized controlled trial for liver cancer screening feasible or still needed? Hepatology. 2011;54(6):1998–2004.

Prabhu A, Cargill T, Roberts N, Ryan JD. Systematic review of the clinical outcomes of iron reduction in hereditary hemochromatosis. Hepatology. 2020;72:1469–82.

Qi W, Zhang Q, Xu Y, et al. Peg-interferon and nucleos(t)ide analogue combination at inception of antiviral therapy improves both anti-HBV efficacy and long-term survival among HBV DNA-positive hepatocellular carcinoma patients after hepatectomy/ablation. J Viral Hepat. 2020;27(4):387–96.

Qin S, Chen M, Cheng AL, Kaseb AO, Kudo M, Lee HC, Yopp AC, Zhou J, Wang L, Wen X, Heo J, Tak WY, Nakamura S, Numata K, Uguen T, Hsiehchen D, Cha E, Hack SP, Lian Q, Ma N, Spahn JH, Wang Y, Wu C, Chow PKH. IMbrave050 investigators. Atezolizumab plus bevacizumab versus active surveillance in patients with resected or ablated high-risk hepatocellular carcinoma (IMbrave050): a randomised, open-label, multicentre, phase 3 trial. Lancet. 2023;402(10415):1835–47.

Raffetti E, Fattovich G, Donato F. Incidence of hepatocellular carcinoma in untreated subjects with chronic hepatitis B: a systematic review and meta-analysis. Liver Int. 2016;36(9):1239–51.

Ravi S, Axley P, Jones D, Kodali S, Simpson H, McGuire BM, Singal AK. Unusually high rates of hepatocellular carcinoma after TreatmentWith direct-acting antiviral therapy for hepatitis C related cirrhosis. Gastroenterology. 2017;152:911–2.

Razavi-Shearer D, Gamkrelidze I, Nguyen MH, Chen D-S, Van Damme P, Abbas Z, Abdulla M, Rached AA, Adda D, Aho I, et al. Global prevalence, treatment, and prevention of hepatitis B virus infection in 2016: a modelling study. Lancet Gastroenterol Hepatol. 2018;3:383–403.

Reig M, Mariño Z, Perelló C, Iñarrairaegui M, Ribeiro A, Lens S, Díaz A, Vilana R, Darnell A, Varela M, et al. Unexpected high rate of early tumor recurrence in patients with HCV-related HCC undergoing interferon-free therapy. J Hepatol. 2016;65:719–26.

Rinella ME, Neuschwander-Tetri BA, Siddiqui MS, Abdelmalek MF, Caldwell S, Barb D, Kleiner DE, Loomba R. AASLD practice guidance on the clinical assessment and management of nonalcoholic fatty liver disease. Hepatology. 2023;77(5):1797–835.

Roche's Tecentriq plus Avastin is the first treatment combination to reduce the risk of cancer returning in people with certain types of early-stage liver cancer in a Phase III trial. Press Release: https://ml-eu.globenewswire.com/Resource/Download/38c62d81-04f6-47bd-bd88-481bf881f859; January 19, 2023.

Rodriguez-Peralvarez M, Tsochatzis E, Naveas MC, Pieri G, Garcia-Caparros C, O'Beirne J, et al. Reduced exposure to calcineurin inhibitors early after liver transplantation prevents recurrence of hepatocellular carcinoma. J Hepatol. 2013;59:1193–9.

Saran U, Guarino M, Rodríguez S, Simillion C, Montani M, Foti M, et al. Anti-tumoral effects of exercise on hepatocellular carcinoma growth. Hepatol Commun. 2018;2(5):607–20.

Sarin SK, Kumar M, Lau GK, et al. Asian-Pacific clinical practice guidelines on the management of hepatitis B: a 2015 update. Hepatol Int. 2016;10:1–98.

Schnitzbauer AA, Filmann N, Adam R, Bachellier P, Bechstein WO, Becker T, et al. mTOR inhibition is Most beneficial after liver transplantation for hepatocellular carcinoma in patients with active tumors. Ann Surg. 2020;272:855–62.

Setiawan VW, Wilkens LR, Lu SC, Hernandez BY, Le Marchand L, Henderson BE. Association of coffee intake with reduced incidence of liver cancer and death from chronic liver disease in the US multiethnic cohort. Gastroenterology. 2015;148:118–25.

Simonich MT, Egner PA, Roebuck BD, Orner GA, Jubert C, Pereira C, Groopman JD, Kensler TW, Dashwood RH, Williams DE, Bailey GS. Natural chlorophyll inhibits aflatoxin B1-induced multi-organ carcinogenesis in the rat. Carcinogenesis. 2007;8(6):1294–302.

Singal AG, Rich NE, Mehta N, Branch A, Pillai A, Hoteit M, Volk M, Odewole M, Scaglione S, Guy J, et al. Direct- acting antiviral therapy not associated with recurrence of hepatocellular carcinoma in a multicenter north American cohort study. Gastroenterology. 2019;156:1683–92.

Singal AG, Llovet JM, Yarchoan M, Mehta N, Heimbach JK, Dawson LA, Jou JH, Kulik LM, Agopian VG, Marrero JA, Mendiratta-Lala M, Brown DB, Rilling WS, Goyal L, Wei AC, Taddei TH. AASLD practice guidance on prevention, diagnosis, and treatment of hepatocellular carcinoma. Hepatology. 2023;78(6):1922–65.

Singal AG, Pillai A, Tiro J. Early detection, curative treatment, and survival rates for hepatocellular carcinoma surveillance in patients with cirrhosis: a meta-analysis. PLoS Med. 2014;11:e1001624.

Singal AK, Salameh H, Kuo YF, Fontana RJ. Meta-analysis: the impact of Oral anti-viral agents on the incidence of hepatocellular carcinoma in chronic hepatitis B. Aliment Pharmacol Ther. 2013;38(2):98–106.

Singer AW, Reddy KR, Telep LE, Osinusi AO, Brainard DM, Buti M, Chokkalingam AP. Direct-acting antiviral treatment for hepatitis C virus infection and risk of incident liver cancer: a retrospective cohort study. Aliment Pharmacol Ther. 2018;47:1278–87.

Sofowora GG, Choo EF, Mayo G, Shyr Y, Wilkinson GRI. In vivo inhibition of human CYP2A2 activity by olipraz. Cancer Chemother Pharmacol. 2001;47:505–9.

Stine JG, Wentworth BJ, Zimmet A, Rinella ME, Loomba R, Caldwell SH, et al. Systematic review with meta-analysis: risk of hepatocellular carcinoma in non-alcoholic steatohepatitis without cirrhosis compared to other liver diseases. Aliment Pharmacol Ther. 2018;48(7):696–703.

Takeda H, Takai A, Inuzuka T, et al. Genetic basis of hepatitis virus-associated hepatocellular carcinoma: linkage between infection, inflammation, and tumorigenesis. J Gastroenterol. 2017;52:26–38.

Tan RZH, Lockart I, Abdel Shaheed C, Danta M. Systematic review with meta-analysis: the effects of non-steroidal antiinflammatory drugs and anti-platelet therapy on the incidence and recurrence of hepatocellular carcinoma. Aliment Pharmacol Ther. 2021;54:356–67.

Tan DJH, Ng CH, Lin SY, Pan XH, Tay P, Lim WH, Teng M, Syn N, Lim G, Yong JN, Quek J, Xiao J, Dan YY, Siddiqui MS, Sanyal AJ, Muthiah MD, Loomba R, Huang DQ. Clinical characteristics, surveillance, treatment allocation, and outcomes of non-alcoholic fatty liver disease-related hepatocellular carcinoma: a systematic review and meta-analysis. Lancet Oncol. 2022;23:521–30.

Terrault NA, Hassanein TI. Management of the patient with SVR. J Hepatol. 2016;65:S120–9.

Terrault NA, Lok ASF, McMahon BJ, et al. Update on prevention, diagnosis, and treatment of chronic hepatitis B: AASLD 2018 hepatitis B guidance. Hepatology. 2018;67:1560–99.

Tran KT, McMenamin ÚC, Coleman HG, Cardwell CR, Murchie P, Iversen L, et al. Statin use and risk of liver cancer: evidence from two population-based studies. Int J Cancer. 2020;146:1250–60.

Tsan YT, Lee CH, Wang JD, Chen PC. Statins and the risk of hepatocellular carcinoma in patients with hepatitis B virus infection. J Clin Oncol. 2012;30:623–30.

Tsan YT, Lee CH, Ho WC, Lin MH, Wang JD, Chen PC. Statins and the risk of hepatocellular carcinoma in patients with hepatitis c virus infection. J Clin Oncol. 2013;31:1514–21.

Tu T, Budzinska MA, Shackel NA, Urban S. HBV DNA integration: molecular mechanisms and clinical implications. Viruses. 2017;9:75.

Turati F, Trichopoulos D, Polesel J, Bravi F, Rossi M, Talamini R, et al. Mediterranean diet and hepatocellular carcinoma. J Hepatol. 2014;60(3):606–11.

Turner PC, Sylla A, Gong YY, Diallo MS, Sutcliffe AE, Hall AJ, Wild CP. Reduction in exposure to carcinogenic aflatoxins by post harvest intervention measures in West Africa: a community-based intervention study. Lancet. 2005;365:1950–6.

Vilar-Gomez E, Martinez-Perez Y, Calzadilla-Bertot L, Torres-Gonzalez A, Gra-Oramas B, Gonzalez-Fabian L, et al. Weight loss through lifestyle modification significantly reduces features of nonalcoholic steatohepatitis. Gastroenterology. 2015;149(2):367–378.e5.

Vogel A, Cervantes A, Chau I, et al. Hepatocellular carcinoma: ESMO clinical practice guidelines for diagnosis, treatment and follow-up. Ann Oncol. 2018;29(Suppl 4):238–55.

Wang JS, Shen X, He X, Zhu YR, Zhang BC, Wang JB, Qian GS, et al. Protective alterations in phase 1 and 2 metabo¬lism of aflatoxin B1 by oltipraz in residents of Qidong, People's Republic of China. J Natl Cancer Inst. 1999;91:347–54.

Wichajarn K, Kosalaraksa P, Wiangnon S. Incidence of hepatocellular carcinoma in children in Khon Kaen before and after national hepatitis B vaccine program. Asian Pac J Cancer Prev. 2008;9:507–9.

Wild CP, Gong YY. Mycotoxins and human disease: a largely ignored global health issue. Carcinogenesis. 2010;31:71–82.

Williams JH, Phillips TD, Jolly PE, Stiles JK, Jolly CM, Aggarwal D. Human aflatoxicosis in developing countries: a review of toxicology, exposure, potential health consequences, and interventions. Am J Clin Nutr. 2004;80:1106–22.

WHO. Global hepatitis report 2017. Geneva: WHO; 2017.

WHO. Hepatitis B Fact Sheet No. 204 (revised October 2000). 2000. Available at www.who.int

Wong GL, Hui VW, Yip TC, Liang LY, Zhang X, Tse YK, Lai JC, Chan HL, Wong VW. Universal HBV vaccination dramatically reduces the prevalence of HBV infection and incidence of hepatocellular carcinoma. Aliment Pharmacol Ther. 2022;56(5):869–77.

Yang JD, Roberts LR. Hepatocellular carcinoma: a global view. Nat Rev Gastroenterol Hepatol. 2010;7:448–58.

Yang JD, Addissie BD, Mara KC, Harmsen WS, Dai J, Zhang N, Wongjarupong N, Ali HM, Ali HA, Hassan FA, Lavu S, Cvinar JL, Giama NH, Moser CD, Miyabe K, Allotey LK, Algeciras-Schimnich A, Theobald JP, Ward MM, Nguyen MH, Befeler AS, Reddy KR, Schwartz M, Harnois DM, Yamada H, Srivastava S, Rinaudo JA, Gores GJ, Feng Z, Marrero JA, Roberts LR. GALAD score for hepatocellular carcinoma detection in comparison with liver ultrasound and proposal of GALADUS score. Cancer Epidemiol Biomarkers Prev. 2019;28(3):531–8.

Yip TC, Lai JC, Wong GL. Secondary prevention for hepatocellular carcinoma in patients with chronic hepatitis B: are all the nucleos(t)ide analogues the same? J Gastroenterol. 2020;55(11):1023–36.

Yuan J-M, Govindarajan S, Arakawa K, Yu MC. Synergism of alcohol, diabetes, and viral hepatitis on the risk of hepatocellular carcinoma in blacks and whites in the US. Cancer. 2004;101(5):1009–17.

Zhou YY, Zhu GQ, Liu T, Zheng JN, Cheng Z, Zou TT, Braddock M, Fu SW, Zheng MH. Systematic review with network meta-analysis: antidiabetic medication and risk of hepatocellular carcinoma. Sci Rep. 2016;6:33743.

Zou B, Odden MC, Nguyen MH. Statin use and reduced hepatocellular carcinoma risk in patients with nonalcoholic fatty liver disease. Clin Gastroenterol Hepatol. 2023;21(2):435–44.

Prospects and Unmet Needs of HCC Management

11

Reda Elwakil and Mohamed Kamal Shaker

Abstract

Hepatocellular carcinoma (HCC) is the most common type of liver cancer in adults. A significant proportion of HCC cases arise in individuals with cirrhosis caused by hepatitis B virus (HBV) or hepatitis C virus (HCV) infections. These infections are especially widespread in low- and middle-income countries (LMICs), making the prevention, early detection, and treatment of HCC particularly challenging in resource-limited settings. Many patients in these regions present at advanced stages of the disease, often with impaired liver function due to underlying chronic liver conditions, resulting in poor treatment outcomes despite available therapies.

Recent advancements have improved early detection techniques and expanded treatment options for HCC. Approvals of new therapies for advanced stage disease have extended patient survival and enhanced quality of life through better symptom management. However, significant barriers to effective HCC management remain. Challenges in screening and diagnosis include the silent nature of early-stage disease, limited healthcare infrastructure, and financial barriers to accessing diagnostic services, particularly in LMICs. Educational barriers are also evident, stemming from both patient illiteracy and gaps in healthcare provider training.

Treatment-related obstacles involve selecting the appropriate therapeutic approach based on disease stage and liver function, ensuring patient acceptance of treatment plans, and securing access to necessary therapies and specialist expertise, issues that are more pronounced in resource-constrained environments. Overcoming these challenges, alongside addressing other unmet needs, is

R. Elwakil (✉) · M. K. Shaker
Tropical Medicine Department, Ain Shams University, Cairo, Egypt

R. Elwakil et al. (eds.), *Approach to Hepatocellular Carcinoma (HCC) Management in Low/Middle-Income Countries*,
https://doi.org/10.1007/978-981-96-3894-9_11

essential for optimizing HCC care. This chapter aims to explore current and emerging strategies for HCC diagnosis and treatment, with a particular focus on addressing gaps in care in low- and middle-income countries.

Keywords

HCC · HCC treatment prospects · HCC unmet needs · HCC diagnosis

Abbreviations

ACT	Adoptive cell transfer
AFP	Alfa fetoprotein
AFP-L3	Lens culinaris agglutinin-reactive AFP
AI	Artificial intelligence
APCs	Antigen-presenting cells
AUC	Area under curve
CAR-T cells	Chimeric antigen receptor T cells
cfDNA	Circulating free DNA
CIKCs	Cytokine-induced killer cells
CT	Computed tomography
CTCs	Circulating tumor cells
ctDNA	Circulating tumor DNA
CTLA- 4	Cytotoxic T-lymphocyte-associated protein 4
DCP	des-γ-carboxyprothrombin
DCs	Dendritic cells
DNA	Deoxynucleic acid
EVs	Extra cellular vesicles
FDA	USA Food and Drug Administration
Gal-9	Galectin 9
GPC 3	Glypican 3
HCC	Hepatocellular carcinoma
ICIs	Immune-check inhibitors
ICD	Immunogenic cell death
LAG-3	Lymphocyte-activation gene 3
LDL	Low-density lipoprotein
LLR	Laparoscopic liver resection
LMICs	Low/middle-income countries
lncRNAs	Long non-coding RNAs
MHC	Major histocompatibility complex
MRI	Magnetic resonance imaging
MDSCs	Myeloid-derived suppressor cells
NKC	Natural killer cell

OS	Overall survival
PBMNCs	Peripheral blood mononuclear cells
PD1	Programmed death- 1
PD-L1	Programmed death ligand-1
PFS	Progression-free survival
PUFAs	Polyunsaturated fatty acids
RECIST	Response evaluation criteria in solid tumors
RNA	Ribonucleic acid
ROC curve	Receiver operating characteristic curve
TCR	T cell chain receptor
TIL	Tumor-infiltrating lymphocytes
TKIs	Tyrosine kinase inhibitors
TNF	Tumor necrosis factor
US	Ultrasonography
USA	United States of America
VEGF	Vascular endothelial growth factor
VSV	Vesicular stomatitis virus
WHO	World Health Organization

11.1 Introduction

In 2020, liver cancer ranked as the third leading cause of cancer-related mortality worldwide (WHO International Agency for Research on Cancer 2022). Hepatocellular carcinoma (HCC) represents the most common subtype of liver cancer in adults. Approximately, 80–90% of HCC cases arise in the context of cirrhosis, predominantly caused by chronic hepatitis B or C virus infections (Li et al. 2019a, b). The persistent difficulty in managing hepatitis infections across many developing regions continues to hinder efforts to lower the global incidence of HCC (Zampino et al. 2015; Averhoff et al. 2012). Notably, over 72% of HCC cases are reported from Asia, where these viral infections are endemic (Singal et al. 2020).

HCC typically develops against a background of chronic liver disease (Kanwal and Singal 2019). Thus, patients with HCC face the dual challenge of malignancy alongside often severely impaired liver function. The extent of liver dysfunction independently affects survival outcomes (Shiani et al. 2017). Given the complexity of managing both liver disease and cancer, multidisciplinary team (MDT) discussions are critical for selecting appropriate treatment pathways. Management strategies must consider not only tumor stage but also the degree of underlying liver impairment. Moreover, the etiological factors leading to HCC can influence therapeutic responses, further complicating clinical decision-making.

Treatment planning for HCC is particularly challenging, as impaired liver function can limit the feasibility of several therapeutic interventions (National Comprehensive Cancer Network 2023). For instance, patients with early-stage tumors may not qualify for surgical resection if liver function is significantly compromised. Similarly, those with more advanced disease may not tolerate systemic treatments. Therefore, thorough liver function assessment is essential to tailor therapy appropriately (Vogel 2021).

Recent approvals of new treatments for advanced HCC have extended patient survival and improved symptom management and quality of life. Available first- and second-line therapies now include tyrosine kinase inhibitors (TKIs) and immunotherapy, though the optimal sequencing of these treatments remains under investigation (Coffman-D'Annibale et al. 2023).

Ongoing research is actively evaluating the efficacy of combining immune checkpoint inhibitors (ICIs) with systemic or locoregional therapies across various stages of HCC. This is based on emerging evidence of increased immune exhaustion at the tumor-stroma interface (Pinter et al. 2021). HCC cells employ multiple mechanisms to evade immune detection, and ICIs function by reversing this immunosuppression, targeting receptors on T cells or their ligands on antigen-presenting cells (Zhou et al. 2017).

Recent discoveries have identified key drivers of anti-tumor immune responses, opening new avenues for immunotherapy. Targeting molecules such as cytotoxic T-lymphocyte-associated protein 4 (CTLA4) and programmed death-1 (PD1) has shown promising results across multiple malignancies, including HCC (Pardoll 2012). Nonetheless, monotherapy targeting single immune pathways in HCC has yielded limited response rates, suggesting that combination strategies targeting multiple pathways may enhance therapeutic efficacy (Llovet et al. 2022).

Looking ahead, novel combinations of TKIs and ICIs, as well as next-generation immunotherapies, are under investigation for use in advanced HCC. Understanding mechanisms of resistance to ICIs and pathways of immune escape has driven the development of these innovative approaches (Luo et al. 2021; Llovet et al. 2022).

The utility of biomarkers in oncology is increasingly recognized. Although targeting specific molecular mutations has not yet produced major advances in HCC, ongoing studies in tumor genetic sequencing may identify new diagnostic and prognostic markers (Coffman-D'Annibale et al. 2023).

However, several challenges persist in the management of HCC, particularly in LMICs. Barriers to effective screening and early diagnosis include the asymptomatic nature of early disease, low public awareness, limited healthcare infrastructure, and patients' inability to afford diagnostic services. Additional difficulties stem from low health literacy among patients and gaps in healthcare providers' expertise. Selecting the most appropriate treatment strategy based on liver function and disease stage also presents a significant hurdle (Kumari et al. 2018). Addressing these barriers, along with other unmet clinical needs, is critical for improving outcomes in HCC, especially in resource-constrained settings.

This chapter focuses on exploring current and future directions in the diagnosis and treatment of HCC, with particular emphasis on overcoming the unmet challenges in its management.

11.2 Prospects of HCC Management

11.2.1 Prospects of Diagnosis

11.2.1.1 Early Diagnosis of HCC

The Use of Artificial Intelligence (AI) in Early Diagnosis of HCC

In 2021, the National Cancer Centre of Singapore (NCCS) initiated a four-year, multi-center project known as the ELEGANCE study. This study aims to enroll 2000 individuals who are at elevated risk of developing hepatocellular carcinoma (HCC), including those with liver cirrhosis, hepatitis B or C, non-alcoholic fatty liver disease (NAFLD), or non-alcoholic steatohepatitis (NASH). Its primary objectives are to enhance early detection of HCC and improve the ability to predict disease onset.

The ELEGANCE study comprises three major components: firstly, it evaluates the effectiveness of a microRNA (miRNA) diagnostic kit for HCC in collaboration with MiRXES; secondly, it focuses on the development of an artificial intelligence (AI) algorithm utilizing quantitative magnetic resonance imaging (MRI) to identify individuals at high risk for HCC; and thirdly, it investigates microbiome and metabolome alterations associated with HCC development. Overall, the study seeks to facilitate earlier diagnosis, improve patient outcomes, and discover novel therapeutic targets (Duke-NUS Medical School, Media Release 2021).

Combined Biomarker Scores for Early HCC Diagnosis

One promising approach to the early detection of HCC is the use of combined biomarker scoring systems. The GALAD Score, developed by Roche, exemplifies this strategy. It recently received breakthrough device designation from the U.S. Food and Drug Administration (FDA) to aid in the early diagnosis of HCC. The GALAD model integrates five variables: gender, age, levels of Lens culinaris agglutinin-reactive alpha-fetoprotein (AFP-L3), total alpha-fetoprotein (AFP), and des-gamma-carboxy prothrombin (DCP). This combination predicts the likelihood of HCC in patients with chronic liver disease (Roche Media Release 2020). Furthermore, evidence suggests that the GALAD Score can effectively detect HCC in patients with NAFLD, both with and without cirrhosis (Best et al. 2020).

A validation study conducted in China by Huang et al. (2022) involved 602 patients with HCC and 923 control participants across five hospitals. The study also assessed the GALAD Score's surveillance capabilities among 204 patients who underwent curative surgery and further evaluated its performance for early HCC detection in a separate prospective cohort. Findings demonstrated that the GALAD Score outperformed individual biomarkers like AFP, DCP, and AFP-L3 in identifying early-stage HCC. Moreover, it proved capable of stratifying patients by risk of overall survival and recurrence. Remarkably, the GALAD Score could detect HCC up to 24 to 48 weeks prior to clinical diagnosis, leading the authors to advocate for its early adoption in clinical practice to enhance prognostic evaluation (Huang et al. 2022).

Additionally, a recent study by Cagnin et al. (2023) reinforced the potential of the GALAD Score, suggesting that its application could significantly refine treatment planning strategies for HCC.

Circulating microRNAs (miRNAs) for Early Diagnosis of HCC

Recent research by Zhang et al. demonstrated that a specific panel of three microRNAs—miR-92-3p, miR-107, and miR-3126-5p—exhibited excellent diagnostic performance for hepatocellular carcinoma (HCC). This panel achieved an area under the receiver operating characteristic curve (AUC) of 0.98 for early-stage HCC detection and an AUC of 0.97 among patients with low serum alpha-fetoprotein (AFP) concentrations. Complementary findings by Yamamoto et al. (2020) further underscored the diagnostic promise of circulating microRNA panels, reporting a sensitivity of 97.7%, specificity of 94.7%, and an AUC of 0.99 for early HCC identification.

In parallel, long non-coding RNAs (lncRNAs) have emerged as additional promising biomarkers, with several studies, including that by Huang et al. (2022), highlighting their potential utility in the early detection and diagnosis of HCC.

The Role of Liquid Biopsy in HCC Surveillance

Methylation Profiling of Circulating Tumor DNA (ctDNA)

Recent advances have highlighted the significance of hypermethylated and hypomethylated cell-free DNA (cfDNA) markers in the pathogenesis of cancer (Liu et al. 2021). In a large-scale study involving 1098 patients with hepatocellular carcinoma (HCC) and 835 healthy individuals, Xu et al. (2017) proposed a diagnostic prediction model utilizing cfDNA biomarkers, demonstrating high sensitivity and specificity for early-stage detection. Moreover, Kisiel et al. (2019) identified 302 methylated DNA candidates exhibiting area under the curve (AUC) values exceeding 0.75, further emphasizing the diagnostic potential of methylation profiling in HCC.

Mutation Profiling of cfDNA

Emerging evidence supports the utility of cfDNA mutation analysis in HCC detection. Mutations in commonly altered genes, such as tumor protein p53 (TP53), have been frequently observed in HCC (Dhanasekaran et al. 2019). Detection of these mutations within cfDNA offers a non-invasive approach for early diagnosis (Mody et al. 2019). Comprehensive genomic profiling of blood samples from 206 patients with HCC revealed that 88% harbored at least one detectable genetic alteration, with frequent mutations in TP53 and the epidermal growth factor receptor (EGFR) genes (Kaseb et al. 2019).

Extracellular Vesicles (EVs)

Extracellular vesicles (EVs), comprising lipid bilayer structures secreted by cells, encapsulate a variety of biologically active molecules, including proteins, DNA, and microRNAs (Margolis and Sadovsky 2019). The role of EVs as potential biomarkers for HCC surveillance is an area of active investigation (Sukowati et al.

2021). Preliminary studies have suggested that EV-derived components may serve as promising prognostic indicators in HCC (Sun et al. 2020).

Circulating Tumor Cells (CTCs)
Circulating tumor cells (CTCs), particularly those expressing the epithelial cell adhesion molecule (EpCAM), have been explored for their diagnostic and prognostic value in HCC. A meta-analysis encompassing 20 studies and 1191 patients reported that CTC assays achieved a sensitivity of 95% and a specificity of 60% in detecting HCC (Cui et al. 2020), highlighting their potential application in clinical practice.

11.2.2 Prospects of HCC Surgery

11.2.2.1 Minimally Invasive Surgery for HCC

The feasibility, safety, and clinical benefits of laparoscopic liver resection (LLR) have been well established. In Japan, approximately 25% of all liver resections are now performed using a laparoscopic approach (Ban et al. 2020). Since 2014, laparoscopic partial hepatectomy has been recognized as a standard treatment option for hepatocellular carcinoma (HCC) located in the anterolateral segments of the liver (Cho et al. 2018). Nevertheless, LLR demands substantial surgical expertise, a steep learning curve, and careful preoperative assessment of procedural complexity (Nakajima et al. 2021).

11.2.2.2 New Expansion Criteria for Liver Transplantation for HCC

The Japanese Liver Transplantation Society recently introduced expanded criteria for liver transplantation, known as the "5–5-500 rule," based on a retrospective analysis of a nationwide survey (Shimamura et al. 2019). This new guideline was evaluated in a cohort of 965 patients undergoing living donor liver transplantation for hepatocellular carcinoma (HCC). Patients meeting the criteria—defined as having no more than five nodules, each measuring 5 cm or less in diameter, and an alpha-fetoprotein (AFP) level of 500 ng/mL or lower, with no evidence of vascular invasion or extrahepatic spread—achieved a five-year recurrence rate of 7.3%. Furthermore, the application of the 5–5-500 rule expanded transplant eligibility by approximately 19% compared to the traditional Milan criteria (Nakajima et al. 2021).

11.2.3 Interventional Radiology New Therapies for HCC

Interventional radiology has seen significant progress in the treatment of HCC by introducing novel intra-arterial delivery systems. Among these, biomimetic drug delivery platforms offer promising results by facilitating targeted treatment at the tumor site (Parodi et al. 2017). These systems mimic biological mechanisms to effectively reach malignant cells and initiate cytotoxic effects within them (Sutphin et al. 2019).

11.2.3.1 Natural Killer Cell-Based Approaches

Natural killer (NK) cells are essential components of the innate immune system, known for their capacity to detect and destroy abnormal cells, including cancerous ones (Vivier et al. 2011). In a study using a rat model of HCC, Sheu et al. (2013) explored the trans arterial infusion of NK cells labeled with superparamagnetic iron oxide (SPIO), enabling their non-invasive visualization and tracking through magnetic resonance imaging (MRI). Su et al. (2018) confirmed that these labeled cells localized to tumors within 24–48 hours post-infusion, with their accumulation validated by histological findings.

11.2.3.2 Viral Vector Therapies

Emerging viral-based therapies for HCC involve arterial infusion of oncolytic and gene-carrying viruses to enhance local therapeutic action.

Vesicular Stomatitis Virus (VSV)

Tumors often have compromised antiviral defenses, particularly in interferon signaling, which allows for selective replication of viruses like VSV within malignant tissues (Stojdl et al. 2000). The replication process disrupts tumor cell integrity, leading to cell lysis and tumor reduction (Ebert et al. 2003). In preclinical experiments, hepatic infusion of engineered VSV led to pronounced viral activity in tumors and improved survival outcomes compared to control animals ($p < 0.028$) (Ebert et al. 2003).

Adenovirus

Adenoviral vectors have been modified to deliver therapeutic genes by replacing native viral components with functional genetic material. Shiba et al. (2008) investigated the efficiency of administering these vectors via the hepatic artery, followed by embolization to restrict blood flow and enhance tumor uptake. Anderson et al. (1998) reported that delivering a p53-expressing adenovirus repeatedly over several days significantly reduced tumor progression in animal models. Furthermore, combining this technique with transarterial chemoembolization (TACE) in clinical settings has shown encouraging results in patients with inoperable HCC (Shen et al. 2015).

11.2.3.3 Omega-3 Fatty Acid Transport Via Lipoproteins

Reynolds et al. (2014) introduced a technique to administer docosahexaenoic acid (DHA), an omega-3 fatty acid, complexed with low-density lipoproteins (LDL) through transarterial injection. This approach enhances tumor-specific delivery by leveraging the LDL receptor-mediated uptake mechanism (Wáng et al. 2015). The nanoscale LDL-DHA particles (approximately 22 nm) readily infiltrate the tumor vasculature, are absorbed by cancer cells, and exert cytotoxic effects. Preclinical studies demonstrated significant tumor destruction following this treatment in rodent models (Wen et al. 2016). Given its biocompatibility and selectivity, LDL-DHA may serve as a suitable alternative for patients unable to undergo conventional TACE procedures (Gonzalez-Periz et al. 2006).

11.2.4 Future Prospects of Systemic Therapy

11.2.4.1 New Paradigms in Systemic Therapy

Immunotherapy as a First-Line Treatment

Tislelizumab, a humanized IgG4 monoclonal antibody targeting PD-1, has been studied as a standalone treatment and in combination regimens for various solid and hematologic malignancies. The RATIONALE 301 Phase 3 trial, a global, randomized, open-label study, evaluated tislelizumab against sorafenib as an initial therapy in adults with unresectable hepatocellular carcinoma (HCC). This trial included 674 participants and was designed to assess whether tislelizumab was not inferior in terms of overall survival (OS) compared to sorafenib. Findings showed that tislelizumab maintained OS non-inferiority, had an improved safety profile, achieved better response rates, and was associated with better quality of life outcomes (Finn et al. 2024).

Combination Therapy Approaches for HCC

The Phase III IMbrave150 trial established that the combination of atezolizumab and bevacizumab significantly surpassed sorafenib in improving OS, progression-free survival (PFS), and objective response rates. This combination has since been recognized as the preferred first-line regimen for advanced HCC (Kudo et al. 2023). The FDA acknowledged its therapeutic promise by granting it breakthrough therapy designation for untreated metastatic or advanced HCC (Lee et al. 2020). Real-world evidence from a Korean study involving 111 patients confirmed its efficacy and tolerability in clinical practice (Song et al. 2024).

In the HIMALAYA Phase III trial, tremelimumab combined with durvalumab extended median OS over sorafenib alone (Abou-Alfa et al. 2022). Another trial assessing lenvatinib with pembrolizumab showed potential; however, it did not meet predefined statistical thresholds for OS or PFS benefit compared to lenvatinib plus placebo, and thus was not deemed practice-changing (Llovet et al. 2023).

Current clinical investigations continue to explore strategies to enhance immune checkpoint inhibitors (ICIs) therapeutic effect through combination approaches as follows:

Dual Immune Checkpoint Inhibition in HCC

- **Nivolumab and Ipilimumab:**

The FDA granted accelerated approval in 2020 for nivolumab plus ipilimumab in HCC patients previously treated with sorafenib, based on the CheckMate-040 Phase I/II trial results (El-Khoueiry et al. 2017).

- **Tremelimumab and Durvalumab:**

This ICI combination received FDA approval in late 2022 as a first-line therapy for patients with advanced unresectable HCC, supported by results from the HIMALAYA trial (Abou-Alfa et al. 2022).

ICIs Combined with Tyrosine Kinase Inhibitors (TKIs)

The CARES-310 Phase III trial was the first to demonstrate notable improvements in both PFS and OS with a regimen combining the PD-1 inhibitor camrelizumab and the TKI rivoceranib versus sorafenib. The interim data showed significantly extended OS with camrelizumab–rivoceranib (22.1 months) compared to 15.2 months with sorafenib (Qin et al. 2023).

11.2.4.2 Dual ICIs in the Neoadjuvant Setting

Emerging findings from early-phase clinical trials suggest that dual checkpoint blockade may hold promise in the neoadjuvant context, potentially reshaping treatment paradigms. This approach appears to offer enhanced anti-tumor responses relative to monotherapies (Mangla et al. 2024; Tian et al. 2024).

11.2.4.3 Emerging Immunotherapeutic Strategies

Direct Immunological Approaches

Oncolytic Viruses (OVs)

Oncolytic virus therapy (OVT) uses viruses—either natural or engineered—that selectively infect and replicate in tumor cells, leading to tumor lysis. This approach also facilitates anti-tumor immunity by releasing immunogenic signals such as damage-associated molecular patterns (DAMPs), tumor antigens, and viral particles that enhance both innate and adaptive responses (Jin et al. 2021; Lemos de Matos et al. 2020). Additionally, OVs can modify the tumor microenvironment to improve immunogenicity (Martini et al. 2020). DNA and RNA virus platforms are under clinical investigation (Fountzilas et al. 2017; Ferrucci et al. 2021; Minaei et al. 2023; Jebar et al. 2015).

Adoptive Cell Transfer (ACT) Therapy

ACT enhances the immune system's capacity to recognize and eliminate cancer cells by employing modified lymphocytes. Approaches include expansion of tumor-infiltrating lymphocytes (TILs) or engineering T cells to express tumor-targeting receptors such as TCRs or CARs. Several studies have demonstrated the feasibility and effectiveness of these therapies in treating solid tumors, including HCC (Rohaan et al. 2019; Shokoohian et al. 2021).

Tumor-Infiltrating Lymphocytes (TILs)

TILs are isolated from the tumor microenvironment, expanded ex vivo, and administered to patients following lymphodepleting regimens. Challenges remain in applying this strategy to HCC, primarily due to the complexities of TIL culture and adverse effects associated with high-dose IL-2 therapy (Fardis et al. 2020; Zhang et al. 2019).

Genetically Modified T Cells

- **TCR-Engineered T Cells:**

These cells are programmed to express receptors targeting specific HCC antigens such as AFP, glypican-3, and HBsAg. While they show promise in preclinical and early-phase trials, broader application is limited by various technical and immunological hurdles (Singh and McGuirk 2020; Minaei et al. 2023).

- **CAR-T Cells:**

CAR-T therapy has made inroads in HCC, particularly targeting glypican-3 (GPC3). Early-phase clinical trials have demonstrated encouraging safety profiles and preliminary efficacy, especially when combined with TKIs. However, toxicity management, particularly cytokine release syndrome, remains essential (Fu et al. 2023).

Natural Killer (NK) Cells

NK cells eliminate malignancies without the need for antigen presentation. They can be derived from various sources, expanded ex vivo, and administered post-lymphodepletion. Despite initial efficacy, immunosuppression in advanced cancer patients may diminish their function. Research is ongoing into donor-derived and genetically enhanced NK cells (Xie et al. 2020; Kim et al. 2021).

Cytokine-Induced Killer (CIK) Cells

CIK cells, which possess both T cell and NK cell properties, show robust cytotoxicity against cancer with minimal toxicity to normal tissues. Trials have indicated that they may improve survival outcomes, particularly when used as adjuvant therapies post-resection. The Korean-approved product Immuncell-LC has also received FDA orphan drug designation (Lee et al. 2015a, b; Wang et al. 2021).

Indirect Immunological Approaches: Cancer Vaccines

Therapeutic vaccination strategies for HCC utilize various platforms, including whole-cell preparations, peptides, DNA, and dendritic cells (Mougel et al. 2019).

Peptide-Based Vaccines

Peptide vaccines target tumor-associated antigens (TAAs) like AFP and GPC3, which are commonly upregulated in HCC. For instance, an intradermal vaccine comprising AFP peptides presented by dendritic cells prompted antigen-specific T cell responses in all enrolled patients (Butterfield et al. 2006). Likewise, GPC3 peptide-based vaccines have elicited immune activation and demonstrated safety in clinical trials (Tsuchiya et al. 2017).

Dendritic Cell-Based Vaccines

These vaccines harness dendritic cells' antigen-presenting capability to stimulate T cell-mediated tumor destruction. Monocytes from patients are cultured, differentiated, loaded with tumor antigens, and reinfused. Clinical investigations have shown that such vaccines are safe and may be beneficial after primary treatment. Nonetheless, their efficacy in advanced HCC remains modest (Qin et al. 2018; Mastelic-Gavillet et al. 2019; Tada et al. 2012; El Ansary et al. 2013).

11.3 The Unmet Needs in HCC Management

11.3.1 Diagnostic Gaps

11.3.1.1 The Need for Earlier Detection of HCC

Improving early diagnosis of hepatocellular carcinoma (HCC) hinges on strengthening surveillance strategies. This remains a major hurdle for healthcare systems aiming to enhance early-stage detection and ultimately improve the poor outcomes associated with HCC. There continues to be a lack of well-structured and evidence-based implementation of surveillance protocols, particularly in low- and middle-income countries (LMICs), which impairs the effectiveness of current programs (Singal et al. 2020).

11.3.1.2 Ongoing Challenges in Enhancing Surveillance

To advance early diagnosis, further research is needed across multiple fronts. One key issue is the development of reliable biomarkers to assess HCC risk, especially in populations such as individuals with cured hepatitis C or those with significant fibrosis from non-alcoholic steatohepatitis (NASH). These biomarkers must be rigorously evaluated through large-scale phase 3 trials. In addition, new imaging techniques and minimally invasive diagnostic tools are required to catch the disease at earlier stages. Addressing barriers to surveillance uptake and improving adherence among at-risk individuals is another critical need (Adeniji and Dhanasekaran 2021).

Detecting HCC early improves the likelihood of successful treatment, which is why surveillance is strongly recommended for patients with cirrhosis (Global Data Health Care 2020).

Japan offers a model of successful early detection, with systematic surveillance beginning in the 1980s. As a result, most cases there are caught at early stages—only 5.7% are found at BCLC stage C, while 62% are diagnosed at stage A. In contrast, in the USA, 31% of diagnoses occur at the more advanced stage C, and only 28% at stage A (Global Data Health Care 2020).

11.3.1.3 The Need for Better Surveillance Promotion Methods

Improving HCC surveillance uptake requires active collaboration between healthcare providers, systems, and patients. Educational tools—such as trained personnel, digital platforms, support groups, and mobile applications—can help raise awareness and promote patient participation. Integrating evaluations into streamlined, single-visit "one-stop" clinics may also encourage better follow-up (Singal et al. 2020). Outreach strategies like mailed invitations have shown success in boosting screening rates (Singal et al. 2017, 2019). Additionally, involving primary care physicians through targeted training could facilitate broader implementation of surveillance practices (McGowan et al. 2015).

11.3.2 Treatment Gaps

11.3.2.1 Insufficient Pain Management Strategies

Pain relief in HCC patients is complicated by the potential for medications to worsen hepatic encephalopathy. Psychological issues such as anxiety and depression can also contribute to insomnia, which may alternatively be a symptom of worsening liver function. Moreover, narcotic-induced constipation may exacerbate encephalopathy, emphasizing the need for comprehensive symptom management (Cicalese Luca 2022).

11.3.2.2 The Need for Tailored Therapeutic Approaches

Recent developments in systemic therapy have expanded treatment possibilities for advanced HCC, but they also bring new uncertainties. There is a pressing need for randomized controlled trials to clarify how best to use combination regimens, particularly in patient populations traditionally excluded from clinical trials, such as individuals with poor liver function, HIV, or transplants.

Efforts to discover biomarkers that can guide personalized therapy remain a high priority. Comparative trials are essential for refining patient-specific treatment choices. In parallel, real-world data and retrospective analyzes should be harnessed to better inform treatment in second-line and later settings. An especially important goal is identifying predictive markers for immunotherapy efficacy when used alone (Kate Kelly 2020).

Another area needing attention is treatment for patients with severely impaired liver function. Limited studies exist for these groups, aside from some research involving nivolumab in Child-Pugh B7 patients (Minsig Choi 2020).

11.3.3 Prevention Gaps

11.3.3.1 Limited Implementation of Lifestyle-Based Prevention

Evidence remains scarce regarding which lifestyle changes most effectively prevent HCC, especially in terms of the type and amount of physical activity, alcohol intake, and dietary habits. Longitudinal, large-scale studies are needed to assess these effects across various at-risk populations. However, conducting such research poses challenges due to the extensive resources and timeframes required (Zelber-Sagi et al. 2021).

11.3.3.2 The Underuse of Statins and Aspirin for Chemoprevention

Although preclinical and epidemiologic data suggest that statins and aspirin may help prevent HCC, the evidence is limited by retrospective design and methodological inconsistencies. Optimal dosage, duration, and safety profiles are yet to be established. No large randomized prospective trials have yet evaluated these agents' preventive roles, underlining the need for more rigorous research before their routine use in HCC prevention can be endorsed (Goh and Sinn 2022).

11.3.3.3 The Inadequate Measures Against Aflatoxin-Related HCC

Addressing aflatoxin exposure, particularly in LMICs, requires national policy commitment. In many regions, regulations are either lacking or poorly enforced (Magnussen and Parsi 2013).

While the dangers of aflatoxin and ways to mitigate them are known, this information is not widely disseminated to vulnerable populations. If current knowledge and preventive strategies were effectively shared and applied, substantial progress could be made (Wild and Gong 2010).

Additional unmet needs include increased funding for aflatoxin-related research, development of aflatoxin-resistant crops, improved sampling methods, and interdisciplinary collaboration, along with the introduction of competitive fungi to limit contamination (Magnussen and Parsi 2013).

11.3.3.4 The Challenges in Preventing HBV- and HCV-Related HCC

Eliminating viral hepatitis by 2030 faces significant hurdles, especially in LMICs. Comprehensive public health strategies must include widespread HBV testing and targeted HCV screening among high-risk populations (Jaquet et al. 2021).

People who inject drugs remain a major transmission group for HCV, necessitating interventions focused on harm reduction and treatment access (Lazarus et al. 2023). Furthermore, the development of affordable diagnostic tools for liver fibrosis and HCC screening is essential. Ensuring access to antiviral therapies is also critical.

Preventing HBV transmission from mother to child—via prenatal screening, antiviral treatment for high-risk mothers, and universal newborn vaccination—should be a policy priority. Achieving global elimination goals requires strong governmental backing, particularly in the most affected regions. Moreover, current treatment guidelines often rely on data from high-income countries, making local clinical research indispensable for LMICs (Jaquet et al. 2021).

11.4 Conclusion

HCC presents a multifaceted challenge due to its diverse etiologies and variable impact on liver function, which complicate treatment decisions. Detecting HCC at earlier stages through effective screening programs is essential to improving patient outcomes. Innovations in diagnostics, including artificial intelligence and biomarker-based approaches, offer promising tools for early identification.

Treatment progress has improved outcomes and quality of life for patients with advanced HCC. Emerging therapies like oncolytic viruses and engineered T-cells, along with innovations in interventional radiology such as targeted drug delivery, are enhancing care. Minimally invasive surgical techniques like laparoscopic liver resection (LLR) also offer safer options with fewer complications.

Despite these developments, critical gaps remain. Broadening access to surveillance, refining diagnostic markers, and tailoring therapies to individual needs are ongoing priorities. Prevention efforts must address major risk factors like HBV, HCV, and aflatoxin exposure, particularly in LMICs. Public education and equitable access to care remain foundational to improving HCC outcomes. Reducing disparities in diagnosis and treatment, especially among socioeconomically disadvantaged populations, is vital to advancing comprehensive HCC management.

References

Abou-Alfa GK, Chan SL, Kudo M, et al. Phase 3 randomized, open-label, multicenter study of tremelimumab and durvalumab as first-line therapy in patients with unresectable hepatocellular carcinoma: HIMALAYA. J Clin Oncol. 2022;40(4):suppl 379C.

Adeniji N, Dhanasekaran R. Current and emerging tools for hepatocellular carcinoma surveillance. Hepatol Commun. 2021;5(12):1972–86. https://doi.org/10.1002/hep4.1823.

Anderson SC, Johnson DE, Harris MP, et al. p53 gene therapy in a rat model of hepatocellular carcinoma: intra-arterial delivery of a recombinant adenovirus. Clin Cancer Res. 1998;4(7):1649–59.

Averhoff FM, Glass N, Holtzman D. Global burden of hepatitis C: considerations for healthcare providers in the United States. Clin Infect Dis. 2012;55(suppl_1):S10–5. https://doi.org/10.1093/cid/cis361.

Ban D, Tanabe M, Kumamaru H, et al. Safe dissemination of laparoscopic liver resection in 27,146 cases between 2011 and 2017 from the National Clinical Database of Japan. Ann Surg. 2020;274:1043.

Best J, Bechmann LP, Sowa JP, et al. GALAD score detects early hepatocellular carcinoma in an international cohort of patients with nonalcoholic steatohepatitis. Clin Gastroenterol Hepatol. 2020;18(3):728–735.e4. https://doi.org/10.1016/j.cgh.2019.11.012.

Butterfield LH, Ribas A, Dissette VB, et al. A phase I/II trial testing immunization of hepatocellular carcinoma patients with dendritic cells pulsed with four α-fetoprotein peptides. Clin Cancer Res. 2006;12(9):2817–25. https://doi.org/10.1158/1078-0432.CCR-05-2856.

Cagnin S, Donghia R, Martini A, Pesole PL, Coletta S, Shahini E, Boninsegna G, Biasiolo A, Pontisso P, Giannelli G. Galad score as a prognostic marker for patients with hepatocellular carcinoma. Int J Mol Sci. 2023;24(22):16485. https://doi.org/10.3390/ijms242216485.

Cho JY, Han H-S, Wakabayashi G, et al. Practical guidelines for performing laparoscopic liver resection based on the second international laparoscopic liver consensus conference. Surg Oncol. 2018;27:A5–9.

Cicalese Luca. Hepatocellular carcinoma (HCC) Treatment & Management; 2022. Source: Medscape : Hepatocellular Carcinoma (HCC) Treatment & Management: Approach Considerations, Nonoperative Therapy, Surgical Therapy (medscape.com).

Coffman-D'Annibale K, Xie C, Hrones D, et al. The current landscape of therapies for hepatocellular carcinoma. Carcinogenesis. 2023;44(7):537–48. https://doi.org/10.1093/carcin/bgad052.

Cui K, Ou Y, Shen Y, et al. Clinical value of circulating tumor cells for the diagnosis and prognosis of hepatocellular carcinoma (HCC): a systematic review and meta-analysis. Medicine. 2020;99:e22242.

Dhanasekaran R, Nault JC, Roberts LR, et al. Genomic medicine and implications for hepatocellular carcinoma prevention and therapy. Gastroenterology. 2019;156(2):492–509. https://doi.org/10.1053/j.gastro.2018.11.001.
Duke-NUS Medical School, Media Release. Landmark study launched to detect liver cancer early in Singapore; 2021. Source: https://www.duke-nus.edu.sg/allnews/landmark-study-to-detect-liver-cancer-early#:~:text=Singapore%2C%203%20May%202021%20%E2%80%93%20A,likelihood%20of%20developing%20the%20cancer. Accessed: January 2024.
Ebert O, Shinozaki K, Huang TG, et al. Oncolytic vesicular stomatitis virus for treatment of orthotopic hepatocellular carcinoma in immune-competent rats. Cancer Res. 2003;63(13):3605–11.
El Ansary M, Mogawer S, Elhamid SA, et al. Immunotherapy by autologous dendritic cell vaccine in patients with advanced HCC. J Cancer Res Clin Oncol. 2013;139(1):39–48. https://doi.org/10.1007/s00432-012-1298-8.
El-Khoueiry AB, Sangro B, Yau T, et al. Nivolumab in patients with advanced hepatocellular carcinoma (CheckMate 040): an open-label, non-comparative, phase 1/2 dose escalation and expansion trial. Lancet. 2017;389(10088):2492–502.
Fardis M, DiTrapani K, Chartier C, et al. Current and future directions for tumor infiltrating lymphocyte therapy for the treatment of solid tumors. Cell Gene Ther Insights. 2020;6:855–63. https://doi.org/10.18609/cgti.2020.088.
Ferrucci PF, Pala L, Conforti F, et al. Talimogene Laherparepvec (T-VEC): an Intralesional cancer immunotherapy for advanced melanoma. Cancers (Basel). 2021;13(6):1383. https://doi.org/10.3390/cancers13061383.
Finn RS, Kudo M, Barnes G, et al. Tislelizumab versus Sorafenib in first-line treatment of Unresectable hepatocellular carcinoma: impact on health-related quality of life in RATIONALE-301 study. Liver Cancer. 2024;13(5):548–60. https://doi.org/10.1159/000537966.
Fountzilas C, Patel S, Mahalingam D. Review: oncolytic virotherapy, updates and future directions. Oncotarget. 2017;8(60):102617–39. https://doi.org/10.18632/oncotarget.18309.
Fu Q, Zheng Y, Fang W, et al. RUNX-3-expressing CAR T cells targeting glypican-3 in patients with heavily pretreated advanced hepatocellular carcinoma: a phase I trial. E Clin Med. 2023;63:102175. https://doi.org/10.1016/j.eclinm.2023.102175.
Global Data Health Care. Continued demand for hepatocellular carcinoma surveillance; 2020. Source: Continued demand for hepatocellular carcinoma surveillance (pharmaceutical-technology.com) Accessed January 2024.
Goh M, Sinn D. Statin and aspirin for chemoprevention of hepatocellular carcinoma: Time to use or wait further? Clin Mol Hepatol. 2022;28(3):380395. https://doi.org/10.3350/cmh.2021.0366.
Gonzalez-Periz A, Planaguma A, Gronert K, et al. Docosahexaenoic acid (DHA) blunts liver injury by conversion to protective lipid mediators: protectin D1 and 17S-hydroxy-DHA. FASEB J. 2006;20(14):2537–9. https://doi.org/10.1096/fj.06-6250fje.
Huang C, Fang M, Xiao X, et al. Validation of the GALAD model for early diagnosis and monitoring of hepatocellular carcinoma in Chinese multicenter study. Liver Int. 2022;42(1):210–23. https://doi.org/10.1111/liv.15082.
Jaquet A, Muula G, Ekouevi DK, Wandeler G. Elimination of viral hepatitis in low and middle-income countries: epidemiological research gaps. Curr Epidemiol Rep. 2021;8(3):89–96. https://doi.org/10.1007/s40471-021-00273-6.
Jebar AH, Errington-Mais F, Vile RG, et al. Progress in clinical oncolytic virus-based therapy for hepatocellular carcinoma. J Gen Virol. 2015;96(7):1533–50. https://doi.org/10.1099/vir.0.000098.
Jin KT, Du WL, Liu YY, et al. Oncolytic virotherapyin solid tumors: the challenges and achievements. Cancers. 2021;13(4):588. https://doi.org/10.3390/cancers13040588.
Kanwal F, Singal AG. Surveillance for hepatocellular carcinoma: current Best practice and future direction. Gastroenterology. 2019;157(1):54–64.
Kate Kelly. Metastatic HCC Unmet Needs. OncLiv; 2020. Source https://www.onclive.com/view/metastatic-hcc-unmet-needs Accessed January 2024.

Kaseb AO, Sánchez NS, Sen S, et al. Molecular profiling of hepatocellular carcinoma using circulating cell-free DNA. Clin Cancer Res. 2019;25:6107–18.
Kim KS, Kim DH, Kim DH. Recent advances to augment NK cell cancer immunotherapy using nanoparticles. Pharmaceutics. 2021;13(4):525. https://doi.org/10.3390/pharmaceutics13040525.
Kisiel JB, Dukek BA, V.S.R. Kanipakam R., et al. Hepatocellular carcinoma detection by plasma methylated DNA: discovery, phase I pilot, and phase II clinical validation. Hepatology. 2019;69:1180–92.
Kudo M, Tsuchiya K, Shao Y, et al. IMbrave150: exploratory analysis to examine the association between bevacizumab (bev) ever being skipped and bev never being skipped in patients with unresectable hepatocellular carcinoma (HCC) treated with atezolizumab (atezo) + bev in a global phase 3 study. J Clin Oncol. 2023;41:538. https://doi.org/10.1200/JCO.2023.41.4_suppl.538.
Kumari R, Sahu M, Tripathy A, et al. Hepatocellular carcinoma treatment: hurdles, advances and prospects. Hepatic Oncol. 2018;5(2) https://doi.org/10.2217/hep-2018-0002.
Lazarus JV, Picchio CA, Colombo M. Hepatocellular carcinoma prevention in the era of hepatitis C elimination. Int J Mol Sci. 2023;24(18):14404. https://doi.org/10.3390/ijms241814404.
Lee MS, Ryoo BY, Hsu CH, et al. Atezolizumab with or without bevacizumab in unresectable hepatocellular carcinoma (GO30140): an open-label, multicentre, phase 1b study. Lancet Oncol. 2020;21(6):808–20. https://doi.org/10.1016/S1470-2045(20)30156-X.
Lee JH, Lee JH, Lim YS, et al. Adjuvant immunotherapy with autologous cytokine-induced killer cells for hepatocellular carcinoma. Gastroenterology. 2015a;148(7):1383–91. https://doi.org/10.1053/j.gastro.2015.02.055.e6.
Lee JH, Lee Y, Lee M, et al. A phase I/IIa study of adjuvant immunotherapy with tumour antigen-pulsed dendritic cells in patients with hepatocellular carcinoma. Br J Cancer. 2015b;113(12):1666–76. https://doi.org/10.1038/bjc.2015.430.
Lemos de Matos A, Franco LS, McFadden G. Oncolytic Viruses and the Immune System: The Dynamic Duo. Mol Ther Methods Clin Dev. 2020;17:349–58. https://doi.org/10.1016/j.omtm.2020.01.001. PMID: 32071927; PMCID: PMC7015832
Li D, Li X, Zhou WL, et al. Genetically engineered t cells for cancer immunotherapy. Signal Transduct Target Ther. 2019a;4:35. https://doi.org/10.1038/s41392-019-0070-9.
Li D, Sedano S, Allen R, et al. Current treatment landscape for advanced hepatocellular carcinoma: patient outcomes and the impact on quality of life. Cancers (Basel). 2019b;11(6):841. https://doi.org/10.3390/cancers11060841.
Liu S, Galat V, Galat Y, Lee YKA, Wainwright D, Wu J. NK cell-based cancer immunotherapy: from basic biology to clinical development. J Hematol Oncol. 2021;14(7) https://doi.org/10.1186/s13045-020-01014-w.
Llovet JM, Kudo M, Merle P, et al. Lenvatinib plus pembrolizumab versus lenvatinib plus placebo for advanced hepatocellular carcinoma (LEAP-002): a randomised, double-blind, phase 3 trial. Lancet Oncol. 2023;24(12):1399–410. https://doi.org/10.1016/S1470-2045(23)00469-2.
Llovet JM, Castet F, Heikenwalder M, et al. Immunotherapies for hepatocellular carcinoma. Nat Rev Clin Oncol. 2022;19(3):151–72. https://doi.org/10.1038/s41571-021-00573-2.
Luo XY, et al. Advances in drug development for hepatocellular carcinoma: clinical trials and potential therapeutic targets. J Exp Clin Cancer Res. 2021;40:172.
Magnussen A, Parsi MA. Aflatoxins, hepatocellular carcinoma and public health. World J Gastroenterol. 2013;19(10):1508–12. https://doi.org/10.3748/wjg.v19.i10.1508.
Mangla A, Lee C, Mirsky MM, et al. Neoadjuvant dual checkpoint inhibitors vs anti-PD1 therapy in high-risk Resectable melanoma: a pooled analysis. JAMA Oncol. 2024;10(5):612–20. https://doi.org/10.1001/jamaoncol.2023.7333.
Margolis L, Sadovsky Y. The biology of extracellular vesicles: the known unknowns. PLoS Biol. 2019;17:e3000363.
Martini V, D'Avanzo F, Maggiora PM, et al. Oncolytic virotherapy: new weapon for breast cancer treatment. E Cancer Med Sci. 2020;14:1149. https://doi.org/10.3332/ecancer.2020.1149.

Mastelic-Gavillet B, Balint K, Boudousquie C, Gannon PO, Kandalaft LE. Personalized dendritic cell vaccines-recent breakthroughs and encouraging clinical results. Front Immunol. 2019;10:766. https://doi.org/10.3389/fimmu.2019.00766.

McGowan CE, Edwards TP, Luong MU, et al. Suboptimal surveillance for and knowledge of hepatocellular carcinoma among primary care providers. Clin Gastroenterol Hepatol. 2015;13(4):799–804. https://doi.org/10.1016/j.cgh.2014.07.056.

Minaei N, Ramezankhani R, Tamimi A, et al. Immunotherapeutic approaches in hepatocellular carcinoma: building blocks of hope in near future. Eur J Cell Biol. 2023;102(1) https://doi.org/10.1016/j.ejcb.2022.151284.

Minsig Choi. Metastatic HCC unmet needs OncLiv; 2020. Source https://www.onclive.com/view/metastatic-hcc-unmet-needs Accessed January 2024.

Mody K, Kasi PM, Yang JD, et al. Feasibility of circulating tumor DNA testing in hepatocellular carcinoma. J Gastrointest Oncol. 2019;10:745–50.

Mougel A, Terme M, Tanchot C. Therapeutic cancer vaccine and combinations with antiangiogenic therapies and immune checkpoint blockade. Front Immunol. 2019;10:467. https://doi.org/10.3389/fimmu.2019.00467.

Nakajima M, Tokumitsu Y, Shindo Y, et al. The recent development of the surgical treatment for hepatocellular carcinoma. Appl Sci. 2021;11(5):2023. https://doi.org/10.3390/app11052023.

National Comprehensive Cancer Network. NCCN guidelines hepatocellular carcinoma. Version 2. 2023. https://www.nccn.org/professionals/physician_gls/pdf/hcc.pdf Accessed January 2024.

Pardoll DM. The blockade of immune checkpoints in cancer immunotherapy. Nat Rev Cancer. 2012;12(4):252–64. https://doi.org/10.1038/nrc3239.

Parodi A, Molinaro R, Sushnitha M, et al. Biomaterials. 2017;147:155–68. https://doi.org/10.1016/j.biomaterials.2017.09.020.

Pinter M, Jain RK, Duda DG. The current landscape of immune checkpoint blockade in hepatocellular carcinoma: a review. JAMA Oncol. 2021;7(1):113–23. https://doi.org/10.1001/jamaoncol.2020.3381.

Qin S, Chan SL, Gu S, et al. Camrelizumab plus rivoceranib versus sorafenib as first-line therapy for unresectable hepatocellular carcinoma (CARES-310): a randomised, open-label, international phase 3 study. Lancet. 2023;402:1133. https://doi.org/10.1016/S0140-6736(23)00961-3.

Qin H, Sheng J, Zhang D, et al. New strategies for therapeutic cancer vaccines. Anti Cancer Agents Med Chem. 2018;19(2):213–21. https://doi.org/10.2174/1871520618666181109151835.

Reynolds L, Mulik RS, Wen X, et al. Low-density lipoprotein-mediated delivery of docosahexaenoic acid selectively kills murine liver cancer cells. Nanomedicine (Lond). 2014;9(14):2123–41. https://doi.org/10.2217/nnm.13.187.

Roche Media Release. FDA grants breakthrough device designation for Roche's Elecsys GALAD score to support earlier diagnosis of hepatocellular carcinoma; 2020. Source: https://assets.roche.com/imported/01_Roche_MediaRelease_04032020_EN.pdf.Accessed January 2024.

Rohaan MW, Wilgenhof S, Haanen J. Adoptive cellular therapies: the current landscape. Virchows Arch. 2019;474(4):449–61. https://doi.org/10.1007/s00428-018-2484-0.

Shen A, Liu S, Yu W, et al. p53 gene therapy-based transarterial chemoembolization for unresectable hepatocellular carcinoma: a prospective cohort study. J Gastroenterol Hepatol. 2015;30(11):1651–6. https://doi.org/10.1111/jgh.13009.

Sheu AY, Zhang Z, Omary RA, Larson AC. MRI-monitored transcatheter intraarterial delivery of SPIO-labeled natural killer cells to hepatocellular carcinoma: preclinical studies in a rodent model. Investig Radiol. 2013;48(6):492–9. https://doi.org/10.1097/RLI.0b013e31827994e5.

Shiani A, Narayanan S, Pena L, Friedman M. The role of diagnosis and treatment of underlying liver disease for the prognosis of primary liver cancer. Cancer Control. 2017;24(3):1073274817729240.

Shiba H, Misawa T, Iida T, et al. Adenovirus vector-mediated gene therapy using iodized oil esters for hepatocellular carcinoma I n rats. Anticancer Res. 2008;28(1a):51–3.

Shimamura T, Akamatsu N, Fujiyoshi M, et al. Expanded living-donor liver transplantation criteria for patients with hepatocellular carcinoma based on the Japanese nationwide survey: the 5-5-500 rule—a retrospective study. Transpl Int. 2019;32:356–68.

Shokoohian B, Negahdari B, Aboulkheyr EH, et al. Advanced therapeutic modalities in hepatocellular carcinoma: novel insights. J Cell Mol Med. 2021;25(18):8602–14. https://doi.org/10.1111/jcmm.16875.

Singal AG, Lampertico P, Nahon P. Epidemiology and surveillance for hepatocellular carcinoma: new trends. J Hepatol. 2020;72(2):250–61. https://doi.org/10.1016/j.jhep.2019.08.025.

Singal AG, Tiro JA, Murphey CC, et al. Mailed outreach invitations signicantaly improve HCC surveillance rates in patients with cirrhosis: a randomized clinical trial. Hepatology. 2019;69:121–30.

Singal AG, Tiro JA, Marrero JA, et al. Mailed outreach program increases ultrasound screening of patients with cirrhosis for hepatocellular carcinoma. Gastroenterology. 2017;152(3):608–615.e4. https://doi.org/10.1053/j.gastro.2016.10.042.

Singh AK, McGuirk JP. CAR T cells: continuation in a revolution of immunotherapy. Lancet Oncol. 2020;21(3):e168–78. https://doi.org/10.1016/S1470-2045(19)30823-X.

Song BG, Goh MJ, Kang W, et al. Analysis of factors predicting the real-world efficacy of Atezolizumab and bevacizumab in patients with advanced hepatocellular carcinoma. Gut Liver. 2024;18(4):709–18. https://doi.org/10.5009/gnl240085.

Stojdl DF, Lichty B, Knowles S, et al. Exploiting tumor-specific defects in the interferon pathway with a previously unknown oncolytic virus. Nat Med. 2000;6(7):821–5. https://doi.org/10.1038/77558.

Sutphin P, Lamus D, Kalva S, et al. Interventional radiologic therapies for hepatocellular carcinoma: from where we began to where we are going. In: Hoshida Y, editor. Hepatocellular carcinoma: translational precision medicine approaches [Internet]. Cham: Humana Press; 2019.

Sukowati CHC, Cabral LKD, Tiribelli C, et al. Circulating long and circular noncoding RNA as non-invasive diagnostic tools of hepatocellular carcinoma. Biomedicines. 2021;9:90.

Sun N, Lee Y-T, Zhang RY, et al. Purification of HCC-specific extracellular vesicles on nanosubstrates for early HCC detection by digital scoring. Nat Commun. 2020;11:4489.

Su Z, Wang X, Zheng L, et al. MRI-guided interventional natural killer cell delivery for liver tumor treatment. Cancer Med. 2018;7(5):1860–9. https://doi.org/10.1002/cam4.1459.

Tada F, Abe M, Hirooka M, et al. Phase I/II study of immunotherapy using tumor antigen-pulsed dendritic cells in patients with hepatocellular carcinoma. Int J Oncol. 2012;41(5):1601–9. https://doi.org/10.3892/ijo.2012.1626.

Tian C, Yu Y, Wang Y, et al. Neoadjuvant immune checkpoint inhibitors in hepatocellular carcinoma: a meta-analysis and systematic review. Front Immunol. 2024;15:1352873. https://doi.org/10.3389/fimmu.2024.1352873.

Tsuchiya N, Yoshikawa T, Fujinami N, et al. Immunological efficacy of glypican-3 peptide vaccine in patients with advanced hepatocellular carcinoma. Onco Targets Ther. 2017;6(10):e1346764. https://doi.org/10.1080/2162402X.2017.1346764.

Vogel A. HCC and impaired liver function: systemic treatment options - Medscape - May 27, 2021. https://decisionpoint.medscape.com/oncology/viewarticle/947690

Vivier E, Raulet DH, Moretta A, et al. Innate or adaptive immunity? The example of natural killer cells. Science. 2011;331(6013):44–9. https://doi.org/10.1126/science.1198687.

Wang LLW, Janes ME, Kumbhojkar N, et al. Cell therapies in the clinic. Bioeng Transl Med. 2021;6(2):e10214. https://doi.org/10.1002/btm2.10214.

Wáng YXJ, De Baere T, Idée JM, et al. Transcatheter embolization therapy in liver cancer: an update of clinical evidences. Chin J Cancer Res. 2015;27(2):96–121. https://doi.org/10.3978/j.issn.1000-9604.2015.03.03.

Wen X, Reynolds L, Mulik RS, et al. Hepatic arterial infusion of low-density lipoprotein docosahexaenoic acid nanoparticles selectively disrupts redox balance in hepatoma cells and reduces growth of orthotopic liver tumors in rats. Gastroenterology. 2016;150(2):488–98. https://doi.org/10.1053/j.gastro.2015.10.008.

WHO International Agency for Research on Cancer. World; 2022. Available at: https://gco.iarc.fr/today/data/factsheets/populations/900-world-fact-sheets.pdf. Accessed March 2024.

Wild CP, Gong YY. Mycotoxins and human disease: a largely ignored global health issue. Carcinogenesis. 2010;31(1):71–82. https://doi.org/10.1093/carcin/bgp264.

Xie G, Dong H, Liang Y, Ham JD, Rizwan R, Chen J. CAR-NK cells: a promising cellular immunotherapy for cancer. EBioMedicine. 2020;59:102975. https://doi.org/10.1016/j.ebiom.2020.102975.

Xu R-H, Wei W, Krawczyk M, et al. Circulating tumour DNA methylation markers for diagnosis and prognosis of hepatocellular carcinoma. Nat Mater. 2017;16:1155–61.

Yamamoto Y, Kondo S, Matsuzaki J, et al. Highly sensitive circulating microRNA panel for accurate detection of hepatocellular carcinoma in patients with liver disease. Hepatol Commun. 2020;4:284–97.

Zampino R, Boemio A, Sagnelli C, et al. Hepatitis B virus burden in developing countries. World J Gastroenterol. 2015;21(42):11941–53. https://doi.org/10.3748/wjg.v21.i42.11941.

Zelber-Sagi S, Noureddin M, Shibolet O. Lifestyle and hepatocellular carcinoma what is the evidence and prevention recommendations. Cancers (Basel). 2021;14(1):103. https://doi.org/10.3390/cancers14010103.

Zhang R, Zhang Z, Liu Z, et al. Adoptive cell transfer therapy for hepatocellular carcinoma. Front Med. 2019;13(1):3–11. https://doi.org/10.1007/s11684-019-0684-x.

Zhou G, Sprengers D, Boor PPC, et al. Antibodies against immune checkpoint molecules restore functions of tumor-infiltrating T cells in hepatocellular carcinomas. Gastroenterology. 2017;153(4):1107–1119.e10. https://doi.org/10.1053/j.gastro.2017.06.017.

MIX
Papier aus verantwortungsvollen Quellen
Paper from responsible sources
FSC® C105338
FSC
www.fsc.org

If you have any concerns about our products,
you can contact us on
ProductSafety@springernature.com

In case Publisher is established outside the EU,
the EU authorized representative is:
Springer Nature Customer Service Center GmbH
Europaplatz 3, 69115 Heidelberg, Germany

Printed by Libri Plureos GmbH
in Hamburg, Germany